Vitamins and Minerals in the Prevention and Treatment of Cancer

MARYCE M. JACOBS

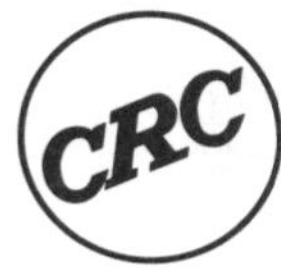

CRC Press
Boca Raton Ann Arbor Boston London

Library of Congress Cataloging-in-Publication Data

Vitamins and minerals in the prevention and treatment of cancer / editor, Maryce M. Jacobs.
p. cm.
based on the first Annual Conference of the American Institute for Cancer Research, held in Pentagon City, Virginia, Oct. 11-12, 1990.
Includes bibliographical references and indexes.
ISBN 0-8493-4259-7
1. Vitamins--Therapeutic use--Congresses. 2. Trace elements--Therapeutic use--Congresses. 3. Cancer--Treatment--Congresses. 4. Cancer--Prevention--Congresses. I. Jacobs, Maryce M. II. American Institute for Cancer Research. Conference (1st : 1990 : Pentagon City, Arlington, Va.)
[DNLM: 1. Minerals--therapeutic use-congresses. 2. Neoplasms-drug therapy--congresses. 3. Neoplasms--prevention & control--congresses. 4. Vitamins--therapeutic use-congresses. QZ 267 V8367 1990]
RC 271.V58V59 1991
616.99'4061--dc20
DNLM/DLC
for Library of Congress 91-19362
CIP

This book represents information obtained from authentic and highly regarded sources. Reprinted material is quoted with permission, and sources are indicated. A wide variety of references are listed. Every reasonable effort has been made to give reliable data and information, but the author and the publisher cannot assume responsibility for the validity of all materials or for the consequences of their use.

Direct all inquiries to CRC Press, Inc., 2000 Corporate Blvd., N.W., Boca Raton, Florida, 33431.

International Standard Book Number 0-8493-4259-7

Library of Congress Card Number 91-19362

Printed in the United States of America 2 3 4 5 6 7 8 9 0
Printed on acid-free paper

Preface

The American Institute for Cancer Research (AICR) sponsored the first of a series of Annual Conferences on nutrition and cancer. The theme was "Vitamins and Minerals in the Prevention and Treatment of Cancer." The Conference was held October 11–12, 1990 at the Ritz Carlton Hotel in Pentagon City, Virginia. The proceedings of this conference contains manuscripts from each platform presentation and abstracts from each poster presentation. Based on research in humans, animals and cell culture the data presented in this conference helped to elucidate the preventive roles of vitamins and micronutrients in carcinogenesis.

The focus of the proceedings in this volume is on the protective interactions of vitamins and micronutrients in carcinogenesis. Epidemiological associations of low dietary intake of several vitamins, lipotropes, and selenium with human cancers at different sites have been made. Adequate or greater intakes of Vitamin A, retinoids and carotenoids, have been associated with decreased human cancers of the bladder, breast, cervix, colorectum, esophagus, gastrointestinal tract, larynx, lung, oral cavity, pancreas, prostate, skin, and stomach; vitamin C with human cancers of the breast, cervix, colorectum, esophagus, larynx, lung, oral cavity, prostate, and stomach; vitamin E with human cancers of the bladder, breast, colorectum, lung, and stomach; lipotropes (folic acid, choline, methionine, and vitamin B12) with human cancers of the bone marrow, cervix, esophagus, gastrointestinal tract, liver, respiratory tract, and liver; and selenium with human cancers of the breast, colorectum, leukemia, lung, lymphoma, mouth, pharynx, and skin. Experimental animal studies and *in vitro* models have been used to validate these associations and to establish specific mechanisms of protection against carcinogenesis.

Cancer is a multistage process of initiation, promotion, and progression that can be influenced by permissive and protective factors. An estimated 35% of all cancer deaths have been related to diet and an estimated 80% to 90% of all human cancers appear to be due to environmental causes, including diet. Some exogenous factors (*e.g.*, diet) and endogenous factors (*e.g.*, hormones) may be permissive promoting agents by acting on initiated cells to elicit neoplasms. In contrast, other dietary factors may protect against genetically predisposed and intentionally induced cancers. Important among these are the vitamins and micronutrients that act as anticarcinogens, altering cancer incidence, differentiation, and growth.

Dietary intervention studies in individuals with inherited cancer-prone disorders have suggested involvement of interactions between environmental (*e.g.*, dietary) and genetic factors in the multistage process of carcinogenesis. Studies in inbred strains of animals differing in selected genes that confer cancer susceptibility, and studies of cell culture systems and transformation *in vitro* have helped to elucidate the mechanisms of dietary and genetic interactions that affect the course and frequency of neoplasia. Epidemiological, animal, and cell culture data suggest the possibility that certain vitamins and micronutrients may prove to be useful in cancer prevention and in cancer treatment as adjuncts to conventional therapy. For example, studies are discussed in which dietary supplementation with calcium carbonate decreased proliferation of colon epithelium in people with a genetic predisposition to develop colon polyps and cancer; in them, the morphology of the colon approached that of persons with a low risk for colon cancer.

Several chapters in this volume discuss epidemiological investigations, primarily dietary intervention studies, that help to elucidate the interactions among diet, genetics, and human cancers. Dietary intervention studies in persons with genetic susceptibilities that predispose them for certain cancers have suggested possible synergism between diet and genetics in modulating human cancers of the colon, gallbladder, and esophagus.

Based on one epidemiological study in the Chinese population, a deficiency of riboflavin had the strongest correlation with the high-risk population for esophageal cancer. In an intervention study the combined supplement of riboflavin, retinol and zinc did not reduce precancerous lesions but did reduce the prevalence of micronucleated cells—possibly an early indicator of the carcinogenic process.

In experiments using hamster embryo and mouse C_3H 10T½ cells under conditions of chemical- or radiation-enhanced cell transformation, vitamins A, C, and E, ß-carotene, and selenium protected against excess oxidative stress, suppressing free radical damage. Protective systems affected by these antioxidants included enzyme induction (e.g., catalase, peroxidases, dismutase), supply of thiols, and interference with free-radical mechanisms in the initiation and promotion of malignant transformation.

The epidemiological links between selenium intake or blood levels and human cancers at various sites are discussed. A review of the inhibition of spontaneous, transplantable and chemically-induced tumors in experimental animal studies that suggests selenium inhibits initiation, promotion and progression by a broad variety of mechanisms is presented. Interactions between vitamins or between a vitamin and selenium suggest that either the reversal or enhancement of the independent chemopreventive actions of either vitamins or selenium may occur with the concurrent supplements.

A review of the literature is presented that reviews the suppression of tumorigenesis by the organosulfur compounds, diallyl sulfide and S-allyl-cystine, from allium vegetables. Several possible mechanisms of action are discussed. In large part these involve the apparent inhibition of P450-related activation enzymes and the apparent enhancement of detoxification enzymes. Via these mechanisms the metabolic disposition of carcinogens might be altered, resulting in inhibition of carcinogenesis.

One mechanism of modulating gene expression is by site-specific binding of Zn-finger domains to double-stranded DNA. This research area is reviewed in detail. Zn-finger domains of certain transcription factors, hormone receptors, oncogenes, and tumor-suppressor genes may be potential targets for metal ions. The effects of substituting Ni^{2+} in the finger-loop domains for Zn^{2+} on the conformation and stability of the DNA are discussed.

The relationships between methyl deficiencies and carcinogenesis are presented in several chapters. Deficiencies in choline, methionine, or folate increase susceptibility to spontaneous and chemically induced carcinogenesis. Folate deficiency-induced biochemical and morphological changes are reported in human cancer patients as well as in experiments from animal and cell culture systems. Associated with dietary methyl deficiency are observed alterations in xenobiotic metabolism, nucleic acid methylation, purine and pyrimidine synthesis, membrane phospholipids, cell adhesive properties, signal transduction pathways, chromosome anomalies (e.g., gaps, breaks, and condensations), and (increased) cell division.

The extent to which physiological methyl insufficiency contributes to the carcinogenic process and alters the transfer of 1-carbon fragments in the folate pool is elucidated. Some of the studies focus on the methotrexate-induced decrease in the bioavailability of methyl groups, perturbed folate metabolism, and enhanced carcinogenesis. Mechanisms associating alcohol consumption, decreased folic acid, and increased risk for certain cancers in humans are proposed.

The controversial issue is raised whereby low serum folic acid levels are observed in cancer patients, yet treatment of the folic acid deficiency might possibly promote tumor growth in these patients. How folate deficiency-induced changes in chromosome stability, cell size, cell cycle distribution, and membrane adherence properties might influence metastatic potential is explored.

Several chapters in this volume present data to elucidate mechanisms by which a number of vitamins might inhibit the carcinogenic process. In one chapter the effects of vitamin D_3 on extrachromosomal oncogene sequences are discussed and a potentially new therapeutic approach is presented. Some episomes, or submicroscopic circular DNA molecules, carry amplified oncogenes as well as amplified drug resistance genes. Studies are described to optimize episome detection and to eliminate episomes from tumor cells. Episome detection is accomplished with alkaline lysis of tumor cells followed by low or high voltage agarose gel electrophoresis, or field-inversion gel electrophoresis. The technique used depends on the topographical state of the episomal DNA. Elimination of the episomes might eventually provide the potential for decreasing tumor progression in patients (by eliminating the amplified oncogenes) or decreasing resistance of a patient's tumor to chemotherapy (by eliminating the drug resistant genes). In preliminary work presented vitamin D_3 is reported to inhibit incorporation of extrachromasomally located amplified c-myc into a chromosomal site, thereby providing a strategy that might make this episome more susceptible to elimination.

Studies with vitamin A metabolites disclose mechanisms by which metabolites of ß-carotene might up regulate gap junctional communication between cells.

Evidence is presented that pyridoxal phosphate, the biologically active form of vitamin B6, can interfere with the ability of the active form of the glucocorticoid receptor to bind DNA. The mechanism of activation/transformation of the cytoplasmic glucocorticoid receptor is proposed. Evidence is presented that specific lysine residues on zinc fingers of the DNA binding domain of the receptor could be targets of pyridoxylation. Experiments in human melanoma cells and mouse B16 melanoma cells suggest that pyridoxal killing of these cells resulted in inhibition of glucocorticoid receptor translocation to the nucleus.

Studies on the antiproliferation activities of vitamin E show that the succinate ester is the most effective form and that tumor cell growth inhibition is probably unrelated to antioxidant functions. In a mechanism similar to active vitamin A and vitamin D metabolites, the antiproliferative activity of vitamin E appears to involve binding of the vitamin to cytosolic receptors followed by translocation to the nucleus where DNA binding domains on the receptor mediate gene regulatory events. Retrovirus-induced tumorigenesis involves transformation of normal cells into tumor cells that exhibit uncontrolled proliferation and that express immune dysfunction. Evidence is presented that suggests vitamin E might ameliorate the immune dysfunction by interacting with macrophages and/or T lymphocytes. This can result in either the down-regulation of PGE_2, a potent immune response inhibitor, or the up-regulation, enhanced production, of IL-2.

The final chapter reviews the influence of potassium on the cancer process. Studies in humans, in experimental animals, and in cell culture systems generally associate increased potassium with decreased tumor cell growth and inhibition of carcinogenesis. Dietary inhibition of colon and other cancers with potassium and elucidating possible mechanisms by which this inhibition is induced are exciting new areas of diet and cancer research. The physiological relationships among potassium and other electrolytes are discussed.

In summary, in this monograph data from human, animal, and cell culture studies are presented that attempt to elucidate the potential roles of vitamins and micronutrients in the prevention and treatment of cancer. These data are reported from both platform and poster presentations at AICR's first Annual Conference.

The Editor

Maryce M. Jacobs, Ph.D., is presently Vice President for Research at the American Institute for Cancer Research in Washington, D.C. She received her Ph.D. in Biological Chemistry in 1970 from the University of California at Los Angeles. Before her present position she was employed five years at The MITRE Corporation in McLean,VA as a Biochemical Toxicologist, six years at the Eppley Institute for Cancer Research in Omaha, NE, as Associate Professor and Industrial Contract Coordinator, and six years at M.D. Anderson Hospital and Tumor Institute in Houston, TX. While in Houston, she also served two years as Cochairman of the Biochemistry Area of the University of Texas Graduate School of Biomedical Sciences.

Her primary research interest is inhibition of chemical carcinogenesis with dietary factors, particularly selenium. She published some of the earliest studies on selenium inhibition of colon carcinogens, as well as of liver and lung carcinogens. Dr. Jacobs has also reported her research findings on antimutagenic, anticlastogenic, and antiangiogenic properties of selenium. In addition, she has described acute, subchronic, and chronic toxicity parameters of selenium in rodents.

Dr. Jacobs is a member of the American Association for Cancer Research, the American Academy of Clinical Toxicology, the American Association for the Advancement of Science, the American Chemical Society, American Men and Women in Science, and the Society of Toxicology, among other organizations. In addition, she has served as Vice President of the National Capital Area Chapter of the Society of Toxicology.

Contributors

Rizwan Akhtar, M.D.
Boston University
School of Medicine and Mallory
Institute of Pathology
Boston City Hospital
Boston, Massachusetts 02118

Allan Baer, Ph.D.
The University of Texas
M.D. Anderson Cancer Center
1515 Holcombe Blvd., Box 78
Houston, Texas 77030

Lu Jian Bang, M.D.
Henan Cancer Institute
Zheng Zhou
PEOPLE'S REPUBLIC OF CHINA

John S. Bertram, Ph.D.
Molecular Oncology Program
Cancer Research Center of Hawaii
University of Hawaii
Honolulu, Hawaii 96813

Carmia G. Borek, Ph.D.
Radiation and Cancer Biology
Tufts University School of Medicine
New England Medical Center
750 Washington Street
Boston, Massachusetts 02111

Richard F. Branda, M.D.
Department of Medicine and
Vermont Regional Cancer Center
University of Vermont
One South Prospect Street
Burlington, Vermont 05405

Mahmut Celiker, M.D.
Fels Institute for Cancer
Research and Molecular Biology
Temple University
School of Medicine
3420 North Broad Street
Philadelphia, Pennsylvania 19140

Massimo Crespi, M.D.
Regina Elena Institute for
Cancer Research
Viale Regina Elena, 291
00161 Rome, ITALY

Sidney M. Hopfer, Ph.D.
Department of Laboratory
Medicine and Pharmacology
University of Connecticut
School of Medicine
Farmington, Connecticut 06030

Osamu Imada, Ph.D.
The University of Texas
M. D. Anderson Cancer Center
1515 Holcombe Blvd., Box 78
Houston, Texas 77030

Maryce M. Jacobs, Ph.D.
American Institute for
Cancer Research
1759 R Street, N.W.
Washington, D.C. 20009

Kimberly Kline, Ph.D.
Division of Nutritional Sciences
University of Texas
WCH-106
Austin, Texas 78712

Contributors (continued)

David Kritchevsky, Ph.D.
The Wistar Institute
36th and Spruce Streets
Philadelphia, Pennsylvania 19104

Gerald Litwack, Ph.D.
Fels Institute for Cancer
Research and Molecular Biology
Temple University
School of Medicine
3420 North Broad Street
Philadelphia, Pennsylvania 19140

Henry T. Lynch, M.D.
Department of Preventive
Medicine/Public Health
Creighton University
School of Medicine
Omaha, Nebraska 68178

Jane F. Lynch, B.S.N.
Department of Preventive
Medicine/Public Health
Creighton University
School of Medicine
Omaha, Nebraska 68178

Gregory S. Makowski, Ph.D.
Department of Laboratory Medicine
University of Connecticut
School of Medicine
Farmington, Connecticut 06030

Andrew B. Maksymowych, Ph.D.
Fels Institute for Cancer
Research and Molecular Biology
Temple University
School of Medicine
3420 North Broad Street
Philadelphia, Pennsylvania 19140

John A. Milner, Ph.D.
Department of Nutrition
The Pennsylvania State University
126 Henderson Building, South
University Pk., Pennsylvania 16803

Nubia Muñoz, M.D.
Unit of Field and
Intervention Studies
International Agency for
Research on Cancer
150 Cours Albert Thomas
69372 Lyon
Cedex 08 FRANCE

Roman J. Pienta, Ph.D.
R. J. Pienta & Associates
Rockville, Maryland 20853

Marilyn C. Plowman, B.S.
Department of Laboratory Medicine
University of Connecticut
School of Medicine
Farmington, Connecticut 06030

Lionel A. Poirier, Ph.D.
National Center for
Toxicological Research
HFT-140
Division of Comparative Toxicology
Jefferson, Arkansas 72079

Noreen M. Robertson, D.D.S.
Fels Institute for Cancer
Research and Molecular Biology
Temple University
School of Medicine
3420 North Broad Street
Philadelphia, Pennsylvania 19140

Contributors (continued)

Adrianne E. Rogers, M.D.
Boston University
School of Medicine and Mallory
Institute of Pathology
Boston City Hospital
Boston, Massachusetts 02118

Bob G. Sanders, Ph.D.
Division of Nutritional Sciences
University of Texas
WCH-106
Austin, Texas 78712

Hiromichi Sumiyoshi, Ph.D.
The University of Texas
M. D. Anderson Cancer Center
1515 Holcombe Blvd., Box 78
Houston, Texas 77030

F. William Sunderman, Jr., M.D.
Department of Laboratory Medicine
University of Connecticut
School of Medicine
P.O. Box G
Farmington, Connecticut 06030

Donald R. VanDevanter, Ph.D.
Tumor Institute
Swedish Hospital Medical Center
1221 Madison Street
Seattle, Washington 98104

Daniel D. Von Hoff, M.D.
Division of Medicine/Oncology
The University of Texas
Health Science Center at
San Antonio
7703 Floyd Curl Drive
San Antonio, Texas 78284

Michael J. Wargovich, Ph.D.
Section of Gastrointestinal
Oncology and Digestive Diseases
The University of Texas
M. D. Anderson Cancer Center
1515 Holcombe Blvd., Box 78
Houston, Texas 77030

Jurgen Wahrendorf, Ph.D.
German Cancer Research Center
Heidelberg
FEDERAL REPUBLIC OF
GERMANY

Steven H. Zeisel, M.D., Ph.D.
Department of Nutrition
The University of North Carolina –
Chapel Hill
School of Public Health
2213 McGavran-Greenberg Hall
Chapel Hill, North Carolina 27599

Table of Contents

Table of Contents (continued)

Chapter 1

Epidemiologic Linkage: Diet, Genetics, and Cancer

Henry T. Lynch and Jane F. Lynch

Table of Contents

I. Introduction

Host factors, in interaction with the environment, inclusive of diet, are etiologic in many of the common tumors (*e.g.*, breast, colon) affecting man. There are more than 200 Mendelian inherited cancer-prone syndromes. Persons with these syndromes may provide an unparalleled resource for studying the effects of dietary interventions. It is important to realize that the oft-quoted statement "80-90% of human cancers are due to environmental factors" does not address the fact that only a fraction of those **exposed** will develop cancer. Do host factors determine who **will** *vs.* **will not** develop cancer, given a specific exposure? Do environmental factors, including diet, modulate the process of carcinogenesis in persons with an inherited cancer-prone disorder? Studies of inbred animal strains, differing only in a gene known to confer high susceptibility to liver cancer, showed that carcinogenesis in the rats carrying the susceptibility genes was enhanced by a choline-deficient diet compared to rats without these genes, suggesting synergism between genetics and diet. The role of diet and genetics in human cancer, with particular attention to carcinoma of the colon, gallbladder, and esophagus, have been discussed. In addition, preliminary evidence for oral supplementation of calcium carbonate to conventional diets and its effect on proliferating epithelial cells lining colonic crypts in subjects at high risk for familial colon cancer has been discussed as a model for further study.

Carcinogenesis is a multistage process involving the environment and genetics in concert with the activation of proto-oncogenes and the inactivation of tumor suppressor genes. Surprisingly, there is a paucity of well-designed studies in man wherein the etiologic role of both genetics and environment, and their interaction, have been systematically investigated in an attempt to elucidate the mechanisms involved in carcinogenesis. A crucial detriment to the understanding of genetic-environmental (G-E) interaction in cancer etiology is the fact that cancer geneticists often totally disregard the contributory role of the environment, while their cancer epidemiology colleagues neglect genetics. Needed is the involvement of cancer geneticists and cancer epidemiologists in the design of cancer etiologic studies.

In reviewing the literature on cancer etiology in man, one would be led to the belief that the environment is the **only** important factor contributing to cancer occurrence and that host factors play only a minuscule role in this equation. For example, the epidemiologic literature is replete with the statement that "80-90% of human cancers are due to environmental factors." However, statistically, only a small fraction of those exposed to any given environmental factor (including diet) develop cancer. Clearly, an exceedingly important question is "Are host factors important in determining who **will** *vs.* who **will not** develop cancer, given a specific exposure?" A question germane to this report is "Does diet modulate genetic susceptibility to cancer?" The answer remains elusive due to the scarcity of research involving nutritionists working hand-in-hand with cancer epidemiologists and geneticists.

Hereditary forms of cancer can provide powerful models for testing G-E interactive hypotheses involving dietary factors in the search for these answers. There is no shortage of cancer-prone families which could qualify for such multidisciplined research, given the recent, veritably explosive attention to the discipline of cancer genetics.[1] For example, prior to the 1950s and 60s, one could count **hereditary** forms of cancer on the fingers of one's hand; e.g., xeroderma pigmentosum, familial polyposis coli, von Recklinghausen's neurofibromatosis, tuberous sclerosis, and retinoblastoma. However, during the past several decades, the list has grown remarkably and includes more than 200 hereditary cancer-prone syndromes.[1-6] These disorders impact heavily on the common cancers of man, including those which have been the subject of extensive nutritional research; namely, carcinomas of the breast and colon.[3,5]

II. Limitations of Animal Studies and Their Implications to Man

Hill[7] has stressed that when interpreting dietary effects in cancer etiology, one must always carefully consider the manner in which dietary factors may vary in context with the particular carcinogen and its effect on a specific animal strain. In addition to the effect of dietary manipulation in concert with the carcinogen and the animal strain, he has emphasized the importance of the "...nature of the baseline diet, the age of the animals, the temporal relation between the dietary manipulation and the administration of initiator, and the method of termination of the study (*e.g.*, age at death of the animal compared with a predetermined time). All of this means that for any given dietary hypothesis, there is at least one animal model which confirms it and at least one which resoundingly refutes it. In setting up the model, there are usually built-in preconceptions..." Thus, the experimental design becomes exceedingly important. Herein, when interpreting data from a particular model, one must consider the likely extant heterogeneity of the particular animal strain. Hill goes on to comment that those protocols which are valid for etiologic studies require that their standardization should be made in terms of "...a) strain and sex of rodent used; b) age of rodents at the start of the experiment; c) the type and dose of carcinogen to be given; d) the regime of the administration of the carcinogen (*e.g.*, single dose, 12-weekly doses, etc.); e) the dietary regime during carcinogen administration and that given afterward; f) type of feeding (ad-lib vs. meals)...."

These issues are important to ponder when interpolating animal data to man. As in animals, there is also immense environmental as well as genetic heterogeneity in man. Pertinent to this chapter will be an appreciation of the distinct differences and heterogeneity evidenced in the many hereditary forms of human cancer.[2]

Our purpose is to review some of the existing research dealing with attempts to elucidate the etiologic role of diet in concert with hereditary factors in human cancer.

III. A Genetic-Environmental (G-E) Interactive Model

Research in pharmacogenetics provides an important rationale for the significance of G-E interaction in cancer etiology. For example, there are countless drugs which are metabolized by enzymatic reactions that are under genetic control. Indeed, knowledge of the marked hereditary variability in drug reactions is crucial to the practice of medicine.[8] Chemoprevention studies also provide fodder for G-E interaction in malignant neoplastic diseases. Finally, selected hereditary forms of cancer provide clinical examples of G-E interaction in high relief. One of the more classical examples is that of xeroderma pigmentosum wherein patients manifest an exquisite hereditary sensitivity of their skin to the effects of solar radiation so that squamous and basal cell carcinomas as well as malignant melanoma may flourish.[9-13]

In order to understand the putative interaction between genetics and environment in human carcinogenesis, a model (Figure 1) has been proposed to depict the etiology of cancer occurrence in man. Note that cancer expression ranges from individuals who are profoundly cancer **resistant** to those whose **susceptibility** to cancer is determined almost exclusively by primary Mendelian genetic factors (cancer predisposing single gene defects). In order to emerge above the cancer threshold, those who are strongly cancer **resistant** require a relatively enormous quantitative exposure to a given carcinogen when compared to their **susceptible** counterparts harboring cancer-prone genes, such as familial adenomatous polyposis (FAP), Lynch syndromes I or II, or retinoblastoma. In these latter disorders, little or perhaps no detectable environmental exposure may be required for cancer expression.

There is a solid experimental basis for the rationale depicted in Figure 1. For example, at the laboratory level, Harris *et al.*[14] have shown that binding levels of benzo(a)pyrene to DNA vary 50- to 100-fold in cultured human tissues and cells. This enormous variation in carcinogen metabolism in humans may be attributed to the fact that the majority of chemical carcinogens require enzymatic activation. Herein, host factors play a major etiologic role. These observations provide a firm basis for testing an hypothesis dealing with the role of primary genetic factors in concert with diet for the elucidation of cancer etiology. It has been postulated that the ratio of metabolic activation to deactivation of carcinogens may determine the individual's cancer risk.

IV. Cardinal Aspects of Cancer Genetics in Man

Certain facets of hereditary cancer's natural history appear with sufficient frequency among putative carriers of the deleterious cancer-prone gene(s) as to lead to their characterization as "cardinal principles of cancer genetics." These features include the following: a) early age of cancer onset, often 15-20 years earlier than its sporadic counterpart.[2,3,6,15] However, early onset is not an invariable finding in that we are now learning that an unknown fraction of hereditary cancer patients may show a later age of cancer onset; b) an excess of bilaterality when paired organs are of concern,[2] such as the breast and ovary in hereditary breast/ovarian cancer syndrome;[3,16] c) integral patterns of multiple primary cancer in specific hereditary cancer syndromes,[17] such as in Lynch syndrome II; d) the occurrence of premonitory physical signs, as in the cancer-associated genodermatoses,[4] and/or biomarkers which associate with the respective cancer-prone genotypes;[18] e) Mendelian inherited patterns of cancer transmission within kindreds wherein the majority of such disorders appear to be consonant with an autosomal dominant mode of genetic transmission;[2-6] and finally, f) in certain hereditary cancers, such as carcinoma of the breast and in colon cancer in Lynch syndromes I and II, there appears to be improved survival when these lesions are compared by appropriate staging with historical controls.[19]

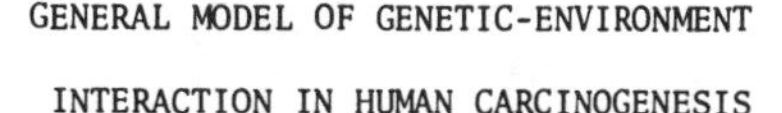

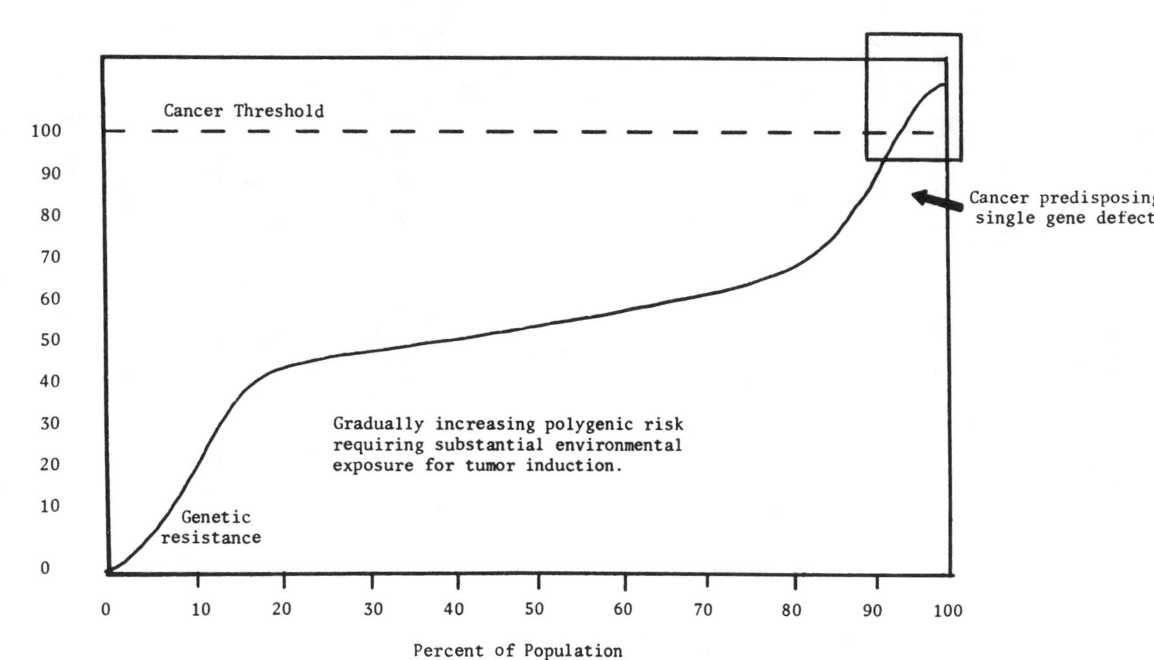

Figure 1. Polygenic and simple genetic model for cancer resistance and cancer proneness in concert with environmental interaction (from HT Lynch, Genetics, etiology, and cancer, *Prev. Med.*, 9, 231, 1980).

These cardinal principles of cancer genetics are clearly depicted in Figures 2-4. Figure 2 is a pedigree of a family showing autosomal dominantly inherited carcinoma of the breast and ovary. This hereditary breast/ovarian cancer kindred shows extraordinarily early age of onset (V-1, V-12, V-17), multiple primary cancer (II-2, III-8, V-1), and the occurrence of cancer through 4 generations in accord with an autosomal dominant mode of inheritance.

Figure 3 depicts an extended family with Lynch syndrome II. As in Figure 2, we see numerous examples of extraordinarily early onset of colorectal carcinoma (III-6, III-9, III-26), multiple primary cancer (III-8, III-24, III-38), and autosomal dominant inheritance, with cancer through 4 generations.

Figure 4 depicts an extraordinary hereditary cancer aggregation, transmitted through 5 generations. This disorder is characterized by an excess of Sarcomas, Brain tumors, Leukemias, and carcinomas of the breast, larynx, lung, and Adrenal cortex.[20,21] In accordance with the predominant tumors in this and similar families, we have called this hereditary tumor complex of adult and childhood tumors the SBLA syndrome.

Review of the pedigrees in Figures 2-4 shows hereditary cancer-prone lineages vs. relatively cancer-free lineages. These kindreds and many others like them provide models which would admirably qualify for prospective studies of G-E investigations, with particular focus on dietary factors. Members of these kindreds would also be candidates for chemoprevention studies employing variable nutritional factors, as discussed subsequently.

V. Migrant Studies

Epidemiologic studies of cancer in migrant populations have stressed changes in **dietary** patterns as a cancer link, particularly among Japanese immigrants to Hawaii and the West Coast of the United States. These migrants showed **increased** rates of cancer of the breast and colon, but **decreased** occurrences of gastric cancer. Unfortunately, these migrant studies paid virtually no attention to the role of **genetics** in concert with **environment** (diet) in cancer occurrence. This failure to systematically collect data to evaluate genetic hypotheses has been a severe shortcoming of these migrant studies. This is pertinent in that the overwhelming majority of cancer occurrences undoubtedly result from the interaction of **both** genetics and environmental determinants, given the fact that the range of host susceptibilities to environmental effects is so extensive.[14]

VI. Inbred Animal Studies

Melhem *et al.*[22] studied male-carrying genes controlling growth and reproduction (grc) in the R-16 strain and compared them with rats without grc genes (ACP strain). By manipulation of the diet of grc rats, hepatocarcinogenesis induced by another carcinogen was shown to be altered. The availability of congenic grc strains and their wild-type counterparts, coupled with the promotion of hepatic cancer by a choline-deficient (CD) diet provided an opportunity to study the interaction of dietary influences and genetic predisposition to development of cancer.[23] Male rats with the grc gene (R-16) and wild-type (ACP)

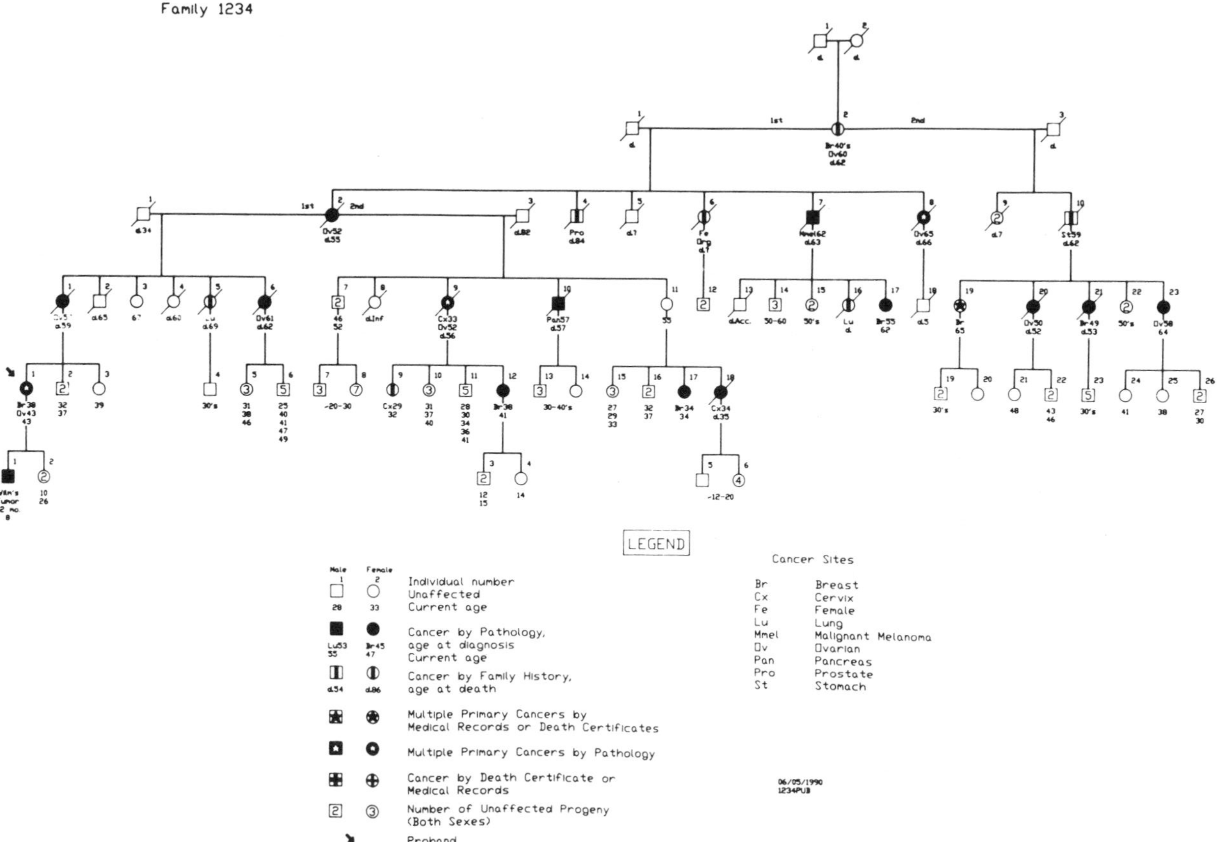

Figure 2. Updated pedigree of an extended hereditary breast/ovarian cancer family (originally published in HT Lynch *et al.*, Hereditary carcinoma of the ovary and associated cancers: A study of two families, *Gyn. Onc.*, 36, 48, 1990).

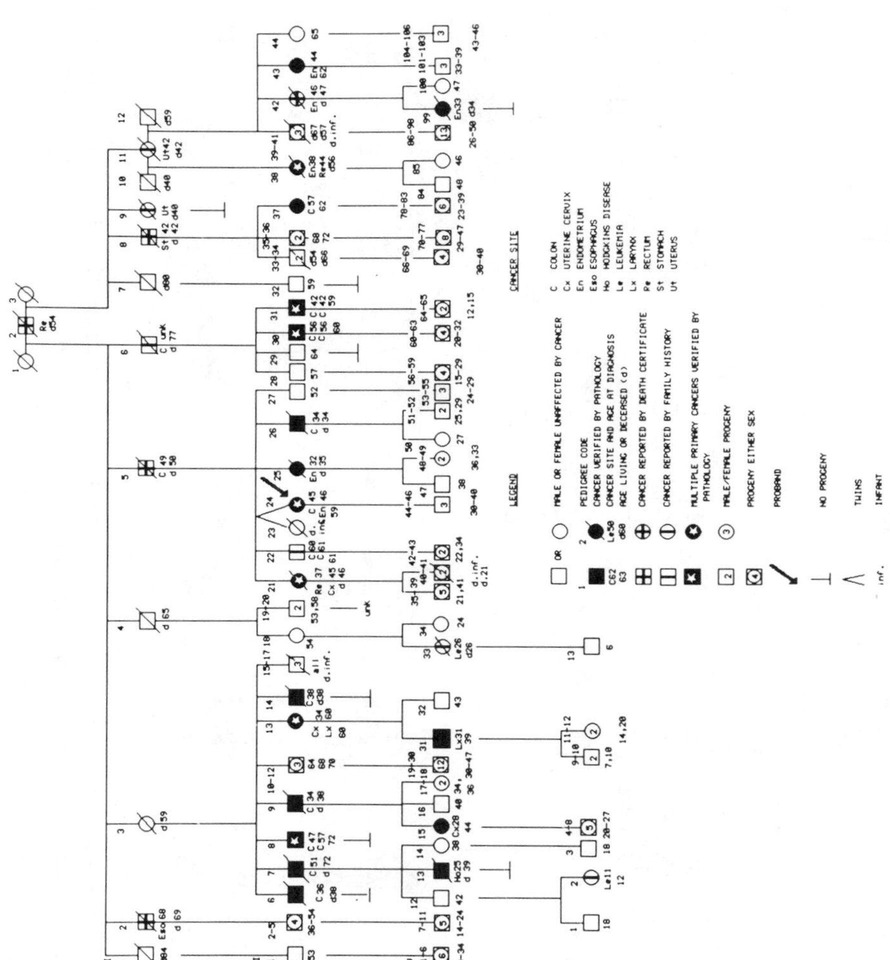

Figure 3. Pedigree of a Lynch syndrome II kindred. Note the occurrence of early onset colon and endometrial carcinoma (from HT Lynch *et al.*, Laryngeal carcinoma in a Lynch syndrome II kindred, *Cancer*, 62, 1007, 1988).

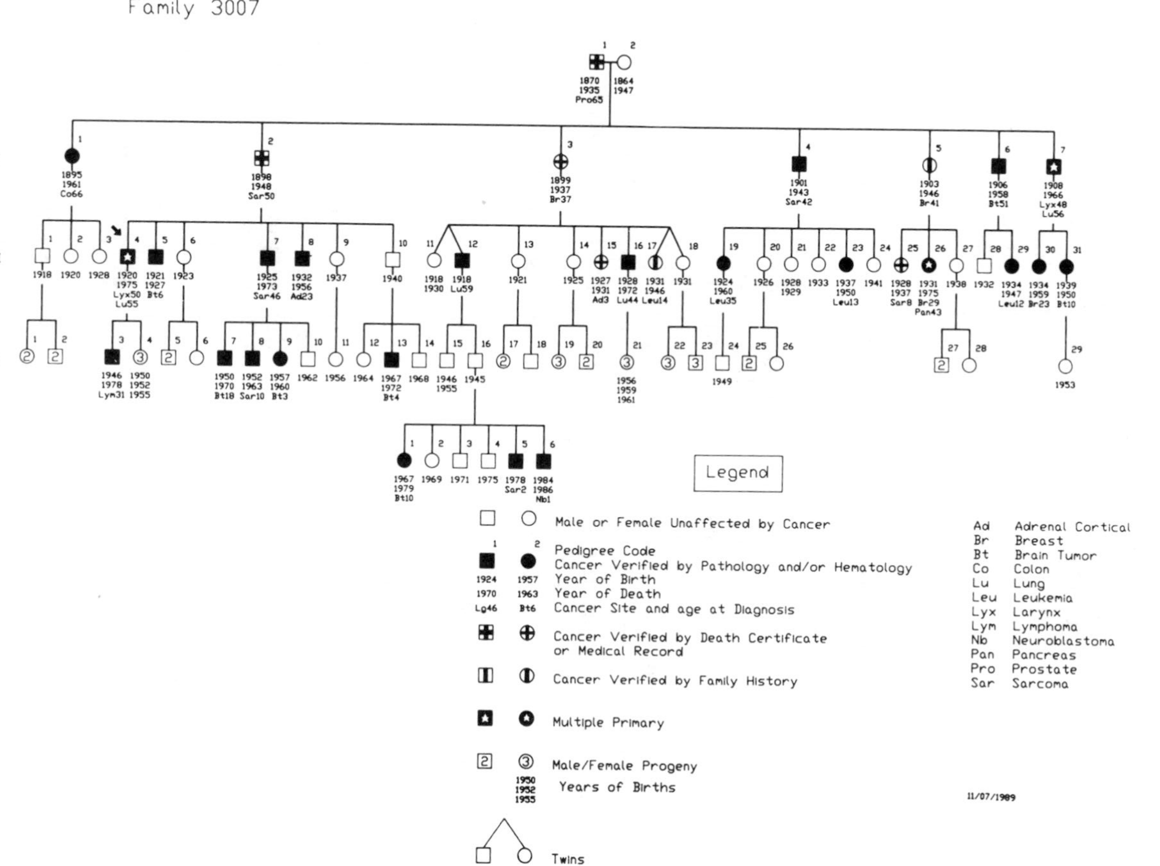

Figure 4. Updated pedigree of an SBLA cancer syndrome family (originally published in HT Lynch *et al.*, *A.J.D.C.*, 139, 134, 1985).

were initiated with diethylnitrosamine (DEN). Some were fed laboratory chow (LC) for 9 months; others were fed a choline-supplemented (CS) or CD diet.

The results after 9 months on an LC diet showed the livers of R-16 animals to be of greater size and to show a higher number of bile duct proliferations, cellular atypia, cirrhosis, and nodular hyperplasia than the ACP counterparts. The first hepatocellular carcinoma in R-16 fed animals on either a CS or LC diet was observed at 9-10 months. One R-16 rat fed a CD diet manifested liver cancer at 4 months. At 12 months, 15 of 22 (68%) of the R-16 rats on a CD diet had liver cancer, as did 7 of 24 (29%) of the R-16 animals on a CS diet. Of the ACP rats, 0 of 15 (0%) on CS and 1 of 18 (6%) on CD diet had liver tumors. It was concluded that the results clearly showed that grc genes confer a high susceptibility to liver cancer which is enhanced by a CD diet, suggesting **synergism** between genetics and diet.

VII. Colorectal Cancer

Dietary factors have been extensively investigated in the etiology of colorectal cancer. Trock *et al.*[24] reviewed the literature pertinent to whether colon cancer risk could be modified by a diet rich in vegetables, grains, and fruit. If this proved to be the case, then appropriate concern was given to whether the protective factor is the dietary fiber or other biologically active components correlated with a high fiber diet. This review assessed evidence from 37 observational epidemiologic studies and meta-analysis of data from 16 of 23 case/control studies. Both types of analyses indicated support for a **protective** effect associated with fiber-rich diets. However, the data did not allow discrimination between effects due to fiber and nonfiber effects of vegetables. Furthermore, the review did not provide any information about the protective role of diet in a **hereditary** colorectal cancer setting.

Lipkin and Newmark[25] studied the frequency and distribution of proliferating epithelial cells lining colonic crypts in 10 subjects at high risk for familial colorectal cancer before and after supplementation of their conventional diets with 1.25 g of calcium carbonate. Prior to dietary supplementation with calcium, the profile of proliferating cells in the colonic crypts was comparable to that previously observed in subjects who had had familial colonic cancer. Two to three months following calcium supplementation, proliferation was significantly reduced, and the profile of the colonic crypts approached that previously observed in subjects at low risk for colonic cancer. These investigators concluded that supplementation of oral calcium induces a more quiescent equilibrium in epithelial cell proliferation in the colonic mucosa of subjects at high risk for colon cancer, similar to that observed in subjects at low risk.

Newmark *et al.*[26] investigated this same phenomenon in a rodent model. They studied the effects of specific nutritional modifications; namely, increased fat and phosphate and decreased calcium and Vitamin-D, on colonic epithelial cell proliferation in mice and rats. Dietary exposure was begun at 3 weeks of age and continued for 12 weeks. The findings showed hyperproliferation in the sigmoid colon of mice and rats, and in the ascending colon of rats, with increased [^{3}H]-thymidine labeling of epithelial cells. It was concluded that in colonic mucosa, the nutritional stress diet, which included risk factors of a Western diet, induced changes that occur in carcinogen-induced rodent models and in humans who are at increased risk for colonic neoplasia.

DeCosse *et al.*[27] performed a randomized, double-blind, placebo-controlled, chemoprevention trial (over a 4-year period) on large bowel neoplasia in 58 patients with familial adenomatous polyposis (FAP.) Treatment comprised 4 g ascorbic acid (Vitamin C) per day plus 400 mg of alpha-tocopherol (Vitamin E) per day alone or with a grain fiber supplement (22.5 g/day). The study parameter pertained to the effects of these supplements on rectal polyps in these patients. The results showed that the high-fiber supplement had a limited effect. Analysis adjusted for patient compliance showed a stronger benefit during the middle 2 years of the trial. There was inhibition of benign large bowel neoplasia by grain fiber supplements in excess of 11 g/day in the study population. These investigators concluded that the findings from their study were consistent with the hypothesis that dietary grain fiber and total dietary fat act as competing variables in the genesis of large bowel neoplasia in these FAP patients.

Stemmerman *et al.*[28] studied 163 Hawaiian Japanese autopsy subjects from a cohort comprised of 8006 men who had participated in a prospective study from 1965-1968 and who had died from 1969-1984. Adenomas were found in 79 of the autopsy subjects, but not in the remaining 84. Results of this study showed an absence of any significant differences between subjects **with** and **without** adenomas with respect to dietary fat, proteins, carbohydrates, serum cholesterol, body mass index, level of physical activity, and cigarette smoking history. The only significant association was an increase in the mean number of polyps with increasing levels of alcohol intake. However, the trend was not monotonic.

Waddell *et al.*[29] evaluated the effect of Sulindac, a non-steroid anti-inflammatory drug, on 7 patients with FAP (or the Gardner's syndrome variant) following subtotal colectomy and ileoproctoscopy, and in 4 patients with intact colons. It was of extreme interest that all of the polyps were eliminated save for a few that arose in the rectal mucosa and the canal. While no cancers appeared in these patients on followup, given the temporal variability in colorectal cancer expression in this disease, one must use extreme caution in interpreting the role of Sulindac as protecting against cancer occurrence. We believe that the use of Sulindac should be subjected to careful clinical trials. Given the life-threatening aspect of FAP, we would not at this time employ the use of Sulindac in the place of prophylactic colectomy.

While dietary factors may be of importance, as evidenced by the studies described above, there is also evidence that cancer expression (phenotype) in certain hereditary forms of cancer may occur regardless of dietary exposure. This phenomenon was evidenced in a study performed by Lynch *et al.*[30] on an American Indian (Navajo) kindred that was prone to colorectal cancer. Specifically, this family (Figure 5) manifested early onset colorectal cancer with proximal predominance, a paucity of colonic polyps, with an inheritance pattern consonant with an autosomal dominant factor.

Of interest is the fact that colorectal cancer is **rare** in American Indians. However, on their reservation in Arizona, multiple occurrences of colorectal cancer were observed. When investigated by us, it was found that many of these cases occurred in this single family. The family resided in dispersed areas on this large reservation. So far as can be determined, their dietary pattern was no different from that of their tribal membership. Yet, in spite of the apparent homogeneity of their dietary exposure, these Indians manifested an excess of early onset proximal predominance of colorectal carcinoma. Thus, we see an

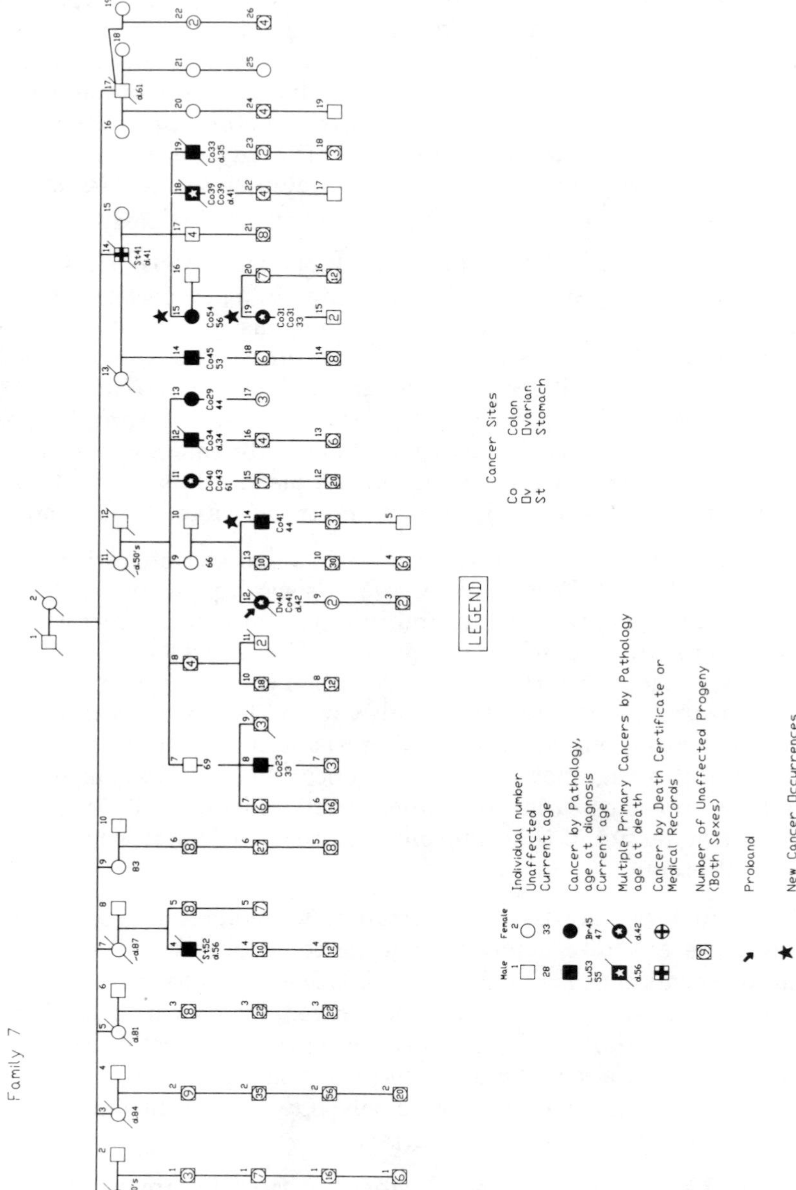

Figure 5. Updated pedigree of a Navajo Indian family showing a preponderance of colorectal cancer (originally published in HT Lynch *et al.*, *Ca. Genet. Cytogenet.*, 15, 209, 1985).

example of a deleterious genetic cancer-predisposing factor which appears to override environmental factors. However, quantitative analysis of the relative strength of primary genetic factors vs. environmental exposure in this particular family would require more elegant studies than the mere descriptive ones employed in this particular investigation. However, what is clear is that the host factor effect was particularly potent in this kindred so far as the colon cancer phenotype was concerned.

VIII. Esophageal Cancer (EC)

Wahrendorf *et al.*[31] studied young men and women (aged 15-26 years) in households in a population from China who were at high risk for EC. This risk was based on whether EC **had** (166 participants) or **had not** (372 participants) occurred in a first-degree relative. An endoscopic survey (43.5% males; 35.9% females) showed histologic signs of chronic esophagitis. These precursor lesions were significantly associated in a multivariate logistic model with: a) consumption of burning hot vegetables; b) family history of EC inclusive of second-degree relatives; c) infrequent consumption of fresh fruit and dietary staples other than maize.

Prospective studies of this cohort would be valuable. It would be important to know whether individuals in this cohort with chronic esophagitis might show resolution of chronic esophagitis with specific dietary modification. It would also be valuable to know whether those patients **lacking** chronic esophagitis develop EC. Formal genetic studies of chronic esophagitis are indicated.

In a similar investigation, Li *et al.*[32] performed a case/control study of EC and cancer of the gastric cardia in Linxian, China. Linxian is a rural county located in north central China which shows one of the world's highest mortality rates for these malignant neoplastic lesions. This involved 1244 patients (758 males, 486 females) with cancer of the esophagus or gastric cardia, and 1314 population-based controls (789 males, 525 females). The findings from this study showed that an increasing intake of wheat and corn was associated with a rise in cancer risk. However, there was no association observed with adult intake of pickled vegetables, which interestingly, had been the leading *a priori* suspect factor. In addition, cancer risks were not elevated among those individuals consuming low quantities of fresh vegetables or fruits. There was no apparent excess of consumption of alcoholic beverages. Smoking appeared to be a mild risk factor which was related to a greater extent to cancer of the cardia as opposed to EC. Of particular interest was the finding that risk "...was increased by 70% among those whose parents had esophageal or stomach cancer, but only slightly among those whose spouses had such cancers, suggesting that exposure early in life and/or genetic factors may be involved."

IX. Gallbladder Disease and Gallbladder Cancer

Among American Indians (Amerinds) there has been a recent "epidemic" of gallbladder disease (GBD). There is a consistent gradient of GBD from more-admixed to less-admixed Amerind populations which cannot be explained by any known aspects of the diet or environment. These observations, when coupled with additional epidemiologic data, suggest that there is a genetic susceptibility in New World (NW) peoples distinct from that which attaches generally to westernization.

Weiss *et al.*[33] suggest that the pattern of GBD among the Amerinds is more consistent with genotype-by-environment interaction than simply with the effects of a changed environment. If this assessment is correct, the bearers of susceptible genotypes may be at much higher risk of GBD, including cancer, than has been previously thought. The most strongly associated risk factor for gallbladder cancer (GBCA) in all populations is the presence of cholesterol stones. However, the carcinogenic mechanism remains elusive in NW peoples. The incidence of coexisting gallstones has approached 100% in some NW studies. Females are more often affected than males in NW populations. However, the reverse of this sex ratio occurs in Japan.

There is evidence that GBCA in NW peoples may be more than just a reflection of their higher prevalence of gallstones. In Caucasians, the frequency of asymptomatic GBCA or carcinoma in-situ (CIS) of the GB discovered at cholecystectomy performed for symptomatic gallstones is about 0.5 - 1.5%. In contrast, studies in Mexico where gallstones occur often and at young ages in females, the rate of cancerous or precancerous lesions in GBs removed for gallstones has been found to range between 3-5%. In Amerinds, cancerous or precancerous lesions have been found in 2-4.5% of GBs removed for stones.[33]

Certain epidemiologic considerations are important. Specifically, obesity can lead to gallstone formation. Diabetes mellitus is associated with GB disease. In other populations of the world, a rise in GBD has resulted from "westernization" which has been attributed to the consumption of a high calorie, high fat, low fiber diet and insufficient exercise.

In NW peoples, GBD is associated with high rates of obesity and non-insulin dependent diabetes mellitus in a manner which is consistent with a shared genetic etiology. Diseases of westernization also include elevated rates of ischemic heart disease and cancers of the breast, endometrium, colon, rectum, and prostate. However, it is of keen interest that these diseases occur at a **lower** frequency in NW peoples who, to judge by GBD and diabetes rates, have been exposed to these relevant environmental risk factors for at least 40 years. The association between rates of colon cancer and cholecystectomy with GBA and GBCA, which has been reported in some but not all studies in other populations, does not occur in NW peoples. Therefore, the pattern of response to those risk factors, whatever they may be, appears to differ in NW peoples. The lower GBD rates in blacks, who have typically shared similar socioeconomic status with NW peoples, suggests that this is not a problem which can be ascribed to poverty. For example, Weiss *et al.*[33] consider it unlikely that NW peoples share with each other, on a continental scale, exposures that they do not also share with blacks and Europeans. It remains unclear whether NW peoples typically have the kind of diet and lifestyle that has been suggested as a cause of GBD.

Weiss *et al.*[33] suggest that the pattern of GBD and GBCA in native peoples of the new world, including Amerinds and admixed Latin Americans such as Mexican-Americans, differs from that which is generally consistent with "westernization." They suggest that there exists "...a gene/environment interaction, and that within an admixed population, there is a subset whose risk is underestimated when admixture is ignored." The risk that an individual of a susceptible new world genotype will undergo cholecystectomy by age 85 can approach 40% in Mexican-American females and the risk of gallbladder cancer can reach several percent. These are heretofore unrecognized levels of risk, especially of the latter, because previous studies have not accounted for admixture or for the loss of at risk individuals due to cholecystectomy. A genetic susceptibility may, thus, be as "carcinogenic" in new world peoples as any known major environmental exposure; yet, while the risk has a genetic basis, its expression as gallbladder cancer is so delayed as to lead only very rarely to multiply-affected families. "It is also possible that this NW susceptibility has evolved as a function of genetic drift. It is not clear if a biocomponent is unusually carcinogenic in NW peoples or if this is simply due to very high rates of subclinical gallstones. Therefore, it is not currently possible to suggest practical preventive measures for GBC or GBCA."

Early detection of gallstones by ultrasonography may at least indicate those who would be at risk for GBA and GBCA. GBD in NW peoples provides a unique opportunity for practicing cancer control by combining approaches to physiology, genetics, epidemiology, and anthropology. This could then contribute to the understanding of a major epidemic of GBD and GBCA in the NW peoples.

X. Summary and Conclusions

It is clear that nutritionally oriented cancer epidemiologists must work more closely with their cancer genetic colleagues in the interest of a more full elucidation of the etiology of carcinogenesis. The studies which we have reviewed relevant to cancers of the colon, esophagus, and gallbladder in man can profit immensely by methodologies which focus heavily on **both** genetic and environmental interaction. In addition to a detailed nutritional evaluation over time, and here (ideally) on a prospective basis, in concert with careful documentation of cancer of all anatomic sites, through at least second degree relatives of the probands, the impact of dietary factors on cancer can then be more clearly elucidated. Such an approach, while time-consuming and expensive, could, in the long-run, provide invaluable knowledge for conducting more focused chemoprevention trials, inclusive of dietary manipulation, in the interest of cancer control.

Acknowledgement

Supported by a grant from the Fraternal Order of Eagles-Nebraska Division.

References

1. Lynch, H.T. and Hirayama, T., *Genetic Epidemiology of Cancer,* C.R.C. Press, Boca Raton, 1989.

2. Lynch, H.T., Ed., *Cancer Genetics,* C.C. Thomas, Springfield, 1976.

3. Lynch, H.T., Ed., *Genetics and Breast Cancer,* V.N. Reinhold Co, New York, 1981.

4. Lynch, H.T. and Fusaro, R.M., Eds., *Cancer-Associated Genodermatoses,* V.N. Reinhold Co, New York, 1982.

5. Lynch, P.M. and Lynch, H.T., Eds., *Colon Cancer Genetics,* V.N. Reinhold, New York, 1985.

6. Lynch, H.T. and Kullander, S., Eds., *Cancer Genetics in Women,* C.R.C. Press, Boca Raton, 1987.

7. Hill, M.J., Experimental studies of fat, fibre, and calories in carcinogenesis, in *Diet and the Aetiology of Cancer,* Miller, A.B., Ed., Springer-Verlag, Berlin, 1989, 31.

8. McKusick, V., *Mendelian Inheritance in Man,* 8th ed., J. Hopk. Un. Press, Baltimore, 1988.

9. Lynch, H.T., Anderson, D.E., Krush, A.J., and Mukerjee, D., Cancer, heredity, and genetic counseling: xeroderma pigmentosum, *Cancer,* 20, 1796, 1967.

10. Lynch, H.T., Anderson, D.E., Smith, J.L., Howell, J.B., and Krush, A.J., Xeroderma pigmentosum, malignant melanoma, and congenital ichthyosis: a family study, *Arch. Derm.,* 96, 625, 1967.

11. Lynch, H.T., Frichot, B.C., and Lynch, J.F., Cancer control in xeroderma pigmentosum, *Arch. Derm.,* 113, 193, 1977.

12. Lynch, H.T., Frichot, B.C., Fisher, J., Smith, J.L., and Lynch, J.F., Spontaneous regression of metastatic malignant melanoma in two siblings with xeroderma pigmentosum, *J. Med. Genet.,* 15, 357, 1978.

13. Lynch, H.T., Fusaro, R.M., and Johnson, J.A., Xeroderma pigmentosum: complementation group C and malignant melanoma, *Arch. Derm.,* 120, 175, 1984.

14. Harris, C.C., Mulvihill, J.J., Thorgeirsson, S.S., and Minna, J.D., Individual differences in cancer susceptibility, *Ann. Int. Med.,* 92, 809, 1980.

15. Lynch, H.T., Guirgis, H.A., Brodkey, F., *et al.*, Early age of onset in familial breast cancer: genetic and cancer control implications, *Arch. Surg.,* 111, 126, 1976.

16. Harris, R.E., Lynch, H.T., and Guirgis, H.A., Familial breast cancer: risk to the contralateral breast, *J.N.C.I.,* 60, 955, 1978.

17. Lynch, H.T. and Lynch, P.M., Tumor variation in the Cancer Family Syndrome: ovarian cancer, *Am. J. Surg.,* 138, 439, 1979.

18. Guirgis, H.A. and Lynch, H.T., Eds., *Biomarkers, Genetics, and Cancer,* V.N. Reinhold, New York, 1985.

19. Albano, W.A., Recabaren, J.A., Lynch, H.T., *et al.*, Natural history of hereditary cancer of the breast and colon, *Cancer,* 50, 360, 1982.

20. Lynch, H.T., Mulcahy, G.M., Harris, R.E., Guirgis, H.A., and Lynch, J.F., Genetic and pathologic findings in a kindred with hereditary sarcoma, breast cancer, brain tumors, leukemia, lung, laryngeal, and adrenal cortical carcinoma, *Cancer,* 41, 2055, 1978.

21. Lynch, H.T., Katz, D.A., Bogard, P.J., and Lynch, J.F., The sarcoma, breast cancer, lung cancer, and adrenocortical carcinoma syndrome revisited: childhood cancer, *A.J.D.C.,* 139, 134, 1985.

22. Melhem, M.F., Kazanecki, M.E., Rao, K.N., Kunz, H.W., and Gill, T.J., Genetics and diet: synergism in hepatocarcinogenesis in rats, *J. Am. Coll. Nutr.,* 9, 168, 1990.

23. Giambarresi, L.I., Katyal, S.L., and Lombardi, B., Promotion of liver carcinogenesis in the rat by a choline-devoid diet; role of liver cell necrosis and regeneration, *Br. J. Cancer,* 46, 825, 1982.

24. Trock, B., Lanza, E., and Greenwald, P., Dietary fiber, vegetables, and colon cancer: critical review and meta-analyses of the epidemiologic evidence, *J.N.C.I.,* 82, 650, 1990.

25. Lipkin, M. and Newmark, H., Effect of added dietary calcium on colonic epithelial cell proliferation in subjects at high risk for familial colonic cancer, *N.E.J.M.,* 313, 1381, 1985.

26. Newmark, H.L., Lipkin, M., and Maheshwari, N., Colonic hyperplasia and hyperproliferation induced by a nutritional stress diet with four components of western-style diet, *J.N.C.I.,* 82, 491, 1990.

27. DeCosse, J.J., Miller, H.H., and Lesser, M.L., Effect of wheat fiber and vitamins C and E on rectal polyps in patients with familial adenomatous polyposis, *J.N.C.I.,* 82, 1290, 1990.

28. Stemmerman, G.N., Heilbrun, L.K., and Nomura, A.M.Y., Association of diet and other factors with adenomatous polyps of the large bowel: a prospective autopsy study, Am. J. Clin. Nutr., 47, 312, 1988.

29. Waddell, W.R., Ganser, G.F., Cerise, E.J., and Loughry, R.W., Sulindac for polyposis of the colon, *Am. J. Surg.,* 157, 175, 1989.

30. Lynch, H.T., Drouhard, T.L., Schuelke, G.S., *et al.*, Hereditary nonpolyposis colorectal cancer in a Navajo Indian family, *Ca. Genet. Cytogenet.,* 15, 209, 1985.

31. Wahrendorf, J., Liang, Q.S., Munoz, N., *et al.*, Precursor lesions of esophageal cancer in young people in a high-risk population in China, *Lancet,* ii, 1239, 1989.

32. Li, J.Y., Ershow, A.G., Chen, Z.J., *et al.*, A case-control study of cancer of the esophagus and gastric cardia in Linxian, *Int. J. Cancer,* 43, 755, 1989.

33. Weiss, K.M., Ferrell, R.E., Hanis, C.L., and Styne, P.N., Genetics and epidemiology of gallbladder disease in New World native peoples, *Am. J. Hum. Genet.,* 36, 1259, 1984.

Chapter 2

Vitamin B6 and Other Inhibitors of Glucocorticoid Receptor Function and Cell Death of B16 Melanoma Cells

Gerald Litwack, Noreen M. Robertson, Andrew B. Maksymowych, and Mahmut Celiker

Table of Contents

I. Introduction

In 1977 and 1978, [1-6] we provided the first evidence that pyridoxal phosphate, the biologically active form of vitamin B6, interfered with the ability of the activated (DNA-binding form) glucocorticoid receptor to interact with DNA, thus opening the possibility that the cellular level of pyridoxal phosphate might regulate the functioning of the receptor mechanism. The precursor or pyridoxal phosphate is dietary vitamin B6, pyridoxine. This is metabolized to pyridoxal phosphate in two steps, the phosphorylation of pyridoxine to form pyridoxine phosphate and its subsequent oxidation to pyridoxal by a riboflavin catalyzed enzymic reaction.[7] Pyridoxal, an alternative form of vitamin B6 can enter the cell and be converted to pyridoxal phosphate by pyridoxal kinase and ATP in a single step. Classically, pyridoxal phosphate is known to form a Schiff base with proteins through a side chain amino group of a lysine residue.[8] Thus, it appeared that not only was pyridoxal phosphate able to form a Schiff base with lysine residues in the DNA binding domain and at or near the steroid binding site of the glucorticoid receptor, but it was likely that the dietary level of vitamin B6 could influence the cellular level of pyridoxal phosphate and exert some control over the glucocorticoid receptor mechanism that mediates stress adaptation at the cellular level.

II. Specificity of Pyridoxal Phosphate Interaction with the Glucocorticoid Receptor

In vitro experiments showed that pyridoxal phosphate inhibited the interaction of activated transformed glucocorticoid receptor with DNA.[6] This was not a consequence of interaction of the vitamer with DNA but rather directly with the receptor.[6] Further experiments showed that a lysine residue at or near the steroid binding domain was also a target and these two sites could be studied independently by virtue of different temperature dependencies.[9] In contrast to pyridoxal phosphate, pyridoxine, pyridoxamine and pyridoxamine phosphate were without activity while pyridoxal had only partial activity.[6] Later experiments showed that a non-specific aldehyde had very low activity indicating that the activity of pyridoxal phosphate was specific.

III. The Glucocorticoid Receptor Activation/Transformation Mechanism

In order to appreciate the significance of vitamin B6 control over the functioning of the glucocorticoid receptor, the activation/transformation mechanism must be introduced (Figure 1). The reaction proceeds from left to right and, as depicted in this scheme, involves three forms of the glucocorticoid receptor. The left hand form represents the unactivated non-DNA-binding form of the receptor. This appears to be an oligomer with one molecule of the steroid (G) receptor, a molecule of modulator (M), a dimer of 90 kDa heat shock protein (HSP90), an RNA noncovalently attached to the DNA binding domain and a 57 kDa protein attached to HSP90. Evidence for the presence of some of these components is more impressive than for others. The rate-limiting step for the

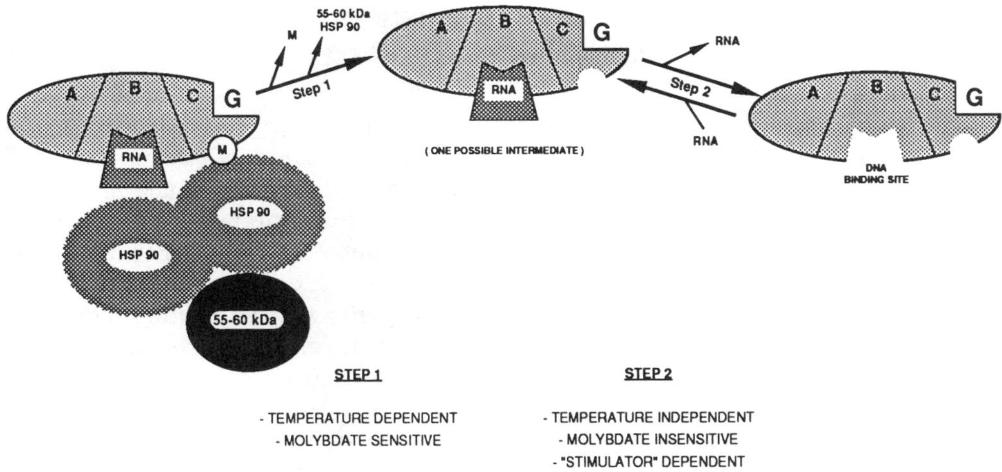

	UNACTIVATED	INTERMEDIATE(S)	ACTIVATED
SEDIMENTATION COEFFICIENT:	8 - 10 S	5 - 7 S	4 - 5 S
STOKES RADIUS:	70 - 80 Å	60 - 80 Å	50 - 60 Å
MOLECULAR WEIGHT:	300,000 - 310,000	130,000 - 180,000	94,000
DNA BINDING:	5 %	10 - 20 %	30 - 40 %
DEAE ELUTION POSITION:	250 mM KP	50 mM KP	50 mM KP

Figure 1. Speculative mechanism of activation/transformation of the cytoplasmic glucocorticoid receptor.

progression of this mechanism appears to be the dissociation of the modulator[10-13] which concurrently releases the nonhomologous proteins. This only occurs in the presence of bound glucocorticoid (G) and it is this non-DNA-binding form that serves productively to bind the steroidal ligand. Although many conditions are known to cause the dissociation of modulator from the unactivated form[10-13] *in vitro*, there is a paucity of information on what exactly drives this process in the intact cell. Probably it is more than the association of the ligand with the unactivated receptor complex, although this step alone must produce some significant alteration in the conformation of the receptor molecule. Following this step, there may be generated an intermediate form of the receptor still bound noncovalently to an RNA molecule. Three laboratories report the association of an RNA with the unactivated receptor.[14-16] Finally, the RNA molecule is removed to generate the DNA-binding activated receptor which can translocate from the cytoplasm, where these events have occurred, to the nucleus to ultimately interact with the glucocorticoid responsive element[17] and affect transcription. With regard to the actions of pyridoxal phosphate we will be concerned with the unactivated, non-DNA-binding form and the activated DNA-binding form.

IV. Effects of Pyridoxal Phosphate on Glucocorticoid Binding

Pyridoxal phosphate in the micromolar to millimolar range inhibits the specific binding of glucocorticoid ([^{3}H] triamcinolone acetonide) to the unactivated receptor complex. If pyridoxal phosphate is added before steroid, the inhibition of steroid binding is substantially more intense so that a preferred target is the unactivated steroid hormone receptor in the absence of steroid (Figure 1; left hand figure but in the absence of G). There is little effect of pyridoxal phosphate on the activated DNA binding form of the receptor with respect to steroid binding under these conditions. Here this measurement is made on the radioactive steroid retained by the activated receptor as measured by hydroxylapatite binding. These measurements can be represented by a double reciprocal plot creating a series of lines with origins in the second quadrant. When the slopes of these lines are replotted as a function of pyridoxal phosphate concentration, a curve of parabolic inhibition results. This curve can be evaluated at each concentration point according to the equation: K_i slope = $K_i^2 / 2K_i + [I]$. When this is done the K_i with respect to pyridoxal is in the range of 1-4 µM, a concentration considered to be well within the limits of "free" or dissociable pyridoxal phosphate in the cell.[18]

V. Effects of Pyridoxal Phosphate on DNA Binding by the Activated Glucocorticoid Receptor

As indicated above, pyridoxal phosphate did not reduce the amount of radioactive steroid bound to the activated glucocorticoid receptor under our test conditions up to 1000 µM. However, DNA binding was inhibited. By separate determinations we had concluded that this inhibition was not due to interaction of pyridoxal phosphate with DNA but rather directly with the receptor.[5,18] DNA binding was completely eliminated in the mM range of pyridoxal phosphate. When inhibition is arranged as a double reciprocal plot, a family of lines emerges and when a secondary replot of slopes as a function of pyridoxal phosphate concentration is prepared, once again a parabola is developed. The K_i is evaluated by the same equation as shown above for each concentration of pyridoxal phosphate and the K_i with respect to pyridoxal phosphate as a function of inhibition of nonspecific DNA binding is on the order of 9 µM, in good agreement with the values obtained for inhibition of steroid binding to the unactivated, unoccupied glucocorticoid receptor complex. Once again, this value seems compatible with the "free" or dissociable concentration of pyridoxal phosphate in the cell. Thus, the function of the glucocorticoid receptor in terms of its translocation will be impaired by pyridoxal phosphate in its effect on the DNA binding domain of the activated receptor and an even greater effect will occur if the level of the steroid in the cell is low or absent.

A. Pyridoxal Phosphate and the Purified Activated Glucocorticoid Receptor

An important aspect of the inhibition by pyridoxal phosphate was to determine whether the vitamer interacts directly with the receptor molecule or with another molecule in the system that regulates receptor function. Our approach was to observe the inhibition of DNA binding with activated forms of the receptor in preparations of adrenalectomized rat liver cytosol, subsequently in partially purified receptor preparations and finally in a virtually homogeneous preparation of the activated receptor. In all cases the same phenomena were recorded. In the absence of pyridoxal phosphate a control amount of virtually homogeneous receptor was recovered on DEAE-cellulose columns. When the activated receptor was treated with calf thymus double stranded DNA, and then subjected to ion exchange chromatography the amount of specifically bound (with [^{3}H] triamcinolone acetonide) recovered was reduced to about 32% indicating that about 60-70% had interacted with DNA. When pyridoxal phosphate in mM amount was mixed with the activated receptor and DNA, recovery on the ion exchange column was increased to about 76% indicating that pyridoxal phosphate inhibited the ability of the activated receptor to bind to DNA by about 40-45%. These results were found to align with those obtained with activated receptor in cytosol or in partially purified preparations. This agreement in results between crude and purified receptors strongly suggests that pyridoxal phosphate interacts directly with the receptor molecule and is not interacting with some other regulator of receptor activation.

B. Effect of Pyridoxal Phosphate on Specific DNA Binding of the Glucocorticoid Receptor

The glucocorticoid responsive element, a 15 mer, has been shown to be the specific enhancer sequence with which the activated glucocorticoid receptor interacts to activate transcription.[17] A synthetic glucocorticoid response element:

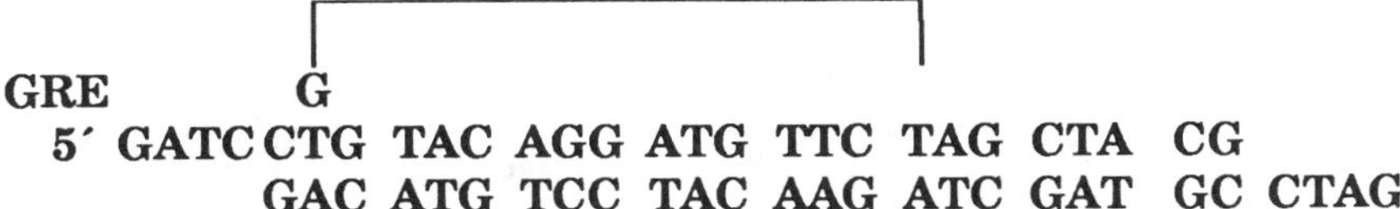

was prepared[18] and utilized in gel retardation assays after end labeling with [^{32}P]. For these experiments, semi-purified receptor was used. This preparation included chromatography of adrenalectomized rat liver cytosol using phosphocellulose and DNA-cellulose. The eluate from DNA-cellulose was bound with [^{3}H] triamcinolone acetonide for 18 hours at 4°C and gel filtered through a column of Sephadex G-25 followed by heating at 25°C for 30 minutes to activate the receptor complex.[18] The activated receptor complex was further purified by DEAE-cellulose chromatography and the peak fractions corresponding to the activated form of the receptor were pooled and concentrated 10 fold using an Amicon centricon for this experiment. The results are shown in Figure 2.

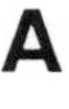

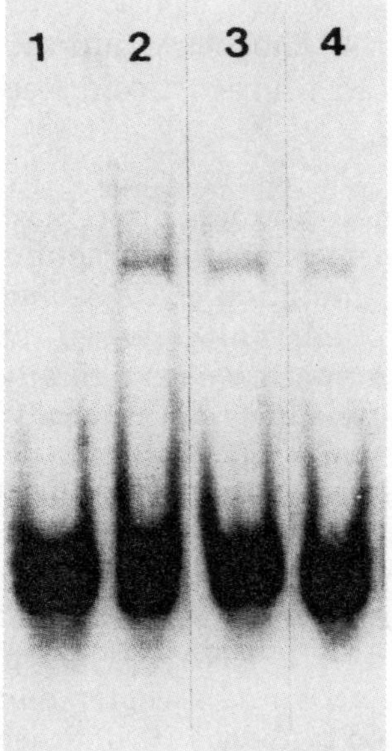

B

	RELATIVE BAND INTENSITY	%	(Δ)	SPECIFIC BINDING TO DNA-CELLULOSE	%	(Δ)
LANE 2	1,932.0	100		74,422.67 [a]	100	
LANE 3	1,236.5	64	(– 36)	ND [b]	ND	
LANE 4	933.8	48	(– 52)	40,136.67	54	(– 46)

[a] dpm

[b] Not determined

Figure 2. Pyridoxal 5′-phosphate inhibition of activated receptor binding to a specific GRE. Partially purified receptors were used directly or preincubated at 20°C for 30 minutes with 2 mM pyridoxal phosphate. Receptors were then allowed to bind to specific ^{32}P end-labeled GRE for 30 minutes at room temperature. The reaction mixtures were loaded onto a nondenaturing polyacrylamide gel and electrophoresis proceeded until the tracking dye just about reached the end of the gel. The gel was dried and autoradiographed with Kodak X-OMAT™ AR film for 20 hours at -80°C. Developed films showed a mobility shift dependent on receptor binding to the specific GRE. (**A**) *Lane 1* contained GRE only. *Lane 2* contains 16 nM activated glucocorticoid-receptor complexes + GRE. *Lane 3* contains 16 nM activated glucocorticoid-receptor complexes preincubated with 200 µM pyridoxal phosphate + GRE. *Lane 4* contains 16 nM activated glucocorticoid-receptor complexes preincubated with 2 mM pyridoxal phosphate + GRE. (**B**) This table summarizes the soft laser quantification of the bands shown in **A** and includes DNA-cellulose binding data for the same receptor preparation. (Reproduced from ref. 18 by permission from the New York Academy of Sciences.)

Clearly, pyridoxal phosphate in µM or mM concentrations was able to inhibit the association of the partially purified receptor with the glucocorticoid responsive element, confirming that the DNA binding domain was affected by pyridoxal phosphate whether interacting with nonspecific or specific DNA. Since the two zinc fingers of the DNA binding domain of the receptor have been shown to interact with the glucocorticoid responsive element, the lysine residues of the DNA binding domain, especially lysines 449, 453, 474, 478 and 487 (mouse sequence) are possible targets of pyridoxal phosphate in this domain. In particular, lysines 474 and 478 reside near the tip of the right hand zinc finger and could be targets for pyridoxylation. Now that the full-length human[19] and rat[20] glucocorticoid receptors have been overproduced in the baculovirus system, it should not be long before this pyridoxylation site is identified directly by peptide sequencing.

VI. Effects of Vitamin B6 on Proliferation of Cells in Culture

The realization that pyridoxal phosphate was an important inhibitor of the glucocorticoid receptor,[5] shown subsequently to be important for other steroid receptors[21] and the function of the glucocorticoid receptor is certainly essential for life of the organism, led us to test the effects of elevated levels of vitamin B6 (pyridoxine) and later pyridoxal on cells in culture. We demonstrated that the vitamin was able to reduce cell growth and kill a number of cell types in culture. These results are briefly summarized in Table 1. Although MCF-7 cells were not killed in these experiments[22] other tumor and some nontransformed cells were.

By far the most interesting effect we observed was with B16 mouse melanoma cells. This cell line was readily killed by pyridoxine or pyridoxal. Later, we used pyridoxal thinking that it required only one enzymatic step to form pyridoxal phosphate and, in most cases, pyridoxal seemed more effective than pyridoxine probably for the reason just mentioned. More recently, we have worked with human pigmented melanoma cells in culture and with human metastatic melanoma cells in culture. In all cases, the cells were readily killed by pyridoxal in the medium and in all cases pyridoxal resulted in inhibition of glucocorticoid receptor translocation to the nucleus.

TABLE 1
Some Cells Killed in Culture by PN/PL

Cell type	Killing[b]
Fu5-5	+
MCF-7	-
Glioma	+
Kidney	+
B16 melanoma[a]	+++
Human melanoma[a]	+++
Human melanoma, mestastatic[a]	+++

[a] pigmented
[b] trypan blue uptake/cell counts

A. Receptor Function and Pyridoxal Treatment in Melanoma Cells. Studies in Intact Cells Using Indirect Immunofluorescence

For this work we have used two monoclonal antibodies: 3A6 developed by our laboratory[23] with an epitope between the DNA binding domain and the steroid binding domain, but closer to the latter, based on the data that steroid binding is quantitatively more affected by the antibody than DNA binding;[23] we also use BUGR-2 developed by the Harrison laboratory[24] with an epitope to the N-terminal side of the DNA binding domain such that the antibody does not interfere with DNA binding. The general technique of indirect immunofluoresence in intact cells has been described.[25] Mouse B16 melanoma cells are grown adherently on microscope slides in media containing phenol red-free, charcoal-stripped bovine fetal serum which removes glucocorticoid and some other growth factors as well. In the absence of triamcinolone acetonide treatment, indirect immunofluorescence with a second antibody conjugated with rhodamine reveals most of the fluorescence in the cytoplasm of B16 melanoma cells. Incubation of the cells with 1 μM triamcinolone acetonide for 30-60 minutes at 37°C results in a shift of fluorescence from the cytoplasm to the nucleus reflecting the translocation process. Control experiments either when the cells were treated with triamcinolone acetonide or not were run in exactly the same manner except that the first antibody was pretreated with partially purified glucocorticoid receptor. This treatment resulted in virtually no fluorescence in both cases. The same experiment was repeated in the presence of 1 mM pyridoxal for one hour at 37°C prior to triamcinolone or vehicle addition. In this case, in the absence of added triamcinolone acetonide, the fluorescence appeared in the cytoplasm, as expected. When cells were pretreated with pyridoxal and then given triamcinolone acetonide the fluorescence was perinuclear concentrating around the nucleus, but clearly not associated directly with the nucleus, leading to the conclusion that pyridoxal prevented the translocation of the receptor. Obviously pyridoxal was converted to pyridoxal phosphate which bound to the DNA binding domain, containing the nuclear translocation signal and prevented movement through the perinuclear membrane into the nucleus. Once again, the controls in which the primary antibody was neutralized with partially purified receptor showed no fluorescence.

Similar experiments were carried out with human WM983A pigmented melanoma cells and also with human WM983C metastatic melanoma cells in culture. In the absence of triamcinolone acetonide treatment fluorescence was located primarily in the cytoplasm, whereas after treatment with triamcinolone acetonide fluorescence was located in the nucleus. When the cells were pretreated with 1 mM pyridoxal, the fluorescence, as in the case of B16 melanoma cells, was concentrated around the periphery of the nucleus indicating that pyridoxal, in the form of pyridoxal phosphate, prevented nuclear translocation of the steroid receptor.

B. Effects of Inhibitors of Glucocorticoid Receptor Function on Melanoma Cell Proliferation

Because the glucocorticoid receptor function, specifically nuclear translocation, is prevented by treatment with pyridoxal and several cell lines are killed by this treatment, we reasoned that if the dysfunction were a major part of the killing effect, other, more specific inhibitors of glucocorticoid receptor function should have the same effect. Initial experiments were carried out with B16 melanoma cells grown to 90% confluency. Test substances were added in a single dose at the beginning of the experiment and viable cell numbers were determined for 4-5 days using trypan blue exclusion and counting live cells microscopically in a hemocytometer.

Cortexolone (11-deoxycortisol) is a well-known glucocorticoid receptor antagonist. By indirect immunofluorescence using B16 melanoma cells, we determined that cortexolone is an inhibitor of the nuclear translocation process.[26] Cortexolone at 100, 150 and 200 μM was added in a single dose to cultures of B16 melanoma cells at 90% confluence. All doses resulted in complete killing of the cells by four days and the highest dose caused complete cell killing in approximately 1.5 days while the intermediate dose killed all the cells by 2-2.5 days. It was noted that, at lower doses than reported here, there was partial killing and the cell growth curve rebounded, suggesting that cortexolone was being metabolized or otherwise voided from the cell at low doses. Although we do not know of alternative effects of this drug other than to antagonize the glucocorticoid receptor, it is possible that it may be exerting effects about which we are unaware. In any case, in the previously described work with pyridoxal phosphate, the glucocorticoid receptor and cell killing predicted that a receptor antagonist such as cortexolone should have these effects and they have been observed, albeit at high concentrations.

We performed similar experiments with RU 38486, a specific antagonist of the glucocorticoid receptor. Again the protocol was similar to that used for cortexolone with B16 melanoma cells. Although a 1 μM single dose of RU 38486 killed a few cells and subsequently stimulated cell growth, higher levels of 10 and 20 μM resulted in total or nearly total killing by about 90 hours of culture. Although we do not understand why 1 μM was ineffective in these experiments it may be that melanoma cells somehow process or secrete RU 38486 at low concentrations. Interestingly, RU 38486 also acts as a translocation inhibitor of the glucocorticoid receptor.[25]

Experiments have been started with human primary melanoma cells (WM983A) as well as with human metastatic melanoma cells (WM983C). In these experiments the serum was stripped with charcoal which removes steroids and some other factors. In the experiments described above with B16 melanoma cells, serum was not stripped with charcoal. Another difference was that with human cells, the medium was changed daily to correct for metabolism or other processes which might cause lower levels of reagents to be ineffective. Under such conditions 1.5 mM pyridoxal had a small effect for 2 days and then precipitously killed all the cells by the fourth day of culture. Of great interest is the observation with WM983A cells that the addition of 2.5 nM triamcinolone acetonide together with 1.5 mM pyridoxal doubled the rate of cell killing so that by 2 days all of the cells had been killed compared to four days with pyridoxal alone. This suggests that pyridoxal is more effective when the cells have a functional receptor (ligand present) than with a poorly functional receptor (ligand nearly absent). Clearly, in the case of the human melanoma cells the basic observation that pyridoxal kills the cells confirms the results observed with mouse B16 melanoma cells. Experiments on cortexolone and RU 38486 are being conducted with human cells as well. However, since there is so much variety in melanoma cell lines, we realize that these kinds of experiments will have to be done with many lines and in alternative modes testing cells in log phase, confluence, synthetic media, etc.

VII. Speculations on Potential Mechanisms

Millimolar levels of pyridoxine and pyridoxal kill melanoma cells and other cell types as well. We have established in intact cells that this treatment interferes with the function of the glucocorticoid receptor blocking the nuclear translocation step by forming a Schiff base with a lysine residue in the DNA binding domain. There is information in the literature suggesting that glucocorticoids induce tyrosinase,[27,28] the key enzyme in the synthesis of melanin which is a major differentiated phenotype of pigmented melanoma cells. We plan to investigate this relationship by testing the capacity of glucocorticoids to specifically up-regulate mRNA tyrosinase. If this relationship is true then it is entirely possible that the actions of glucocorticoids, mediated by the glucocorticoid receptor are an important site of inhibition by pyridoxal phosphate derived from pyridoxal. This inhibition of receptor function could down-regulate tyrosinase and curtail the production of melanin which could be deleterious to a pigmented melanoma cell. On the other hand, other essential proteins could also be pyridoxylated by pyridoxal phosphate to modify their activities and in concert with changes in the function of the glucocorticoid receptor could bring about the demise of the cell. It is still a possibility that the changes in function of the glucocorticoid receptor are not lethal but toxicity develops from alteration of other essential proteins. Also to be considered is the possibility that the alteration of the glucocorticoid receptor plays a key role but that it functions in other pathways in addition to the formation of melanin and the interference in these other pathways may contribute to cell death. Necessarily these questions will have to be answered before melanoma cell death induced by pyridoxal is understood.

Acknowledgements

Work related to this subject in the Litwack Laboratory is supported by Research Grants DK13531 from the NIH, 87A19 from the American Institute for Cancer Research and by Core Grant CA12227 to the Fels Institute from the NIH. Andrew B. Maksymowych is a trainee on training grant T32DK07162 from the National Institutes of Health to the Department of Biochemistry. Noreen M. Robertson is a trainee on training grant T32CA09637 from the National Institutes of Health to the Fels Institute.

References

1. Cake, M.H. and Litwack, G., Interaction of pyridoxal phosphate with the DNA binding site of activated glucocorticoid receptor from rat liver, *Proc. Austral. Biochem. Soc.*, 10, 51, 1977.

2. Litwack, G. and Cake, M.H., DNA binding site of activated glucocorticoid receptor, *Fed. Proc.*, 36, 911, 1977.

3. DiSorbo, D.M. and Litwack, G., Pyridoxal-5′-phosphate is involved in the regulation of the glucocorticoid receptor, *Endocrine Proc.*, 60th Meeting, 131, 1978.

4. Dolan, K.P. and Litwack, G., Stabilization of the glucocorticoid receptor by pyridoxal-5′-phosphate, *Endocrine Proc.*, 60th Meeting, 308, 1978.

5. Cake, M.H., DiSorbo, D.M., and Litwack, G., Effect of pyridoxal phosphate on the DNA binding site of the activated hepatic glucocorticoid receptor, *J. Biol. Chem.*, 253, 4886, 1978.

6. Cake, M.H. and Litwack, G., Effect of methylxanthines on binding of the glucocorticoid receptor to DNA cellulose and nuclei, *Eur. J. Biochem.*, 82, 97, 1978.

7. Merrill, Jr., A.H. and Henderson, J.M., Vitamin B6 metabolism by human liver, in *Vitamin B6*, Dakshinamurti, K., Ed., Annals New York Acad. of Sciences, New York, 1990, 110.

8. Snell, E.E., Fasella, P.M., Braunstein, A., and Rossi Fanelli, A., *Chemical and Biological Aspects of Pyridoxal Catalysis*, Pergamon Press, New York, 1963.

9. DiSorbo, D.M., Phelps, D.S., and Litwack, G., Probes of basic amino acid residues affect active sites of the glucocorticoid receptor, *Endocrinology*, 106, 922, 1980.

10. Goidl, J.A., Cake, M.H., Dolan, K.P., Parchiman, L.G., and Litwack, G., Activation of the glucocorticoid receptor complex, *Biochemistry*, 16, 2125, 1977.

11. Bodine, P.V. and Litwack, G., Evidence that the modulator of the glucocorticoid-receptor complex is the endogenous molybdate factor, *Proc. Nat. Acad. Sci.*, 85, 1462, 1988.

12. Bodine, P.V. and Litwack, G., Purification and structural analysis of the modulator of the glucocorticoid receptor complex. Evidence that the modulator is a novel phospholipid, *J. Biol. Chem.*, 263, 3501, 1988.

13. Bodine, P.V. and Litwack, G., Regulators of the glucocorticoid-receptor complex, *Receptor*, 1, 83, 1990.

14. Webb, M.L., Schmidt, T.J., Robertson, N.M., and Litwack, G., Evidence for an association of a ribonucleic acid with the unactivated glucocorticoid receptor, *Biochem. Biophys. Res. Commun.*, 140, 204, 1986.

15. Sablonniere, B., Economidis, I.V., Lefebere, P., Place, M., Richard, C., Formstecher, P., Rousseau, G.G., and Dautrevaux, M., RNA binding to the untransformed glucocorticoid receptor. Sensitivity to substrate-specific ribonucleases and characterization of a ribonucleic acid associated with the purified receptor, *Eur. J. Biochem.*, 177, 371, 1988.

16. Unger, A.L., Uppaluri, R., Ahern, S., Colby, J.L., and Tymoczko, J.L., Isolation of ribonucleic acid from the unactivated rat liver glucocorticoid receptor, *Molec. Endocrinol.*, 2, 952, 1988.

17. Beato, M., Gene regulation by steroid hormones, *Cell*, 56, 335, 1989.

18. Maksymowych, A.B., Daniel, V., and Litwack, G., Pyridoxal phosphate as a regulator of the glucocorticoid receptor, in *Vitamin B6*, Dakshinamurti, K., Ed., Annals of the New York Acad. of Sciences, New York, 1990, 438.

19. Srinivasan, G. and Thompson, E.B., Overexpression of full-length human glucocorticoid receptor in *Spodoptera frugiperda* cells using the baculovirus expression vector system, *Molec. Endocrinol.*, 4, 209, 1990.

20. Alnemri, E.S., Maksymowych, A.B., Robertson, N.M., and Litwack, G., Characterization and purification of a functional rat glucocorticoid receptor overexpressed in a baculovirus system, submitted.

21. DiSorbo, D.M. and Litwack, G., The use of pyridoxal-P as a tool in the study of steroid receptors, in *Biochemical Actions of Hormones*, Vol. 9, Litwack, G., Ed., Academic Press, New York, 1982, 205.

22. DiSorbo, D.M. and Litwack, G., Vitamin B6 kills hepatoma cells in culture, *Nutrition and Cancer*, 3, 216, 1982.

23. Robertson, N., Kusmik, W., Grove, B., Miller-Diener, A., Webb, M.L., and Litwack, G., Characterization of a monoclonal antibody that probes the functional domains of the glucocorticoid receptor, *Biochem. J.*, 246, 55, 1987.

24. Gametchu, B. and Harrison, R.W., Characterization of a monoclonal antibody to the rat liver glucocorticoid receptor, *Endocrinology*, 114, 274, 1984.

25. Lindemeyer, R.G., Robertson, N.M., and Litwack, G., Glucocorticoid receptor monoclonal antibodies define the biological action of RU38486 in intact B16 melanoma cells, *Cancer Research*, in press.

26. Robertson, N.M., Lindemeyer, R.G., and Litwack, G., unpublished experiments.

27. Abramowitz, J. and Chavin, N., Interaction of ACTH, corticosterone and cyclic nucleotides in Hardey-Passey melanoma melanogenesis, *Arch. Dermatol. Res.*, 261, 303, 1978.

28. Abramowitz, J. and Chavin, N., Glucocorticoid modulation of adrenocorticotropin induced melanogenesis in the cloudman S91 melanoma, *In Vitro*, 46, 268, 1978.

Chapter 3

Cancer Chemoprevention by Retinoids and Carotenoids: Proposed Role of Gap Junctional Communication

John S. Bertram

Table of Contents

I. Introduction

The prevention of disease should always be the primary goal of medical science, indeed many of the successes of 20th century medicine have come through the prevention of infectious disease rather than treatment. Unfortunately, only recently has serious attention been given to the prevention of neoplasia. This shortcoming is particularly serious since cancer chemotherapy is by no means as benign as antibiotic therapy nor as successful. Two reasons can be presented to explain this lack of interest: first, a poor understanding of cancer etiology; second, an equally poor understanding of the mechanisms of carcinogenesis (i.e. the stages in conversion of a normal cell to one with a malignant phenotype). Recent years have seen remarkable progress in both areas.

Epidemiologic studies have firmly established that diet and tobacco contribute to approximately 70% of excess cancer in the US population.[1] Furthermore, as will be discussed later, not all aspects of the diet are deleterious; consumption of fruits and vegetables rich in carotenoids have frequently been associated with a lower risk of cancer.[2,3] Epidemiologic data of this sort and evidence from studies in experimental systems of carcinogenesis have led to the conclusion that carotenoids, plant pigments some of which possess pro-vitamin A activity, and the retinoids, compounds possessing vitamin A-like activity, offer the best prospects for prevention of human cancer.[3] At present, prospects for prevention seem restricted to cancers of epithelial origin, i.e. the carcinomas.

Advances in molecular biology have allowed spectacular breakthroughs in our understanding of the genetic changes that occur during the process of carcinogenesis. It is now clear that many human cancers require both the activation of genes concerned with proliferation—the oncogenes,[5] and the deletion or inactivation of genes concerned with the control of proliferation or programmed terminal differentiation—the tumor suppressor genes.[6,7] This sequence of events is being elegantly dissected in human colon carcinoma[8] as well as in other diseases. For the purposes of this chapter, it is sufficient to divide the carcinogenic process into 3 stages: initiation, where genetic damage is introduced by a carcinogen or occurs spontaneously; promotion, a process which culminates in this damage becoming expressed phenotypically, and progression where a neoplastically transformed cell grows to form a progressively more malignant tumor, or, in the experimental cell culture system to be described, a transformed focus (Figure 1). As will be demonstrated, retinoids and carotenoids inhibit carcinogenesis in the promotional stage. This statement may be made for both the experimental and clinical application of these compounds.

II. Development of an *in vitro* System for Cancer Chemoprevention Research

In the late 1960s and early 1970s a series of cell culture systems were developed in which neoplastic transformation could be induced reproducibly and quantitatively after exposure to chemical or physical carcinogens. Probably the most widely used of these *in vitro* systems is the C3H/10T1/2 mouse embryo fibroblast cell line developed in the laboratory of the late Charles Heidelberger.[9,10] This line has been used extensively by my group to study the

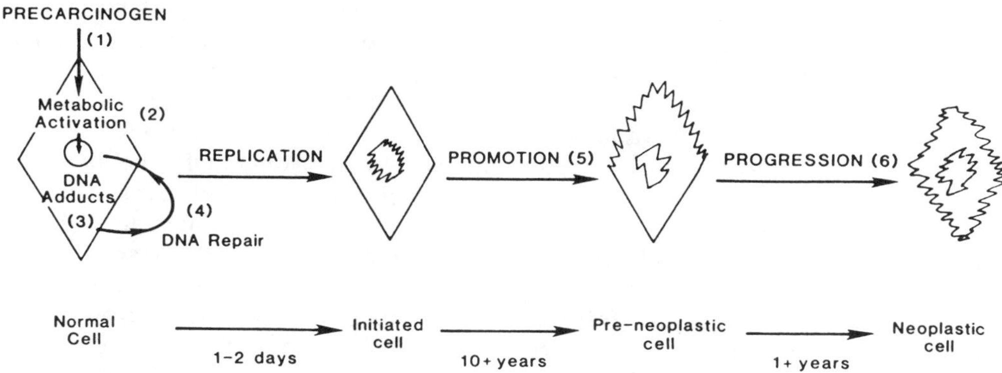

Figure 1. Stages in the induction of neoplasia. In steps 1-3 a carcinogen becomes metabolically activated, reacts with DNA and may be subject to DNA repair. If, however, DNA replication occurs prior to repair, a mutation may result in the formation of an initiated cell. This cell may undergo additional changes causing the eventual production of cells with increasingly neoplastic phenotypes (reproduced from ref. 3).

inhibitory effect of retinoids and carotenoids on the transformation process. While *in vitro* systems clearly have many advantages over established whole animal systems, their use can only be justified if that system will faithfully reproduce events occurring in the whole organism. While it is clear that no single cell culture system can mimic the complex events that may occur in an entire organ, or fully represent the diversity of cell types present in an entire animal (just as the use of laboratory animals can never substitute for a clinical trial), nevertheless certain minimal requirements for fidelity of response must be met. The following criteria we believe are of great importance in the use of any cell line for this type of research:

(a) The different stages of carcinogenesis demonstrated in animals and humans should be fully represented.

(b) Structure/activity relationships determined *in vivo* for known chemopreventive agents should be accurately reproduced.

(c) The system should be responsive to diverse classes of known chemopreventive agents.

Extensive independent studies by many investigators have confirmed that the 10T1/2 cell line satisfies all three criteria.[11]

III. Development and Use of the 10T1/2 Cell Line in Chemopreventive Research

These cells are a subtetraploid line of fibroblasts derived from C3H mouse embryos. They are non-tumorigenic in syngeneic immunosuppressed hosts, have a very low spontaneous transformation rate when properly handled, and were selected to exhibit a high degree of postconfluence inhibition of cell division:[6] a major criterion of the nonmalignant phenotype in fibroblasts. When cultures are treated for 24 hr with carcinogenic hydrocarbons one day after seeding at low cell density, a small portion of the exposed cells (up to 2%) becomes initiated. Cultures generally become confluent and growth is arrested about 10 days after treatment, and at this time no morphological effects of the carcinogen can be detected. After holding for about 3 weeks in the confluent state with weekly refeeding, foci of morphologically transformed cells can be detected microscopically. One week later (i.e. by day 35 after seeding), these foci have reached macroscopic size (Figure 2). At this time some foci can be cloned for further testing, while the majority of the dishes are fixed and stained for determination of transformation frequency (TF). This is expressed as (number of transformants/number of cells at risk) x 100. Injection of morphologically transformed cells into syngeneic mice results in the production of sarcomas at the site of injection. In contrast a 10-fold excess of the parental line is not tumorigenic under these conditions. Our group has introduced small modifications in the assay procedure but it is essentially performed as originally described.[10]

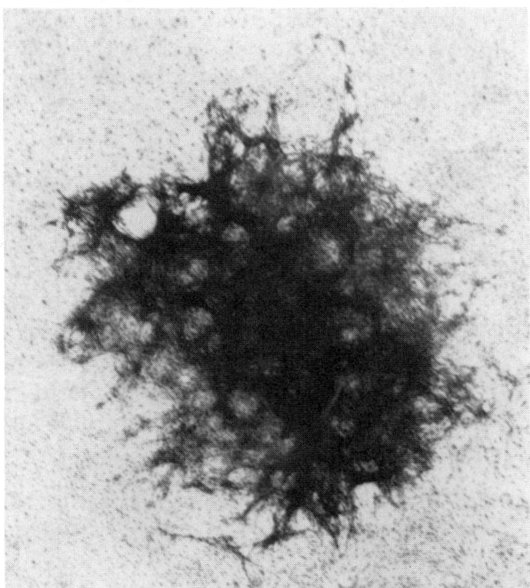

Figure 2. A type III transformed focus within a background monolayer of non-transformed cells. This culture had received methylcholanthrene 1 μg/ml, 35 days prior to fixing and staining with Giemsa; X5.

IV. Activity of Retinoids in Carcinogen-Initiated Cultures of 10T1/2 Cells

Addition of non-toxic concentrations of diverse natural and synthetic retinoids (Figure 3) to 10T1/2 cultures 7 days after removal of the carcinogen (i.e. in the post-initiation phase of carcinogenesis) and maintained in these cultures for the remaining 4 week period of the experiment, caused an inhibition of formation of transformed foci. It was found that those compounds with vitamin A-like activity in epithelial models of differentiation[12] were active in 10T1/2 cells whereas

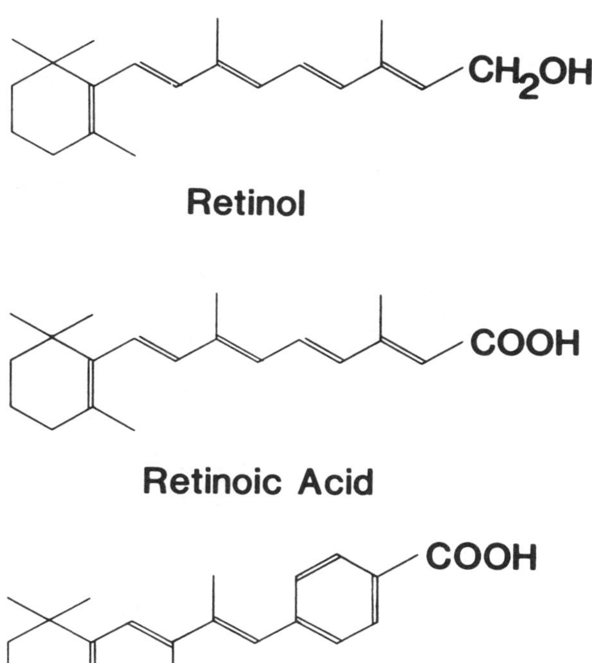

Figure 3. Structures of retinol, the form of vitamin A released from the liver and which circulates in plasma, retinoic acid, an active metabolite of retinol believed responsible for normal growth and differentiation of epithelial tissues, and Ro13-7410 or tetrahydrotetramethylnaphthylenylpropenylbenzoic acid (TTNPB) a highly potent synthetic analog of retinoic acid.

side-chain or ring modified compounds without vitamin A-like activity did not suppress the formation transformed foci.[13] We have recently extended studies to include a novel class of highly potent retinoids—the benzoic retinoids—a typical example of which is TTNPB. This compound is highly active in its ability to inhibit 10T1/2 cell transformation (Figure 4).

In a series of studies we have demonstrated the following:

1. Suppression of transformation is reversible upon drug withdrawal. Three to 5 weeks is then required for expression of foci; this is the same length of time required for expression in carcinogen-only treated cultures.[15]

2. Treatment can be delayed until 21 days post-carcinogen. However, once micro-foci can be detected treatment is ineffective.[15]

3. At concentrations which totally eliminate transformation, retinoids are not antiproliferative when applied to logarithmic phase cultures of non-transformed or transformed cells.[15]

4. When applied to confluent cultures, retinoids reduce the confluent saturation density and reduce proliferation of density-arrested cells.[16]

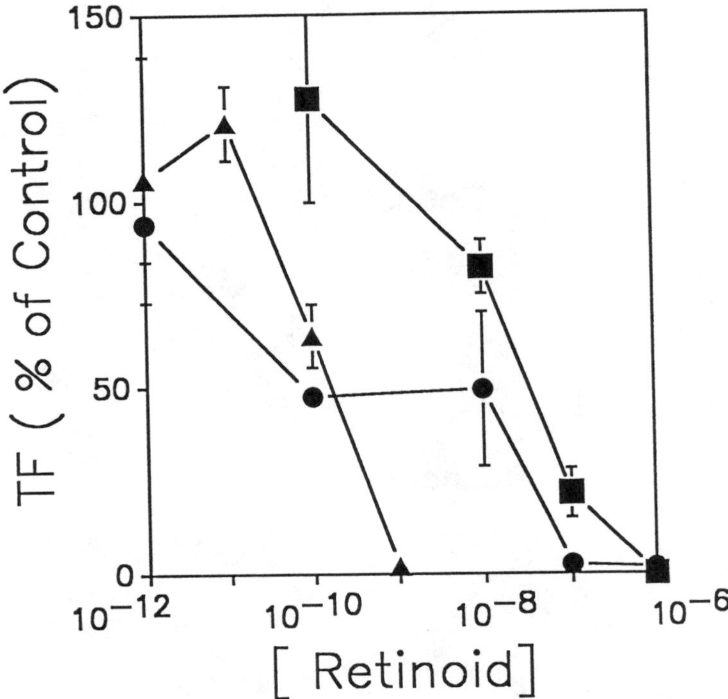

Figure 4. Inhibition of methylcholanthrene induced neoplastic transformation by retinoids. Cultures were initiated by methylcholanthrene then received retinoids 7 days after removal of carcinogen. Retinoid treatment was given every 3 days for the remaining 35 day duration of the experiment. ▲ - ▲, TTNPB; ● - ●, retinol; ■ - ■, retinoic acid. Results are expressed as a % of the transformation observed in cultures exposed to methylcholanthrene then to the acetone vehicle used to deliver the retinoids (from ref. 14).

5. Addition of retinoids to confluent 10T1/2 cultures upon which were seeded transformed cells did not reduce the formation of foci by these cells. Focus formation was in contrast enhanced.[15]

These observations demonstrated that retinoids have a specific action on the ability of initiated cells to undergo neoplastic transformation and that this action is not due to cytotoxicity or antiproliferative effects on transformed cells acting to restrict the production of transformed foci. At this time, we stated that this action was consistent with a retinoid-induced stabilization of the initiated state.[15]

V. Activity of Carotenoids as Chemopreventive Agents in Carcinogen-Initiated 10T1/2 Cultures

We have studied in detail two carotenoids; ß-carotene, the carotenoid with highest pro-vitamin A potential, and canthaxanthin, a carotenoid without pro-vitamin A activity in mammals.[17] The structures of these and other carotenoids studied are shown in Figure 5.

A major problem in the *in vitro* use of carotenoids is their lack of solubility in cell culture medium. Initial attempts to supply ß-carotene in a hexane solution to culture medium resulted in evaporation of the hexane, crystallization of the

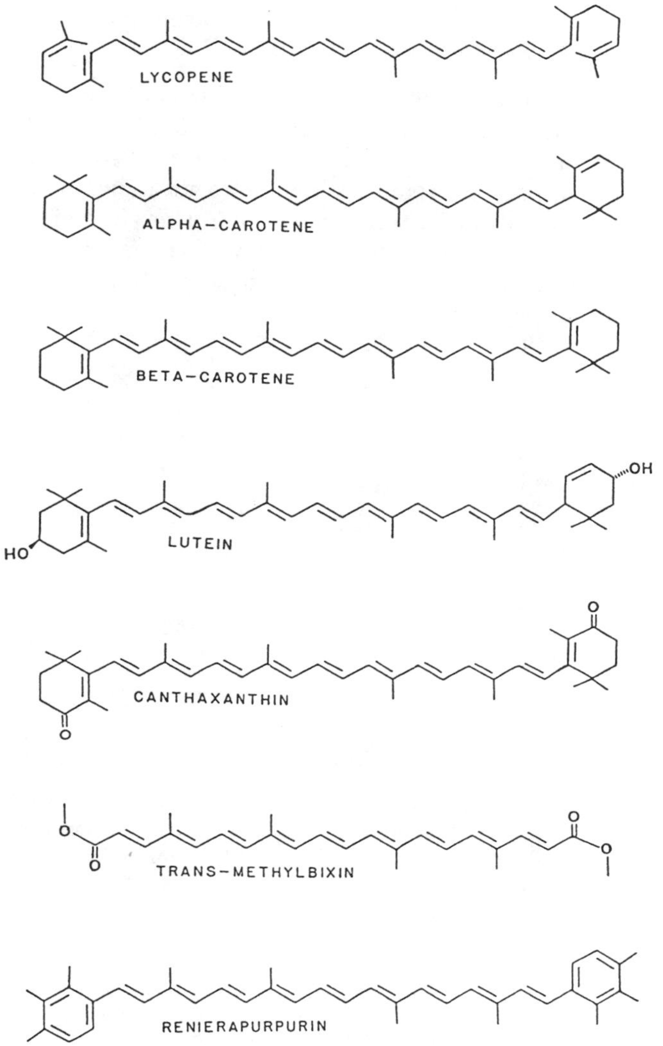

LYCOPENE

ALPHA–CAROTENE

BETA–CAROTENE

LUTEIN

CANTHAXANTHIN

TRANS–METHYLBIXIN

RENIERAPURPURIN

Figure 5. Structures of carotenoids examined for their ability to inhibit carcinogen-induced transformation in 10T1/2 cells. Of the molecules shown only α-carotene and ß-carotene have known pro-vitamin A activities in mammals. Canthaxanthin has activity in fish and perhaps birds. Lycopene and lutein are major dietary carotenoids present in high amounts in tomatoes and green leaves respectively (from ref. 18).

ß-carotene, and poor uptake by 10T1/2 cells. We originally overcame this problem by the use of the "beadlet" form of ß-carotene and of canthaxanthin supplied by Hoffmann-LaRoche for clinical studies. On reconstitution of these beadlets with water, an oil in water emulsion is formed which efficiently delivers carotenoids to the cell. A drawback to this vehicle is that inert constituents and antioxidants constitute 90% of the dry weight of the beads; consequently control cultures must be treated in parallel with the appropriate concentrations of "empty" beadlets not containing carotenoids. Furthermore only two carotenoids are available in this formulation. More recently, we have utilized the excellent solvent properties of tetrahydrofuran (THF) and have demonstrated that upon addition to an aqueous medium, carotenoids are placed in a micelle-like environment. In this form, they are highly bioavailable.[18]

Using a treatment protocol essentially identical to that used previously for the retinoids, ß-carotene and canthaxanthin were added to 10T1/2 cell cultures which had been treated 7 days previously with a transforming concentration of MCA. As shown in Figure 6, both compounds induced a dose-dependent inhibition of focus formation. In control MCA-treated cultures, the yield of transformed foci was usually about two foci/dish to give a calculated transformation frequency of about 1%. At concentrations of 10^{-5} M both ß-carotene and canthaxanthin completely eliminated focus production.[29]

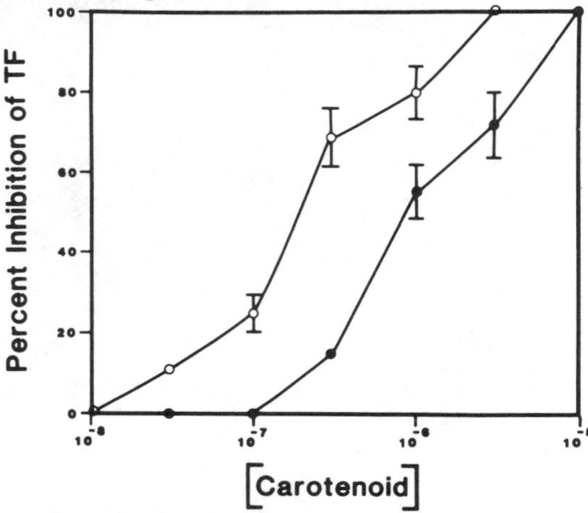

Figure 6. Inhibition of methylcholanthrene induced transformation by ß-carotene and canthaxanthin. The experiment was performed as described for Figure 4. ○ - ○, canthaxanthin; ● - ●, ß-carotene. The carotenoids were delivered in beadlet form. Control cultures received methylcholanthrene then control beadlets. Results are expressed as the % inhibition of transformation observed in these controls (from ref. 17).

VI. Reversibility Studies

Cultures were exposed to MCA and subsequently given weekly treatments of 10^{-5}M ß-carotene or $3x10^{-6}$M canthaxanthin to completely inhibit transformation. After 4 weeks of carotenoid treatment, cultures were divided into two groups; one continued to receive treatment, one had treatment withdrawn. As shown in Figure 7, removal of ß-carotene or canthaxanthin after 4 weeks of treatment allowed the development of foci. As with the retinoids, 2-4 weeks were required for complete reversibility. In cultures maintained in the presence of carotenoids over this time period, a slow increase in focus formation occurred, indicating that the block of transformation was not absolute.

VII. Identification of the Phase of Carcinogenesis Influenced by Carotenoids

As discussed above, the induction of cancer can be divided into (a) the initiation phase, where stable, presumably genetic, damage is produced in a

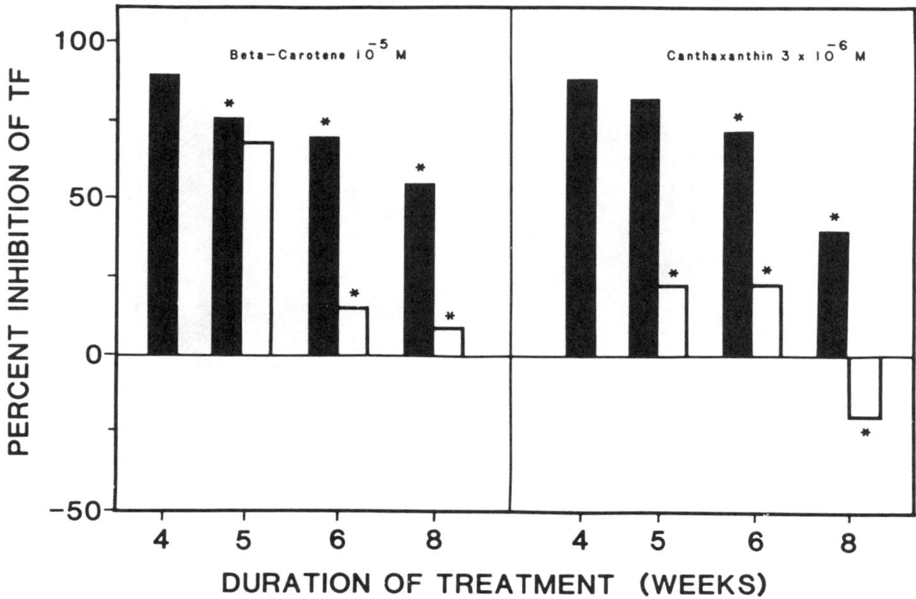

Figure 7. Reversibility of the inhibitory effects of carotenoids on MCA-induced transformation. MCA-exposed cultures were treated with either 10^{-5}M ß-C (left) or CTX ($3x10^{-6}$M) (right) for a period of 4 weeks. Carotenoid was then withdrawn from half the cultures in each group and was maintained in the other half. Twelve cultures were fixed and stained and the numbers of transformed foci evaluated at the indicated times. (solid bars) continued treatment; (open bars) treatment withdrawn. Percentages were calculated as in Figure 6 with reference to dishes treated with MCA and fixed 4 weeks after starting control beadlet treatments. (*) significantly different ($P<0.05$) from 4 week beadlet controls; (*) significantly different from beadlet controls and from respective carotenoid-treated cells (from ref. 17).

target cell but no phenotypic changes occur; (b) the promotion phase, where clones of initiated cells develop in which secondary events leading to neoplastic transformation occur; and (c) the progression/expression phase where the neoplastic cell forms a focus *in vitro* or an identifiable cancer *in vivo*. Data presented in Figures 6 and 7 demonstrate that the carotenoids are probably active during the promotional phase since they function after carcinogen addition, but do not address their potential activities in other phases.

To investigate activity during the initiation phase, we utilized X-irradiation as the transforming agent rather than MCA to eliminate potential interactions among this lipophilic carcinogen, the carotenoids, and the constituents of the beadlets. In these studies, we pretreated cells with carotenoids, exposed them to a transforming dose of X-irradiation then removed the carotenoid. As shown in Figure 8, neither ß-carotene nor canthaxanthin caused a dramatic reduction in transformation. In contrast when added after irradiation and maintained in cultures as in the MCA-transformation protocol, carotenoids were highly efficient inhibitors of focus formation.

To study the potential of carotenoids to inhibit the expression of transformation, reconstruction experiments were performed in which established transformed cells were plated on a confluent monolayer of 10T1/2 cells. The ability of ß-carotene and canthaxanthin to influence the growth of these transformed cells

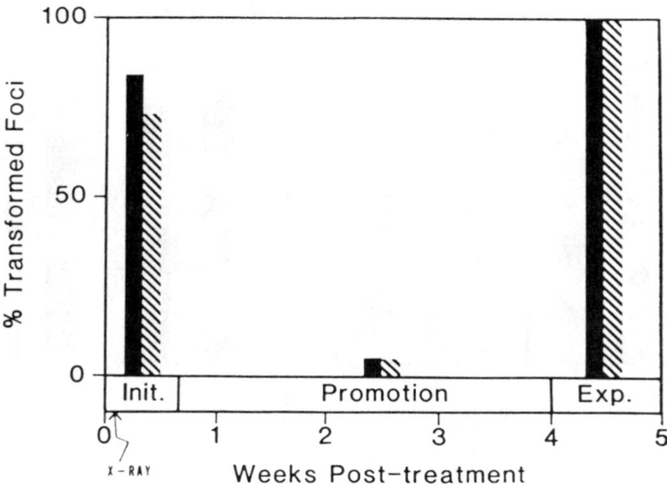

Figure 8. Inhibition of carotenoids of X-ray-induced neoplastic transformation of 10T1/2 cells. Cells were exposed to either ß-carotene (10^{-5}M) (■) or canthaxanthin (10^{-5}M) (▧) at three phases of the transformation process; initiation (Int), 24 hr prior to, during, and 1 hr postirradiation: promotion, 7 days postirradiation to the termination of the experiment 28 days later; and during expression (Exp) of the transformed phenotype. This latter experiment was conducted by plating transformed cells onto a confluent monolayer of 10T1/2 cells and counting transformed foci after 7 days. Results were expressed as a percentage of foci which appeared in beadlet only treated controls. From ref. 17.

was determined. Neither compound inhibited the growth and formation of foci by these transformed cells (Figure 8). In other experiments these carotenoids were also shown not to inhibit the growth rate or colony-forming ability of non-transformed 10T1/2 cells treated under the conditions of the transformation assays (data not shown). Taken together, these results demonstrate that carotenoids do not prevent formation of initiated cells, nor are they selectively cytotoxic to these cells. As with the retinoids, activity seems best described as a stabilization of initiated cells in their progression to cells having the transformed phenotype.

VIII. Activity of Structurally Diverse Carotenoids

The studies described above demonstrated that carotenoids with and without provitamin A activity in mammals could inhibit chemical- and X-ray-induced transformation. However over 600 carotenoids are found in nature,[20] and human serum contains at least 20 different carotenoids of dietary origin.[21] That other carotenoids may also be protective is suggested by epidemiologic studies which show the strongest protection from cancer risk is associated with diets rich in fruits and vegetables—major sources of diverse carotenoids, not just with their ß-carotene content.[22] We have recently concluded studies of the other carotenoids shown in Figure 3. Some, such as lycopene and lutein found in abundance in tomatoes and green leaves respectively, are of major dietary importance; others were of structural interest. For these studies, we utilized the ability of tetrahydrofuran to formulate carotenoids into a bio-available aqueous pseudo-solution.[18] When added to MCA-initiated cultures using the same protocol previously employed for the carotenoids formulated into beads, lutein, lycopene and α-carotene were all found to suppress the formation of transformed foci. However, ß-carotene, canthaxanthin and α-carotene were the most potent of the carotenoids tested in that order. All have the potential for conversion to active retinoids, though in the case of canthaxanthin conversion is not believed to occur in mammals.[23] The activity of lycopene, a straight chain hydrocarbon with strong antioxidant properties,[24] was comparable to that seen after addition of another membrane active antioxidant—α-tocopherol. Bixin and renierapurpurin were without activity.

These studies suggest that chemoprevention by carotenoids has two components: one, a function of bioconversion to active retinoids; second, a function of their intrinsic antioxidant properties. We have so far been unable to detect evidence for the conversion of ^{14}C-labeled ß-carotene to the expected retinoids.[25] This may be explained by the recent discovery of a family of nuclear receptors for retinoids activated by sub-nanomolar concentrations of retinoic acid;[26] concentrations below our level of radiochemical detection. Production of apo-carotenoids by enzymatic or chemical process has been proposed.[27] Low frequency production of biologically active fragments from α-carotene, ß-carotene and canthaxanthin could explain their biological activity and our inability to detect formation of radiolabeled retinoids after incubation with ^{14}C-ß-carotene.

IX. Mode of Action of Retinoids and Carotenoids as Cancer Preventive Agents

The similarity of biological action of retinoids and carotenoids in inhibiting neoplastic transformation suggests that these compounds share similar molecular mechanisms of action. We now have evidence that this is the case: both compounds act to up-regulate gap junctional communication. The potential significance of this observation is that we and others have proposed that gap junctions serve as conduits for growth regulatory signals.[28-30] Conversely, inhibition of junctional communication is associated with carcinogenesis.[31] In the 10T1/2 system, in all cases so far examined, enhanced communication leads to decreased proliferation, whereas a low level of communication is associated with high proliferation rates. As will be described, we propose that enhanced communication induced by retinoids places carcinogen-initiated cells within a network of communicating normal cells and thereby stabilizes them against subsequent transformation.

X. Gap Junctions: Form and Function

Gap junctions are composed of water filled pores which link most cells with their neighbors. The pores are in many cases gated and when open allow the passive diffusion of small molecules and ions up to about 1000 daltons in size. A single channel is called a connexon and is formed by the docking of two hemi-connexons contributed by each of the communicating cells. The structural unit of the connexon is composed of proteins called connexins, six of which are believed to form a hexagonal array surrounding the pore. A family of connexins have been described with tissue and cell type specificity.[32] As shown in Figure 9, each protein has 4 putative trans-membrane domains, the third of which is amphipathic and may line the hydrophobic channel. We have prepared an antibody to the C-terminal region of connexin43 (residues 368 to 382). This protein was first described as a component of the intercalated disc of the heart. It is the only junctional protein known to be expressed in 10T1/2 cells.[33]

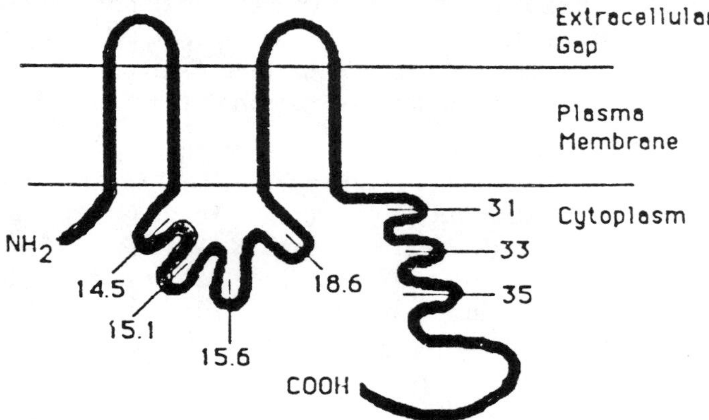

Figure 9. Proposed topology of connexin43 first described as a component of the cardiac intercalated disc. Six of these proteins are believed to form a hemi-connexon. Numbers refer to fragment sizes in kilodaltons. The antibody utilized in these studies recognizes the C-terminal 15 amino acid residues (from ref. 32).

XI. Correlation Between Retinoid-Induced Inhibition of Transformation and Enhancement of Gap Junctional Communication

In the studies described below, we measured junctional communication by a dye injection technique. In this method the spread of a fluorescent, junctionally permeable dye (Lucifer Yellow) from a donor cell to adjacent cells is quantitated under fluorescence optics.[14]

To investigate whether concentrations of retinoids which were equi-potent in transformation assays would have equal effects on communication over the time course of a typical transformation assay, cultures of 10T1/2 cells were treated with maximally effective concentrations of retinoids (i.e. 10^{-6} M for retinol and retinoic acid and 10^{-9} M for TTNPB) using the same 3 day treatment protocol. As shown in Figure 4 above, at these concentrations all three retinoids completely inhibited transformation. At increasing intervals post-treatment junctional communication was assayed. As seen in Figure 11, junctional communication was markedly increased by all three retinoids, and this increase was sustained over the 35-day period of observation. The increases produced by the various retinoids were of comparable magnitude, but required a 1000-fold higher concentration of retinol and retinoic acid than of TTNPB. Enhancement of junctional communication induced by TTNPB (10^{-9}M) required several hours; no effect was detectable after 6 hr, but after 18 hr treatment communication was significantly different ($p<0.001$) from acetone-treated controls and continued to increase thereafter (Figure 11, inset).[14] As is typical of 10T1/2 cells, junctional communication increased as cultures aged; this was observed in both treated and control cultures.

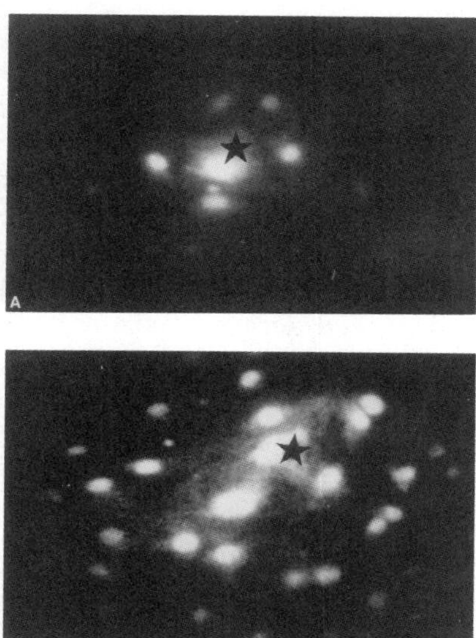

Figure 10. Photomicrographs of cell communication networks. The cell which was part of a confluent 10T1/2 monolayer was injected with Lucifer Yellow. After 10 min the image was recorded digitally under epifluorescent illumination. The image has been digitally processed with background subtraction using the Loats (Westminster, MD) intercellular communication software package. (A) Acetone-treated control; (B) replicate culture treated 3 days previously with 10^{-9}M TTNPB (from ref. 19).

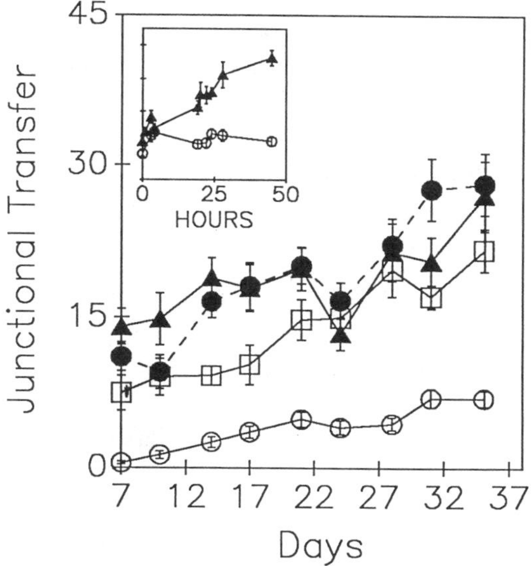

Figure 11. Retinoid effects on homologous junctions in 10T1/2 cells. 10T1/2 cells were seeded and treated with retinoids on day 1 post-seeding and every 3 days thereafter. Junctional transfer was indexed by the number of cells to which Lucifer Yellow was transferred within 10 min of injection into a test cell ("number of communicating cells"). Cultures were probed at intervals shown. Data points are the means ± SE of at least 10 microinjection trials performed in each of two dishes. O - O, acetone control 0.2%; □ - □, retinoic acid 10^{-6}M; ● - ●, retinol 10^{-6}M; ▲ - ▲, TTNPB 10^{-9}M. Inset: Time-course of enhancement of junctional communication by TTNBP 10^{-9}M, and the cultures were probed at the indicated times. Results represent the mean ± SE of at least 20 microinjections in two dishes each (from ref. 14).

We next examined homologous junctional communication in initiated cells, the presumed target of retinoid action, and compared their response to that of parental 10T1/2 cells. As shown in Figure 12A and B, TTNPB and retinol enhanced junctional transfer in a dose-dependent manner in both cell types. Retinoic acid also enhanced junctional transfer at concentrations $>10^{-8}$ M, but it inhibited at 10^{-10} M (Figure 12C). This inhibition of communication correlated with the enhancement of transformation found with this dose (Figure 4). Initiated cells had higher basal levels of communication than did 10T1/2 cells, and this difference was maintained across treatment groups.

XII. The Transformation-Communication Correlation

The enhancement of junctional permeability induced by retinoids correlated with the inhibition of transformation, and vice versa. When the transformation frequency of the retinoid-treated cells (expressed as a percentage of the transformation frequency of carcinogen-only treated control cells) was plotted against junctional transfer (expressed as a percentage of junctional transfer measured in the respective controls) the plot showed a strong negative correlation between the two parameters (Pearson correlation coefficients of -0.86 and -0.89 for initiated and normal cells, respectively), which was statistically highly significant in both cases. Figure 13 demonstrates this relationship in normal and initiated 10T1/2 cells.

XIII. Retinoids Enhance Junctional Communication by Increasing the Formation of Junctional Channels

To investigate the mechanism for the retinoid-enhanced junctional communication we measured by Western blotting the levels of connexin43 in treated and control 10T1/2 cells. As previously mentioned, 10T1/2 cells were found to express the gene connexin43, responsible for the formation of gap junctions in the intercalated disc of the heart.[32] Analysis of total cell proteins isolated from 10T1/2 cells by sodium dodecylsulphate polyacrylamide gel electrophoresis (SDS-PAGE), followed by immunoblotting with the C-terminal rabbit polyclonal antibody to connexin43, revealed that retinoid treatment resulted in a major increase in immunoreactive protein in the appropriate 43-45 kD region of the gel (Figure 14). Suitable controls demonstrated that the antibody was recognizing a specific sequence on connexin43.[33]

When cells were fixed *in situ* and subjected to indirect immunofluorescence microscopy using the rabbit anti-connexin43 antibody, a dramatic increase in fluorescent plaques was seen in regions of cell/cell contact in retinoid-treated cells (Figure 15). This demonstrates that the increased levels of connexin43 became localized in regions of the cell membrane where gap junctions would be expected to form.

XIV. Mechanisms of Carotenoid Action

Recent studies have shown that carotenoids such as ß-carotene and canthaxanthin (i.e. carotenoids with and without pro-vitamin A activity) also

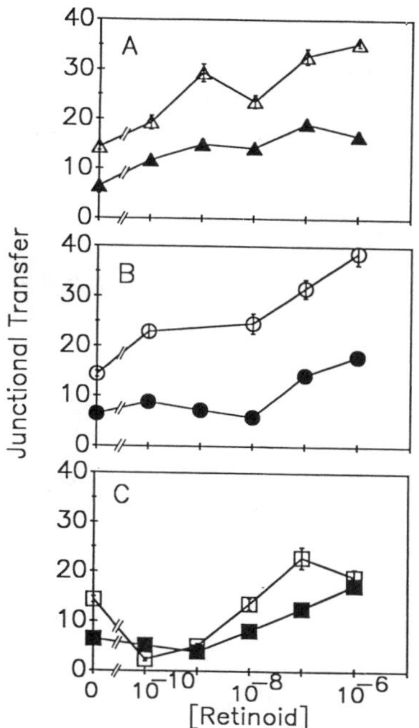

Figure 12. Comparative responses of 10T1/2 cells and INIT/10T1/2 cells to retinoid induced communication. Cultures were seeded and treated as in Figure 11. They were probed for junctional communication 2 days after reaching confluence. (A) TTNPB; (B) retinol; (C) retinoic acid. Closed symbols, 10T1/2; open symbols INIT/10T1/2. Data points represent means ± SE of two experiments each involving approx. 20 microinjections in two separate cultures. Linear regression analysis resulted in r^2 values of 0.99, 0.96 and 0.98 for TTNPB, retinol and retinoic acid respectively. Dose-response relationships were statistically significant for the following groups: TTNPB, 10T1/2: P=0.002; TTTNP, INIT: P=0.004; retinol, 10T1/2: P=0.003; retinol, INIT: of borderline significance at P=0.08. We excluded the zero dose group for the retinoic acid group, since 10^{-10}M retinoic acid inhibited communication. The resulting dose-response relationships were statistically significant: 10T1/2: P=0.0003; INIT: P=0.002. In the case of TTNPB, initiated cells were significantly more responsive than were 10T1/2 cells (P<0.005) (from ref. 14).

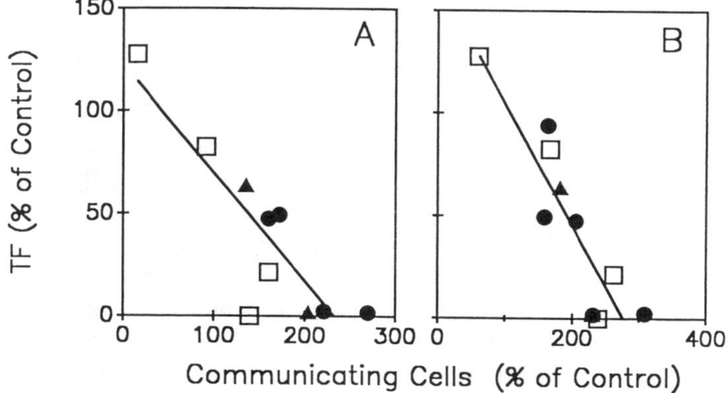

Figure 13. Correlation between transformation and junctional communication. Data taken from Figures 4 and 11. ● - ●, retinol; □ - □, retinoic acid; ▲ - ▲, TTNPB. (A) 10T1/2 cells; (B) initiated cells. The Pearson correlation coefficient was -0.86 and -0.89 for (A) and (B) respectively, indicating a strong negative association between the two events. This was highly statistically significant in both cases: P=0.001 and P=0.007 respectively (from ref. 14).

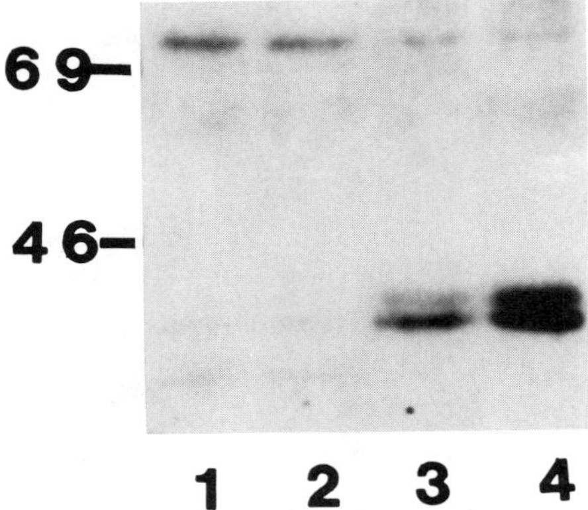

Figure 14. Dose response for induction of connexon43 by TTNPB. Confluent cultures of 10T1/2 cells were treated with TTNPB or acetone vehicle for 96 hrs. Equal amounts of total cell protein were electrophoresed after reduction with 5% 2-mercaptoethanol and Western blotting performed. Lane 1, acetone control; Lane 2, TTNPB 10^{-10}M; Lane 3, TTNPB 10^{-9}M; Lane 4, TTNPB 10^{-8}M. Immunoblotting with pre-immune serum did not give a signal (data not shown). Note the incomplete conversion of connexin43 to monomers. More vigorous denaturation at 50° reduced the immunoreactivity of this antigen. Positions of molecular weight markers (x 10^{-3} daltons) are shown (from ref. 33).

elevate junctional communication as dramatically as do the retinoids. As with the retinoids, this elevation was highly correlated with the ability of carotenoids to inhibit neoplastic transformation, furthermore, enhanced communication was also associated with an elevation of connexin43 detected by Western blotting and by immunofluorescence. A notable difference between these two classes of drugs is that whereas retinoid-induced communication occurred within 24 hr of treatment, carotenoids required 7 days to produce an effect (Zhang *et al.*, submitted). We propose that this apparently identical mode of action of retinoids and carotenoids in 10T1/2 cells is not a coincidence and that it provides additional evidence suggesting that a low rate of conversion of carotenoids to active retinoids can occur in these cells.

XV. Conclusions

We have demonstrated that procedures that modify junctional communication also modify the expression of transformation in 10T1/2 cells. Expression of established transformed cells can be inhibited when cells are forced into communication with non-transformed cells by elevation of cAMP,[28] while elevation of communication between normal and initiated cells by retinoids[14] and carotenoids inhibits initiated cells from progressing to cells expressing the neoplastic phenotype. For reasons that are not yet apparent, retinoids fail to enhance heterologous communication between normal and neoplastic cells. This is consistent with the general lack of action of retinoids on established neoplastic cells. Thus in clinical chemoprevention studies of retinoic acid in head and neck cancer, the occurrence of second primary malignancies was reduced. However no effect on the rate of recurrence of primaries in existence prior to treatment was detected.[34] Similarly in the 10T1/2 cell system, retinoids only suppress neoplastic transformation when applied prior to the onset of phenotypic transformation. Paradoxically when applied after transformation, retinoids act to inhibit

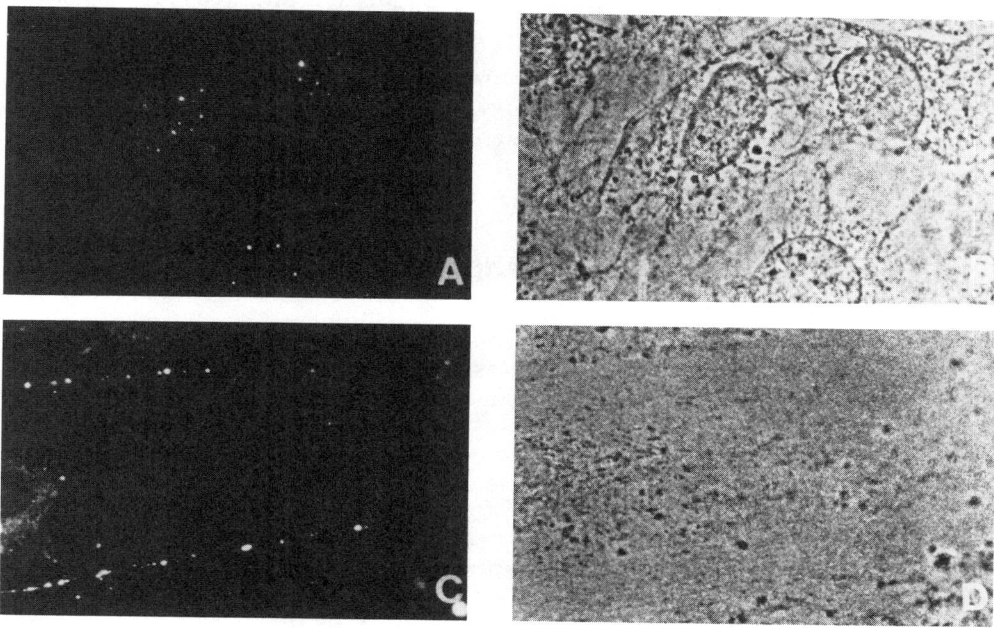

Figure 15. Connexin43 is localized in regions of cell/cell contact. 10T1/2 cells were grown on Permanox culture slides and treated with TTNPB or acetone solvent for 96 hrs. Cultures were then fixed, labeled with connexin43 antiserum then with FITC labeled goat anti-rabbit IgG $(ab)^2$ fragment. A,B acetone control, fluorescent and respective phase image; C,D, TTNPB 10^{-8}M, fluorescent and respective phase image. In all treated cultures, the brightest fluorescence was observed in regions of cell/cell contact, regions which are poorly imaged by phase contrast microscopy. Magnification x 750 (from ref. 33).

communication, explaining the stimulation of growth of transformed cells,[15,29] and perhaps some of the deleterious actions of retinoids noted in experimental animals.[3]

These correlations between gap junctional communication and growth control all support the hypothesis first proposed by Loewenstein[30] that gap junctions serve as conduits for growth regulatory signals. As we have pointed out,[28] these data do not define the chemical nature of these signals, nor whether they are growth inhibitory (being transferred from normal to malignant) or stimulatory (being lost from malignant cells to surrounding normal cells). However, by analogy with tumor suppressor genes which must be deleted in order that neoplasia develop, the concept of transfer of anti-proliferative signals is attractive. Indeed, the re-introduction of junctional communication has many similarities to the effects of tumor suppressor genes.[35] As to the chemical nature of such signals, it may be expected that they would be free to travel only through junctions; they would thus be electrically charged, so as to limit membrane diffusion. This requirement would predict small molecules or ions of less than 1000 daltons, with good solubility in water and low protein binding. An additional expectation is that such signals be capable of rapid generation and efficient destruction or sequestration. Cyclic AMP, inositol trisphosphate and free Ca^{++} have all been shown to transverse gap junctions and would satisfy these criteria.[36,37]

A major focus of current research is directed towards determining if retinoids exert comparable effects in human tissues. Such an action could in part explain many of the diverse effects of retinoids on growth control and differentiation.

Acknowledgements

Research was supported by grants CA39947 and CA39604 from the National Cancer Institute, U.S. National Institutes of Health; BC686 from the American Cancer Society and grant 89B60 from the American Institute for Cancer Research.

References

1. Doll, R. and Peto, R., *The Causes of Cancer*, Oxford University Press, Oxford, 1981.

2. Connett, J.E., Kuller, L.H., Kjelsberg, M.O., Polk, B.F., Collins, G., Rider, A., and Hulley, S.B., Relationship between carotenoids and cancer: the multiple risk factor intervention trial (MRFIT) study, *Cancer*, 64, 126, 1989.

3. Bertram, J.S., Kolonel, L.N., and Meyskens, F.L., Jr., Rationale and strategies for chemoprevention of cancer in humans, *Cancer Res.*, 47, 3012, 1987.

4. Weinberg, R.A., Oncogenes, antioncogenes and the molecular basis of multistep carcinogenesis, *Cancer Res.*, 49, 3713, 1989.

5. Storms, R.W. and Bose, H.R., Jr., Oncogenes, protooncogenes, and signal transduction: toward a unified theory, *Adv. Virus Res.*, 37, 1, 1989.

6. Sager, R., Tumor suppressor genes: the puzzle and the promise, *Science*, 246, 1406, 1989.

7. Green, M.R., When the products of oncogenes and anti-oncogenes meet, *Cell*, 56, 1, 1989.

8. Fearon, E.R., Cho, K.R., Nigro, J.M., Kern, S.E., Simons, J.W., Ruppert, J.M., Hamilton, S.R., Preisinger, A.C., Thomas, G., Kinzler, K.W., and Vogelstein, B., Identification of a chromosome 18q gene that is altered in colorectal cancers, *Science*, 247, 49, 1990.

9. Reznikoff, C.A., Brankow, D.W., and Heidelberger, C., Establishment and characterization of a cloned line of C3H mouse embryo cells sensitive to postconfluence inhibition of division, *Cancer Res.*, 33, 3231, 1973.

10. Reznikoff, C.A., Bertram, J.S., Brankow, D.W., and Heidelberger, C., Quantitative and qualitative studies of chemical transformation of cloned mouse embryo cells sensitive to postconfluence inhibition of cell division, *Cancer Res.*, 33, 3239, 1973.

11. Bertram, J.S., Neoplastic transformation in cell cultures: *in vivo* correlations, *IARC Sci. Pub.*, 67, 77, 1985.

12. Newton, D.L., Henderson, W.R., and Sporn, M.B., Structure-activity relationships of retinoids in hamster tracheal organ culture, *Cancer Res.*, 40, 3413, 1980.

13. Bertram, J.S., Structure-activity relationships among various retinoids and their ability to inhibit neoplastic transformation and to increase cell adhesion in the C3H/10T1/2 CL8 cell line, *Cancer Res.*, 40, 3141, 1980.

14. Hossain, M.Z., Wilkens, L.R., Mehta, P.P., Loewenstein, W.R., and Bertram, J.S., Enhancement of gap junctional communication by retinoids correlates with their ability to inhibit neoplastic transformation, *Carcinogenesis*, 10, 1743, 1748, 1989.

15. Merriman, R.L. and Bertram, J.S., Reversible inhibition by retinoids of 3-methylcholanthrene-induced neoplastic transformation in C3H/10T1/2 clone 8 cells, *Cancer Res.*, 39, 1661, 1979.

16. Mordan, L.J. and Bertram, J.S., Retinoid effects on cell-cell interactions and growth characteristics of normal and carcinogen-treated C3H/10T1/2 cells, *Cancer Res.*, 43, 567, 1983.

17. Pung, A., Rundhaug, J., Yoshizawa, C.N., and Bertram, J.S., ß-carotene and canthaxanthin inhibit chemically- and physically-induced neoplastic transformation in 10T1/2 cells, *Carcinogenesis*, 9, 1533, 1988.

18. Bertram, J.S., Pung, A., Churley, M., Kappock IV, T.J., Wilkens, L.R., and Cooney, R.V., Diverse carotenoids protect from chemically-induced neoplastic transformation, *Carcinogenesis*, in press.

19. Bertram, J.S., Hossain, M.Z., Pung, A., and Rundhaug, J.E., Development of *in vitro* systems for chemoprevention research, *Prev. Med.*, 18, 562, 1989.

20. Pfander, H., Ed., *Key to Carotenoids*, 2nd ed., Basel, Birkhauser, 1987.

21. Parker, R.S., Carotenoids in human blood and tissues, *J. Nutr.*, 119, 101, 1989.

22. LeMarchand, L., Yoshizawa, C.N., Kolonel, L.N., Hankin, J.H., and Goodman, M.T., Vegetable consumption and lung cancer risk: a population-based case-control study in Hawaii, *J. Natl. Cancer Inst.*, 81, 1158, 1989.

23. Bauernfeind, J.C., Carotenoid vitamin precursors and analogs in foods and feeds, *Agric. Food Chem.*, 20, 456, 1972.

24. DiMascio, P., Kaiser, S., and Sies, H., Lycopene as the most efficient biological carotenoid singlet oxygen quencher, *Arch. Biochem. Biophys.*, 274, 532, 1989.

25. Rundhaug, J.E., Pung, A., Read, C.M., and Bertram, J.S., Uptake and metabolism of ß-carotene and retinal by C_3H/10T1/2 cells, *Carcinogenesis*, 9, 1541, 1988.

26. Zelent, A., Krust, A., Petkovich, M., Kastner, P., and Chambon, P., Cloning of Murine α and ß retinoic acid receptors and a novel receptor gamma predominantly expressed in skin, *Nature*, 339, 714, 1989.

27. Olson, J.A., Provitamin A function of carotenoids: the conversion of ß-carotene into vitamin A, *J. Nutr.*, 119, 105, 1989.

28. Mehta, P.P., Bertram, J.S., and Loewenstein, W.R., Growth inhibition of transformed cells correlates with their junctional communication with normal cells, *Cell*, 44, 187, 1986.

29. Mehta, P.P., Bertram, J.S., and Loewenstein, W.R., The actions of retinoids on cellular growth correlate with their actions on gap junctional communication, *J. Cell. Biol.*, 108, 1053, 1989.

30. Loewenstein, W.R., Junctional communication and control of growth, *Biochim. Biophys. Acta*, 560, 1, 1979.

31. Klaunig, J.E. and Ruch, R.J., Role of inhibition of intercellular communication in carcinogenesis, *Lab. Invest.*, 62, 135, 1990.

32. Yancey, S.B., John, S.A., Lal, R., Austin, B.J., and Revel, J.-P., The 43kD polypeptide of heart gap junctions: immunolocalization, topology and functional domains, *J. Cell Biol.*, 108, 2241, 1989.

33. Rogers, M., Berestecky, J.M., Hossain, M.Z., Guo, H., Kadle, R., Nicholson, B.J., and Bertram, J.S., Retinoid-enhanced gap junctional communication is achieved by increased levels of connexin43 mRNA and Protein, *Mol. Carcinogenesis*, in press.

34. Hong, W.K., Lippman, S.M., *et al.*, Prevention of second primary tumors with isotretinoin in squamous-cell carcinoma of the head and neck, *N. Eng. J. Med.*, 323, 795, 1990.

35. Weinberg, R.A., Negative growth controls and carcinogenesis, *Mol. Carcinogenesis*, 3, 3, 1990.

36. Fletcher, W.H., Byus, C.V., and Walsh, D.A., Receptor-mediated action without receptor occupancy: a function for cell-cell communication in ovarian follicles, *Adv. Exp. Med. Biol.*, 219, 299, 1987.

37. Saez, J.C., Connor, J.A., Spray, D.C., and Bennett, M.V.L., Hepatocyte gap junctions are permeable to the second messenger, inositol 1,4,5-trisphosphate and to calcium ions, *Proc. Natl. Acad. Sci. USA*, 86, 2708, 1989.

Chapter 4

The Role of Free Radicals and Dietary Antioxidants in Cellular and Molecular Carcinogenesis *in Vitro*

Carmia G. Borek

Table of Contents

I. Introduction

Summary. Cancer is a multistage process which involves the interaction between endogenous and exogenous factors. The neoplastic process is genetic in origin and is modulated by permissive and protective factors which determine its course and frequency. Thyroid hormone acts as a permissive agent. The hormone which plays a role in oxidative metabolism is a critical cofactor for transformation by radiation and chemicals, viruses and cancer genes. Agents that catalytically scavenge intermediates of oxygen reduction act as protectors and inhibit transformation.

Our findings indicate that dietary antioxidants, such as vitamin E, selenium and vitamin C suppress the transformation by radiation and chemical carcinogens including ozone.

The dietary factors act as protectors by enhancing cellular free radical scavenging systems or modifying lipid peroxidation. The results support the notion that free radicals play an important role in carcinogenesis and that dietary factors can serve as cancer preventing agents.

Neoplastic development is a multistage process. It is determined in part by a genetic predisposition to the disease as well as by interactions between endogenous and exogenous factors which ultimately establish its course and frequency.[1]

Cell culture systems and transformation *in vitro* offer powerful tools to study the process of carcinogenesis.[1] These *in vitro* models of rodent or human cells afford the opportunity to elucidate underlying molecular mechanisms in carcinogenesis. They also make it possible to identify and characterize permissive co-transforming factors, in transformation, or protective factors which serve as potential cancer preventive agents.[2,3]

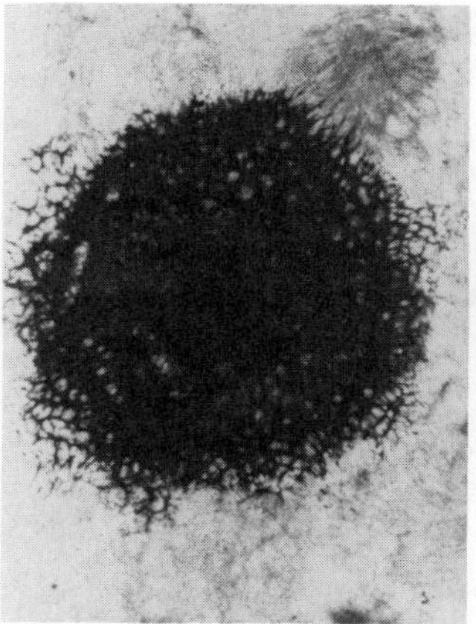
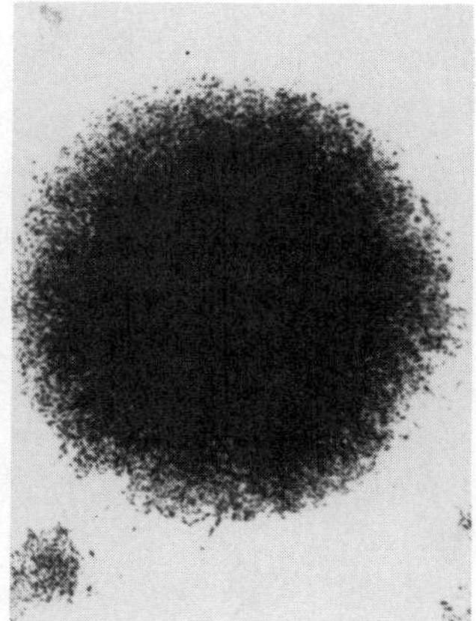
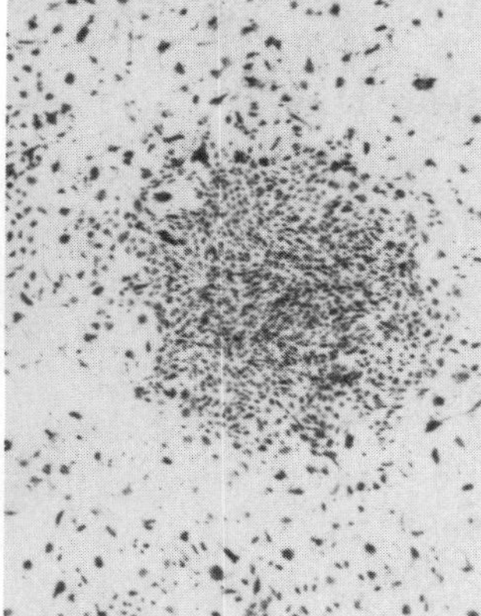

Figure 1. Photographic representation of colonies of normal hamster cells (left); hamster cells transformed by x-rays (middle); and mouse C_3H 10T1/2 cells transformed by x-rays growing over normal cells. Note the multi-layers of the transformed cells.

II. Cellular and Molecular Aspects of Transformation *in Vitro*

Studies in cell cultures have shown that transformation of cells by direct exposure to radiation or chemicals is associated with the activation of dominant transforming genes (oncogenes) which specify many of the malignant traits of the cells.[4,5] When these genes are isolated and reintroduced into normal cells they confer upon the latter many of the phenotypic traits characteristic of the parental transformed cells.[4,5]

The ability of DNA from *in vitro* transformed cells to transform normal cells into malignant cells indicates that DNA is the target in radiation and chemically induced transformation, and that the origin of malignancy induced by these carcinogenic agents is of a genetic nature.[4]

These genetic modifications may code for gene products which act as modulators or transducers of signals that control cell proliferation.

While DNA alterations are essential for malignant transformation of rodent and human cells, susceptibility to transformation and the course and frequency of the neoplastic process are determined by an interplay of a variety of permissive and protective factors in the cell.[1]

Physiological factors as well as cell contact and loss of cell communication between normal and transformed cells may modify the expression of transformation in cells exposed to radiation or chemical carcinogens.[6] A loss of cell communication between normal and transformed cells may lead to growth inhibition of the transformed cells by their normal counterparts.[6] Factors which alter cellular metabolism and gene expression, such as thyroid hormone act as co-transforming factors in the cells and agents which act as antioxidants and modify metabolism, by suppressing free radical cascade reaction, play a role as protective factors and inhibit the oncogenic effects of radiation and a variety of chemicals.[7-9]

III. Thyroid Hormone as a Co-Transforming Factor

The role of thyroid hormone on diverse aspects of cellular metabolism including respiration have long been known.[10]

Our studies, using *in vitro* cell systems have demonstrated that thyroid hormones serve as critical permissive factors for cell transformation by x-rays, chemical carcinogens, tumor viruses and specific transforming sequences of DNA (oncogenes).[7-11] The action of T3 in modulating transformation by oncogenic agents or by specific oncogenes appears to be mediated via more than one route.

Our earlier work has suggested that thyroid hormone may be critical for the synthesis of a transformation associated protein(s) which may alter cell function.[8] This possibility is supported by the fact that the T3 dose response relationship for transformation is similar to the T3 dose dependence for another protein, the enzyme Na/K ATPase, and by recent work showing a high resolution two dimensional electrophoresis, that T3 modulates the expression of specific growth related proteins (in preparation).[8]

An additional mechanism by which thyroid hormone regulates neoplastic transformation may reside in the ability of the hormone to modify the oxidant state of the cells, resulting in the enhanced levels of free radical processes under conditions of oxidant stress (in preparation).[10] These effects must be counteracted by constitutive cellular antioxidants or by induced molecular processes directed at scavenging free radicals and impeding their deleterious action.

IV. Antioxidants as Protecting Factors in Transformation

The interaction of cells with radiation, both x-ray and ultraviolet (UV) light, as well as with a variety of chemicals, results in an enhanced generation of free oxygen species and free radical products and in a modified pro-oxidant state.[13] The result is a loss in the optimal cellular balance between the oxidative challenge, a source of DNA damage, and the inherent mechanisms that protect the cell from excess oxidative stress. These protective systems include enzymes (SOD, catalase, peroxidases, transferases) and thiols. Also included are dietary antioxidants which attenuate processes of peroxidation and autoxidation of macromolecules: vitamin A, β-carotene, vitamin C, selenium and vitamin E.[13]

In recent years, increasing evidence has implicated free radical mechanisms in the initiation and promotion of malignant transformation *in vivo* and *in vitro*. Much of the evidence has come from the fact that the agents that scavenge free radicals directly or that interfere with the generation of free radical-mediated events inhibit the neoplastic process.[9,14,15] We have shown in hamster embryo cells that SOD inhibits transformation by radiation and bleomycin and suppresses the promoting action of a free radical producing tumor promoter.[15] Catalase had no effect as an inhibitory agent in this cell system, perhaps because of the inherent high level of the enzyme in the hamster cells.[15] SOD had a more dramatic inhibitory effect when maintained on the cells throughout the experiment suggesting that later stages in the transformation process are influenced by free radicals.[15]

V. Selenium and Vitamin E

Other agents which qualify as important antioxidants are various examples of nutrients important in controlling free radical damage. These include selenium, a component of glutathione peroxidase, and vitamin E, a powerful antioxidant and a component of the cell membrane.

An important determinant in the efficiency of cellular protection by inherent antioxidants lies in the interaction between various factors. The metabolic functions of vitamin E and selenium are interrelated and selenium plays a role in the transport and storage of vitamin E.[9]

We examined the single and combined actions of selenium and vitamin E on cell transformation induced in C_3H 1OT1/2 cells by x-rays, benzo(a)pyrene, or tryptophan pyrolysate and on the levels of cellular scavenging systems and peroxide destruction.[9] Incubation of C_3H 1OT1/2 cells with 2.5 M Na_2SeO_3 (selenium) or with 7 μM alpha-tocopherol succinate (vitamin E) 24 h prior to exposure to x-rays or the chemical carcinogens resulted in an inhibition of transformation by each of the antioxidants with a super additive action when the two nutrients were combined. Cellular pretreatment with selenium resulted in increased levels of cellular glutathione peroxidase, catalase, and nonprotein thiols (glutathione) and in an enhanced destruction of hydrogen peroxide.[9] Cells pretreated with vitamin E did not show these biochemical effects, and the combined pretreatment with vitamin E and selenium did not augment the effect of selenium on these parameters. The results indicate that free radical-mediated events play a role in radiation and chemically induced transformation, and that selenium and vitamin E act alone and in additive fashion as radioprotecting and chemopreventing agents. Selenium confers protection in part by inducing or activating cellular free-radical scavenging systems and by enhancing peroxide breakdown, thus increasing the capacity of the cell to cope with oxidant stress. Vitamin E appears to confer its protection by an alternate complementary mechanism, e.g., by reducing cellular lipid peroxidation products. Exposure of cells to radiation in the presence and absence of vitamin E (alpha-tocopherol succinate) indicated that the levels of lipid peroxidation products were lowered in the vitamin E pretreated cells.[1]

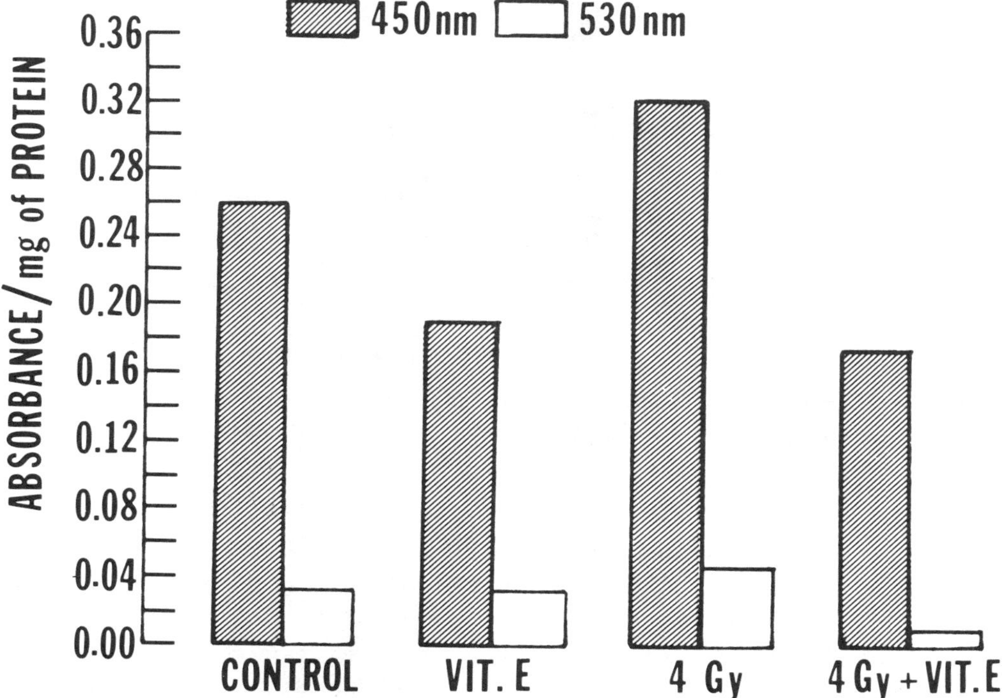

Figure 2. Cells were exposed to 400 rad with and without vitamin E (alpha tocopherol succinate at 7 μM.) TBA products were measured as reported.[20]

VI. Vitamin E and Vitamin C

While vitamin E closely interacts with selenium it also interacts with vitamin C. Vitamin C has been shown to preserve the antioxidant action of vitamin E by reducing oxidized vitamin E.[16,17]

We investigated whether vitamin E would interact with vitamin C in suppressing transformation of C_3H 10T1/2 cells exposed to x-rays.

Our work indicates that vitamin E and vitamin C act in concert to inhibit radiogenic transformation in a manner which appears to be synergistic in nature.[1]

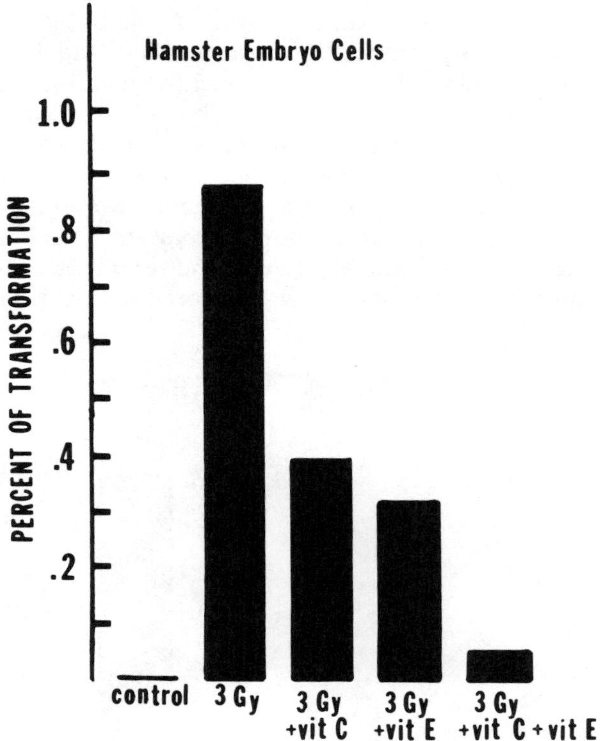

Figure 3. Hamster embryo cells were exposed to 300 rad in the presence and absence of vitamin E (alpha tocopherol succinate 7 μM) and vitamin C 1 μg/ml.[3]

VII. Antioxidant Inhibition of Ozone Carcinogenesis

The role of free radicals in the carcinogenic process can be inferred from the protective action of agents which attenuate free radical reactions at different stages of the oxidative process. However, their role in carcinogenesis can further be evaluated by exposing the cells to the direct action of ozone, an active form of ozone and a powerful oxidant.

Ozone, a key component in smog, is the largest pollutant in our atmosphere. Ozone, though not a free radical by itself, interacts with a wide range of biological molecules to produce free radicals.[20,21] Its toxic action can be inhibited by a variety of antioxidants which prevent its effects in oxidizing proteins or polyunsaturated fatty acids.[20,21]

Our experiments show that treatment of hamster embryo and mouse C_3H 1OT1/2 cells with 5 ppm O_3 for 5 min. resulted in enhancing cell transformation compared to control untreated cells. In addition, we found that O_3 and ionizing radiation act synergistically to induce cell transformation and that O_3 and ultraviolet light act in additive fashion to transfer cell.[19,20]

One of the major actions of ozone resides in its ability to peroxidize polyunsaturated fatty acids and produce malonaldehyde, which reacts with thiols, crosslinks DNA and histones and acts as an initiator in mouse skin carcinogenesis.[19,22] We tested the short term effects of 5 ppm O_3 in producing lipid peroxidation products in the hamster embryo and mouse C_3H 10T1/2 cells compared to air treated controls. Lipid peroxidation as measured by the formation of thiobarbituric acid (TBA) reactive products was assayed within 10 min after O_3 exposure.[20]

We found that malonaldehyde and malonaldehyde-like products were formed at higher levels in O_3 exposed cells as compared to controls.[20]

The finding that lipid peroxidation products are elevated in response to O_3 suggests a partial role for free radical-mediated reactions in O_3 induced neoplastic transformation. Further support comes from our recent results indicating that the antioxidant vitamin E (alpha tocopherol) inhibits O_3 induced transformation in mouse and hamster cells (Figure 1) in a time related manner, and inhibits the single and combined carcinogenic action of O_3 and ultraviolet light (in preparation).

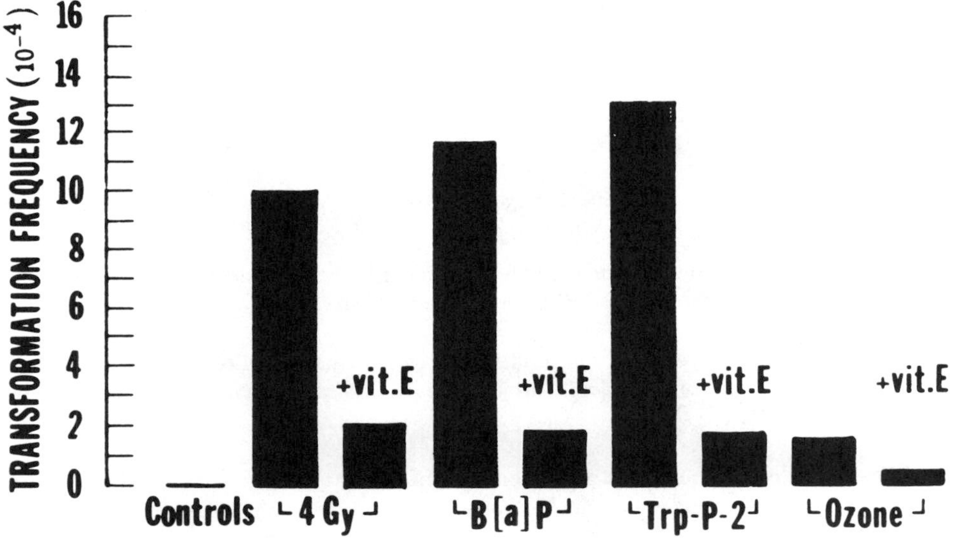

Figure 4. Inhibition of radiation and chemically induced transformation by vitamin E.

VIII. Conclusions

One of the basic conundrums in carcinogenesis evolves from our inability to unequivocally distinguish primary events associated with the induction of malignant transformation from those which function as secondary events. Thus the role of oncogenes, mutations, gene rearrangements, amplification and other

DNA alterations in transformation is yet unclear. The changes which take place give rise to abnormal expression of cellular genes, and altered gene expression.

We must always be cognizant of the fact that a variety of factors may modify the neoplastic process at its various stages of development. These constitute physiological permissive factors such as thyroid hormone which may modify directly or indirectly diverse processes in the cell, provide the cell with new messages and signals which play a role in cell proliferation and transforation.

Transformation takes place following exposure to a variety of free radical producing agents, when permissive factors prevail and protective factors are at a reduced level. By contrast, if permissive factors do not prevail, or protective factors such as free radical scavengers are at a sufficiently high level, the onset and progression of the neoplastic process will be suppressed. These protectors may be inherent cellular factors or those added externally, such as dietary factors which act as anticarcinogens. Thus, the interplay between inherent genetic and physiological factors and lifestyle influences, which either enhance or inhibit the neoplastic process, are critical determinants in the process of multistage carcinogenesis and in establishing the incidence of cancer.

Acknowledgements

This work was supported by Grant No. CA-12536 from the National Cancer Institute, and by a contract from the National Foundation for Cancer Research.

References

1. Borek, C., The induction and control of radiogenic transformation *in vitro*: Cellular and molecular mechanisms, *Pharmac. Ther.*, 27, 99, 1985.

2. Borek, C., Protective factors in malignant transformation of cells in culture, in *The Biochemical Basis of Chemical Carcinogenesis*, Greim, H., *et al.*, Eds., Raven Press, New York, 1984, 175.

3. Borek, C., *In vitro* cell cultures as tools in the study of free radicals and free radical modifiers in carcinogenesis, in *Methods in Enzymology*, Vol. on oxygen radicals in biological systems, Colowick, C.P., *et al.*, Eds., Academic Press, New York, 1984, 464.

4. Shilo, B.Z. and Weinberg, R.A., Unique transforming gene in carcinogen transformed mouse cells, *Nature*, 289, 607, 1981.

5. Borek, C., Ong, A., and Mason, H., Distinctive transforming genes in x-ray transformed mammalian cells, *Proc. Natl. Acad. Sci. USA*, 84, 794, 1987.

6. Borek, C., Higashino, S., and Lowenstein, W.R., Intercellular communication and tissue growth. IV. Conductance of membrane junctions of normal and cancerous cells in culture, *J. Memb. Biol.*, 1, 274, 1969.

7. Guemsey, D.L., Borek, C., and Edelman, I.S., Crucial role of thyroid hormone in x-ray induced transformation in cell culture, *Proc. Natl. Acad. Sci. USA*, 78, 5708, 1981.

8. Borek, C., Guemsey, D.L., Ong, A, and Edelman, I.S., Critical role played by thyroid hormone in induction of neoplastic transformation by chemical carcinogens in tissue culture, *Proc. Natl. Acad. Sci. USA*, 80, 5749, 1983.

9. Borek, C., Ong, A., Mason, H., Donahue, L., and Biaglow, J.E., Selenium and vitamin E inhibit radiogenic and chemically induced transformation *in vitro* via different mechanisms of action, *Proc. Natl. Acad. Sci. USA*, 83, 1490, 1986.

10. Ismail-Beigi, F., Bissell, D.M., and Edelman, I.S., Thyroid thermogenesis in adult rat hepatocytes in primary monolayer culture, *J. Gen. Physiol.*, 73, 369, 1979.

11. Borek, C., Ong. A.,and Rhim, J.S., Thyroid hormone modulates transformation induced by Kirsten murine sarcoma virus, *Cancer Res.*, 45, 1702, 1985.

12. Borek, C., Oncogenes, hormones, and free-radical processes in malignant transformation *in vitro, Ann. NY Acad. Sci.*, 551, 95, 1988.

13. Borek, C., Radiation and chemically induced transformation: Free radicals, antioxidants and cancer, *Br. J. Cancer*, 55, 74, 1987.

14. Doll, R. and Peto, R., The causes of cancer: quantitative estimates of avoidable risks of cancer in the United States, *J. Natl. Cancer Inst.*, 66, 1191, 1981.

15. Cerutti, P.A., Pro-oxidant states and tumor promotion, *Science*, 227, 375, 1985.

16. Borek, C. and Troll, W., Modifiers of free radicals inhibit *in vitro* the oncogenic actions of x-rays, bleomycin, and the tumor promoter 12-0-tetradecanoylphorbol 13-acetate, *Proc. Natl. Acad. Sci. USA*, 80, 1304, 1983.

17. Packer, L., Slater, T.F., and Willson, R.L., Direct observation of a free radical interaction between vitamin E and vitamin C, *Nature*, 278, 737, 1979.

18. Niki, E., Saito, T., Kawakami, A., and Kamiya, Y., Inhibition of oxidation of methyl linoleate in solution by vitamin E and vitamin C, *J. Biol. Chem.*, 259, 4177, 1984.

19. Muller, A., Cadenas, E., Graf, P., and Sies, H., A novel biologically active selno-organic compound-I. Glutathione peroxidase-like activity *in vitro* and antioxidant capacity of PZ 51 (Ebselen), *Biochem. Pharmacology*, 33, 3235, 1984.

20. Borek, C., Ong, A., and Mason, H, Ozone and ultraviolet light act as additive co-carcinogens to induce *in vitro* neoplastic transformation, Teratogenesis, *Carcinogenesis and Mutagenesis*, 9, 71, 1989.

21. Borek, C., Zaider, M., Ong, A., Mason, H., and Witz, G. Ozone acts alone and synergistically with ionizing radiation to induce *in vitro* neoplastic transformation, *Carcinogenesis*, 7, 1611, 1986.

22. Pryor, W.A., Dooley, M.M., and Church, D.F., Mechanisms for the reaction of ozone: Its biological molecules, the source of the toxic effects of ozone, in *The Biomedical Effects of Ozone and Related Photochemical Oxidants*, Lee, S.E., *et al.*, Eds., Princeton Scientific Publishers, Princeton, NJ, 1983, 7.

23. Shamberger, R.J., Andreone, T.L., and Willis, C.E., Antioxidants and cancer. IV. Initiating activity of malonaldehyde as a carcinogen, *J. Natl. Cancer Inst.*, 53, 1771, 1974.

Chapter 5

An Intervention Trial on Precursor Lesions for Oesophageal Cancer in a High Incidence Area of China

Nubia Muñoz, Massimo Crespi, Jurgen Wahrendorf, and Lu Jian Bang

Table of Contents

I. Introduction

Cancer of the oesophagus is the sixth most common cancer in the world; in developing countries it ranks fourth.[1] The disease is rapidly fatal for the majority of those whom it strikes even where medical care meets the highest standards, and the prospect appears poor of reducing this toll through earlier diagnosis or improvements in treatment. Its epidemiological behavior, marked by large differences in incidence within small geographic confines and sharp changes in incidence over time, suggests a predominant role for external environmental factors.

Cancer of the oesophagus, like cancer of the lung, then appears to be a disease whose control will come about by primary prevention utilizing the findings of epidemiologic studies.

The identification and characterization of premalignant lesions are of crucial importance in primary prevention programs since they could be used as early end points to assess the efficacy of the intervention.

Little is known about the precursor lesions of squamous cell carcinoma of the oesophagus in man. Endoscopic surveys in high- and low-risk populations for oesophageal cancer in Iran and China have been instrumental in the characterization of oesophageal lesions different from those associated with reflux oesophagitis and suspected to be precancerous. These lesions include: chronic oesophagitis, epithelial atrophy and dysplasia. Their prevalence in the two high-risk areas (Iran and Linxian County, China) sharply differs from the one found in the low-risk area (Jiaoxian County, China), as seen in Table 1. Of interest is the finding that epithelial atrophy and dysplasia, considered as intermediate steps towards malignancy, are in fact absent in the subjects surveyed in the low-risk area, the basic lesion being chronic oesophagitis, mainly of mild degree.

The precancerous nature of these lesions is suggested by:

- the similar location of these lesions and oesophageal cancer, both involve mainly the middle and lower thirds of the oesophagus.
- the high prevalence of these lesions in populations with high incidence of oesophageal cancer and their lower prevalence in low-incidence areas.[2-4]
- the high progression to cancer in a limited group of subjects with these lesions in China.[3]
- the induction of similar lesions in the oesophagus of non-human primates after treatment with 1-methyl-nitrosourea.[5]

Their precancerous nature can only be confirmed by long-term follow-up studies. In China, follow-up of patients with early oesophageal cancer who refused treatment, suggests that these lesions progress slowly to invasive cancer. The slow pace of changes of frank neoplastic lesions may suggest the opportunity to block the progression of precursor lesions, such as the ones previously described, through intervention studies utilizing the findings from aetiological research.

On the other hand, there is a considerable body of experimental and epidemiological evidence indicating that certain micronutrients have a great potential as protective agents for oesophageal cancer.

TABLE 1
Precursor Lesions of Oesophageal Cancer in High- and Low-risk Populations (Histological Findings)

	Male			Female		
	High-risk		Low-risk	High-risk		Low-risk
	Iran Turkoman	China Linxian	China Jiaoxian	Iran Turkoman	China Linxian	China Jiaoxian
Number of subjects	213	292	152	205	235	100
Oesophagitis						
Mild	58.7%	55.8%	33.5%	57.6%	56.2%	18.0%
Moderate	21.6%	7.5%	0.7%	17.6%	6.4%	0.0%
Severe	2.8%	1.7%	0.0%	1.0%	0.9%	0.0%
Total	83.1%	65.0%	34.2%	76.2%	63.5%	18.0%
Clear cell acanthosis	66.2%	80.8%	82.9%	64.9%	72.4%	85.0%
Atrophy	12.7%	11.6%	0.7%	8.3%	9.8%	0.0%
Dysplasia	4.7%	7.9%	0.0%	2.9%	8.1%	0.0%

Both vitamin A and riboflavin are essential for maintaining the integrity of the squamous epithelium. Experimental studies have shown that severe riboflavin deficiency in the mouse and baboon causes atrophy and ulcerative lesions in the oesophageal mucosa. Concerning the epidemiological evidence, several studies indicate that subpopulations at high risk for oesophageal cancer in Iran, South Africa and China have low intake and/or low plasma levels of vitamins A, C, β-carotene, riboflavin and other micronutrients. Case-control studies have also reported a history of lower intake of vitamins A, C and riboflavin among cases than among controls.[6] The associations with these micronutrients were, however, in general less strong than those observed for the food groups providing them, raising the possibility that other unidentified constituents of these foods might contribute to their protective effect. A further source of difficulty in the assessment of the effect of specific nutrients is the high degree of correlation among them. In a case-control study in France, strong correlations were found between nutrients while between foods the correlations were weak.[7] Studies in China showed that low levels of vitamins A, C, riboflavin and zinc were widespread but that riboflavin deficiency was more severe in the high-risk population.[8]

Intervention studies might help in elucidating the role of certain micronutrients in the development of oesophageal cancer. One of such studies has been carried out in Huixian, a high-risk area for oesophageal cancer in China and will be described below.

II. Vitamin Intervention Study

The results of this study, which is the first controlled nutritional intervention study in cancer epidemiology, have been published elsewhere[9-11] and can be summarized as follows:

The aim of this randomized double-blind intervention trial was to determine whether a combined treatment with retinol, riboflavin and zinc could result, after one year, in a lower prevalence of precancerous lesions of the oesophagus in the group receiving the active treatment as compared to the group receiving a placebo. A random sample of 610 subjects in the age group 35-64, was drawn from two production brigades. These subjects were randomized into two groups of 305 each. One group received the active treatment (15 mg [50,000 IU] of retinol, 200 mg riboflavin and 50 mg of zinc) once a week. A second group of 305 individuals received a placebo, identical looking capsules administered weekly. The capsules were distributed by "barefoot doctors."

At entry into the study and at the end of the treatment, 13.5 months later, the study subjects were interviewed by questionnaire on smoking, drinking and dietary habits; they were examined, looking especially for signs of vitamin A and riboflavin deficiencies; blood samples were drawn for biochemical analysis of riboflavin, retinol, β-carotene and zinc.

Compliance with the treatment, assessed by inspection of follow-up records kept by the "barefoot doctors" and by changes in the blood levels 2 and 13.5 months after initiation of the treatment, was excellent. The final examination of the 567 subjects (93 percent) also included oesophagoscopy with at least two biopsies taken. Histologic slides were read independently and blindly by three pathologists. After a final diagnosis was reached by consensus, the code for treatment assignment was opened. The prevalence of micronuclei was also evaluated. For these studies, smears were prepared from exfoliated cells obtained from the buccal mucosa and oesophagus in subsamples of 200 and 170 subjects respectively. The smears were evaluated for the presence of micronuclei by means of 4^1-6-diamidino-2-phenylindole fluorescent staining.

Two end points were used to evaluate the effect of the treatment: the prevalence of precancerous lesions and the prevalence of micronucleated cells in the oesophageal mucosa.

The main results are summarized in Table 2.

The prevalence of oesophagitis with or without atrophy or dysplasia was 45.3% in the placebo and 48.9% in the vitamin-treated group. Oesophagitis was accompanied by atrophy in 12.7% and dysplasia in 2.2% in the placebo group, and in the vitamin-treated group by atrophy in 12.3% and by dysplasia in 2.5%. Although no reduction in the prevalence of histologically diagnosed precancerous lesions was observed, a significantly lower prevalence of oesophageal micronucleated cells was found in the group receiving a combined treatment of riboflavin, retinol and zinc during 13.5 months as compared to the control group receiving a placebo.[8,9] The reduction of oesophageal micronucleated cells may represent an effect of treatment at an earlier stage of the carcinogenesis process. One difficulty in the final interpretation of this trial arises from the fact that at the end of the trial an increase in blood retinol levels occurred in 47% of subjects

TABLE 2
Effect of Riboflavin, Retinol and Zinc Treatment on the Prevalence of Micronuclei and of Histologically Diagnosed Precancerous Lesions of the Oesophagus

	Placebo	Vitamins
Micronuclei (mean ± SD)	0.31% (± 0.29)	0.19% (± 0.15)
Histological diagnosis		
Normal oeosphagus	53.6%	49.6%
Chronic oesophagitis	30.4%	34.1%
Epithelial atrophy	12.7%	12.3%
Dysplasia	2.2%	2.5%
Squamous cancer	0.7%	1.5%
Adenocarcinoma	0.4%	0.0%
Number of subjects	276	276

Adapted from Muñoz *et al.*, 1985; Muñoz *et al.*, 1987

in the placebo group and in 76% of those receiving the treatment. The corresponding figures for riboflavin were 17% and 66%. These changes in blood levels of the vitamins were probably the result of dietary changes that occurred during the study period.[12] To account for these changes a multivariate analysis was made. There were 462 individuals who had complete information on all variables required for this analysis. Table 3 shows the mean blood levels of retinol, riboflavin and zinc found before the treatment and 13.5 months after treatment. An increase in the retinol levels occurred in both treatment groups, although it was more marked in the vitamin-treated group and in females. For zinc an increase of the same magnitude was seen in both treatment groups, while there was a clear improvement in the riboflavin status in the vitamin treated group and only a slight improvement in the placebo group. Riboflavin status was measured using the erythrocyte glutathione reductase test in which biochemical deficiency is regarded as activation coefficient (AC) values greater than 1.30.

Five models were used to assess the effect of the changes in the blood levels of the three micronutrients on the prevalence of the precancerous lesions. In models 1 and 2 the levels at the initial and final survey were considered, in model 3 the absolute differences between final and initial survey, in model 4, the relative change and in model 5 the relative change was categorized into worse (more than 20% decrease), improvement (more than 20% increase), and unchanged (neither worsening nor improving). The results for model 5 are summarized in Table 4 which shows a reduction in the prevalence of precancerous lesions in those whose blood levels of retinol, riboflavin and zinc improved or remained unchanged as compared to those whose levels got worse during the study period. Although the effect of riboflavin was not statistically significant in this model, it was when the relative changes (model 4) were considered.

TABLE 3
Blood Levels of Retinol, Riboflavin and Zinc (Mean ± SD) Before and After Treatment

	Placebo group		Vitamin group	
	Males (No. = 110)	**Females (No. = 119)**	**Males (No. = 118)**	**Females (No. = 115)**
Retinol:				
Before tx. (µg/l)	408.0±105.7	333.2±95.0	411.7±104.7	333.7±109.6
After tx. (µg/l)	486.1±109.1	412.4±103.6	561.3±127.7	481.4±116.1
Riboflavin:				
Before tx. (AC)	1.65±0.23	1.68±0.27	1.65±0.26	1.67±0.29
After tx. (AC)	1.62±0.31	1.60±0.31	1.22±0.18	1.29±0.24
Zinc:				
Before tx. (µg/l)	0.82±0.19	0.76±0.12	0.83±0.17	0.78±0.13
After tx. (µg/l)	0.94±0.29	0.94±0.27	0.96±0.29	0.95±0.31

AC = Activation Coefficient
Adapted from Wahrendorf *et al.*, 1988

TABLE 4
Effect of Blood Level Changes of Riboflavin, Retinol and Zinc on the Prevalence of Precancerous Lesions of the Oesophagus

Vitamin change	**Odds ratio for precancerous lesions**		
	Retinol	**Riboflavin**	**Zinc**
Worse	1.00	1.00	1.00
Unchanged	0.56	0.76	0.14
Improved	0.41	0.61	0.11
p for linear trend	0.04	0.13	0.001

Adapted from Wahrendorf *et al.*, 1988.

The overall results of this trial suggest a beneficial effect of retinol, riboflavin and zinc on the prevalence of precancerous lesions. The effect of these micronutrients on the occurrence of oesophageal cancer may emerge from the results of large-scale intervention studies being conducted in the same high-risk population in China in which the end points are changes in incidence and mortality of oesophageal cancer.[13]

References

1. Parkin, D.M., Läärä, E., and Muir, C.S., Estimates of the world-wide frequency of sixteen major cancers in 1980, *Int. J. Cancer*, 41, 184, 1988.

2. Crespi, M., Muñoz, N., Grassi, A., Aramesh, B., Amiri, G., and Mojtabai, A., Esophageal lesions in northern Iran: a premalignant condition? *Lancet*, 1, 217, 1979.

3. Muñoz, N., Crespi, M., Grassi, A., Wang, G.-Q., Shen, Q., and Li, Z.C., Precursor lesions of esophageal cancer in high-risk populations in Iran and China, *Lancet*, 1, 876, 1982.

4. Crespi, M., Muñoz, N., Grassi, A., Shen, Q., Wang, K.J., and Lin, J.J., Precursor lesions of oesophageal cancer in low-risk population in China: comparison with high-risk populations, *Int. J. Cancer*, 34, 599, 1984.

5. Adamson, R.H., Krolikowski, J.F., Correa, P., Sieber, S.M., and Dalgard, D.W., Carcinogenicity of 1-methyl-1-nitrosourea in nonhuman primates, *J. Natl. Cancer Inst.*, 59, 415, 1977.

6. Day, N. and Muñoz, N. Oesophagus, in *Cancer Epidemiology and Prevention*, Schottenfeld, D. and Fraumeni, J.F., Jr., Eds., W.B. Saunders Co., Philadelphia, 1982, 596.

7. Tuyns, A.J., Riboli, E., Doornbos, G, and Peguignot, G., Diet and oesophageal cancer in Calvados (France), *Nutr. Cancer*, 9, 81, 1987.

8. Thurnham, D.I., Zheng, S.F., Muñoz, N., Crespi, M., Grassi, A., Hambidge, M., and Chai, T.F., Comparison of riboflavin, vitamin A and zinc status in high- and low-risk regions for oesophageal cancer in China, *Nutr. Cancer*, 7, 131, 1985.

9. Muñoz, N., Wahrendorf, J., Lu, J.B., Crespi, M., Thurnham, D.I., Day, N.E., Zheng, H.J., Grassi, A., Li, W.Y., Liu, G.L., Lang, Y.Q., Zhang, C.Y., Zheng, S.F., Li, J.Y., Correa, P., O'Conor, G.T., and Bosch, F.X., No effect of riboflavin, retinol and zinc on prevalence of precancerous lesions of esophagus, *Lancet*, 2, 111, 1985.

10. Muñoz, N., Hayashi, M., Lu, J.B., Wahrendorf, J., Crespi, M., and Bosch, F.X., Effect of riboflavin, retinol and zinc on micronuclei of buccal mucosa and of oesophagus: (a randomized double-blind intervention study in China), *J. Natl. Cancer Inst.*, 79, 687, 1987.

11. Wahrendorf, J., Muñoz, N., Lu, J.B., Thurnham, D.I., Crespi, M., and Bosch, F.X., Blood, retinol and zinc riboflavin status in relation to precancerous lesions of the esophagus: findings from a vitamin intervention trial in the People's Republic of China, *Cancer Res.*, 48, 2280, 1988.

12. Thurnham, D.I., Muñoz, N., Lu, J.B., Wahrendorf, J., Zheng, S.F., Hambidge, K.M., and Crespi, M., Nutritional and haematological status of Chinese farmers: the

influence of 13.5 months treatment with riboflavin, retinol and zinc, *Eur. J. Clin. Nutr.*, 42, 647, 1988.

13. Li, J.Y., Li, G.Y., Zheng, S.F., *et al.*, A pilot vitamin intervention trial in Linxian, People's Republic of China, *Natl. Cancer Inst. Monogr.*, 69, 19, 1985.

Chapter 6

Chemoprevention of Gastrointestinal Cancer in Animals by Naturally Occurring Organosulfur Compounds in Allium Vegetables

Michael J. Wargovich, Hiromichi Sumiyoshi, Allan Baer, and Osamu Imada

Table of Contents

I. Introduction

Diet has been considered to be the primary lifestyle factor that influences risk for development of several gastrointestinal cancers. While advances in molecular genetics point toward some commonalities in the cellular evolution of inherited forms of GI cancer, migration studies in populations have lent support that some aspects in diet impart a preeminent risk for cancer. The association may be quite positive as is the case for dietary fat in colon cancer in Japanese migrating to North America or the salt content of food for gastric cancer's high prevalence in Asian nations, or, in many cases a negative association is found, that is, ingestion of some foods imparts a protective cellular environment from cancer development. The plant members of the genus *Allium* (members of the lily family) contain a variety of vegetables utilized as food throughout the world. They include onion, garlic, leeks, chives, shallots, amongst others. The flavors and fragrances associated with these vegetables and herbs are generated by chemical compounds distinguished by organosulfur moieties. Our laboratory has studied allium organosulfur agents as possible chemopreventives for gastrointestinal cancer. The results we have obtained suggest that some sulfur chemicals in alliums, strongly associated with characteristic taste and smell of these vegetables are, in fact, also potent inhibitors of carcinogenesis. Our studies to date have concentrated on the preventive effects of these agents in rodent models for esophageal and colon cancer.

II. Organosulfur Compounds in Garlic (*Allium sativum*)

The redolent chemicals associated with the odor of garlic are generated when the bulb is crushed or macerated. A cascade of chemical transformations occurs when the principle compound S-allyl-L-cysteine sulfoxide is acted upon by the enzyme allinase. The reactions conclude with a yield of greater than 16 distinct organosulfur compounds. For more detailed information on these fascinating chemicals generated by allinase reactions excellent reviews by Block[1] and Fenwick *et al.*[2] encompass the chemistry of garlic and onion. The natural breakdown products of the allinase reaction and the distillation processes that have been instrumental to the production of garlic flavorings for the food flavor industry have produced a number of purified agents for testing as chemopreventive compounds. Constitutive organosulfur compounds from garlic are separable into those soluble in organic solvents and those which are water-soluble. Our work has primarily concentrated on diallyl sulfide (DAS) and S-allyl-cysteine (SAC) which are representative of each class of these compounds respectively. Both have been and continue to be available in purified form which allows for testing in experimental chemoprevention protocols.

III. Effects of Garlic and Garlic Derived-Agents in Animal Carcinogenesis Studies

Although the number of studies in which garlic extracts or purified organosulfur compounds have been tested in as inhibitors of carcinogenesis are limited, the results reported are distinguished by the degree of efficacy in their prevention of cancer. The first group of studies has examined the effects of garlic or garlic oil on polycyclic hydrocarbon carcinogenesis in epidermal cells. Belman[3] contributed the original report in this area when it was shown that skin papillomas induced by the carcinogen dimethylbenzanthracene and promoted by phorbol myristate acetate moderately inhibited tumor formation. In the same system this group[4] has found that garlic oil stimulated glutathione peroxidase activity (a protective enzyme) and reduced ornithine decarboxylase activity in carcinogen-stimulated cells. More recently Belman's laboratory found garlic oil to inhibit the conversion of papilloma to carcinoma in the same system.[5] Sadhana *et al.*[6] using benzo[a]pyrene as the carcinogen found that garlic oil application during the initiation phase of skin carcinogenesis was an effective inhibitor of carcinogenesis. Athar *et al.*[7] tested the combination of DAS and nondihydroguaiaretic acid (NDGA) in the mouse skin cancer model and reported that DAS did not greatly increase the inhibition of tumors than that observed with NDGA alone. In the cervix of mice treated with methylcholanthrene oral administration of garlic strongly inhibited the incidence of carcinoma.[8]

In other studies, the hepatotoxic effects of the combination of partial hepatectomy and administration of the carcinogen 1,2-dimethylhydrazine (DMH) were diminished when a prophylactic dose of DAS was given before the carcinogen.[9] SAC and related S-allyl-mercapto-cysteine (SAMC) were suppressive of liver damage induced in rats by paracetamol or carbon tetrachloride-induced toxicosis in mice.[10]

In summary, the experimental evidence in non-gastrointestinal carcinogenesis models supports a specific inhibition of chemical carcinogenesis. Since all of the carcinogens used in these studies require metabolic activation, it may be postulated that garlic or garlic derived substances such as DAS, SAC, or SAMC act by interruption of P450-related carcinogen metabolism. That this is indeed the case is entirely supported by studies where monoalkylating gastrointestinal carcinogens have been used. In most cases suppression by the these same organosulfur agents was observed.

IV. Chemoprevention Studies of Diallyl Sulfide and S-Allyl-Cysteine and Related Agents in Gastrointestinal Cancers

In our laboratory we have surveyed the effects of DAS and SAC in the DMH-induced colon cancer in mice and in nitroso-methylbenzylamine-induced (NMBA) esophageal cancer in rats.[11,12] DMH is a well-studied intestinal carcinogen and the type of cancer that is induced in the rat is indistinguishable from that in man.[13] We have used the model to examine the dose-related inhibitory effects of DAS and a summary of our results is shown in Table 1.

DAS administered orally prior to carcinogen caused a linear reduction in tumor incidence; moreover, at higher concentrations of the agent the number of invasive carcinomas was significantly reduced. DMH is an alkylating carcinogen that is metabolically activated through several oxidation steps mediated by cytochrome P450IIE1.[14] This isoform of cytochrome P450 is also responsible for the metabolizing of a number of xenobiotic chemical compounds including other

TABLE 1
Chemopreventive Efficacy of DAS in DMH Colon Carcinogenesis in Mice

Dose DAS[a]	Tumor[b] incidence	Adenoma incidence per rat	Adenocarcinoma incidence per rat
0	77%	0.50 ± 0.51	0.43 ± 0.51
50	60%	0.51 ± 0.16	0.37 ± 0.10
100	53%	0.50 ± 0.12	0.13 ± 0.06
200	20%	0.17 ± 0.38	0.03 ± 0.19

[a] In mg/Kg by gavage
[b] Total animals with colon tumor

carcinogens. Therefore it is possible that DAS illicits a specific inhibition of this isoform of cytochrome, thus accounting for chemopreventive activity as the most likely mechanism involved. Our studies have now been extended to a water soluble organosulfur compound in garlic, S-allyl-cysteine (SAC). SAC is an effective inhibitor of DMH-induced colon cancer.[15] The doses that achieve this effect are higher than those of DAS but the compound has a much higher toxicity threshold. Recent studies of the toxicological aspects of DAS and SAC suggest that LD_{50}'s for the compounds are in the order of 1.8-2 g/kg for DAS and 8.8-9.3 g/kg for SAC.[16] We have also determined that DAS and SAC are stimulatory for gluatathione-S-transferase in the colon and liver within 24-48 h of administration; however induction of this enzyme, known to aid in the detoxification of carcinogenic substances is not sufficient to totally explain the chemopreventive inhibition observed. Additional studies have examined more pleiotropic effects of DAS. In mice exposed to ionizing radiation DAS has radio-protective properties. Baer *et al.*[17] found that the induction of ornithine decarboxylase in response to radiation-induced injury to the colonic mucosa of mice was attenuated by oral pre-treatment with DAS.

NMBA is a carcinogen long known for its ability to induce squamous cell carcinoma of the esophagus in the rat.[18] Like DMH for the colon, the type of esophageal tumors produced by NMBA in the rat and their growth and development histologically emulate that of squamous cell esophageal cancers in man. The model became of interest to us because of the similarities to the DMH model. As well, NMBA is metabolized by cytochrome P450IIE1.[19] We recently completed a series of chemoprevention experiments with DAS. In the NMBA model we tested several doses of DAS during initiation and one dose post-initiation. Such a protocol is necessary to examine with clarity the full spectrum of activity of a putative chemopreventive agent, since it may happen that while the compound inhibits cancer during the initiation phase of carcinogenesis it may be tumor promoting in the post-initiation phase. The results of these experiments (to be fully reported elsewhere) are shown in Table 2.

It can be readily seen that DAS is an active inhibitor only during the initiation phase of carcinogenesis; its effect in the post-initiation phase is negligible. NMBA is a lipophilic nitrosamine that has been reported to have been isolated from contaminated foodstuffs in China in regions of endemic prevalence

TABLE 2
Chemopreventive Effects of DAS in Initiation/and Post-Initiation Phases of NMBA Esophageal Cancer in Rats

Group	Dose DAS[a]	Tumor Incidence	Tumors TBA	Paps[b] TBA	SSC[c] TBA
DAS	10	-0-	-0-	-0-	-0-
DAS	100	-0-	-0-	-0-	-0-
NMBA	0	96%	3.48	2.65	0.82
NMBA	10	90%	3.34	3.03	0.62
NMBA	100	63%[d]	1.63	1.53	0.10
NMBA[e]	200	96%	3.43	2.60	0.69

[a] In mg/Kg by gavage, once per week for 5 weeks.
[b] Papillomas per tumor bearing animal.
[c] Squamous cell carcinomas per tumor bearing animal.
[d] Significantly different from NMBA alone, $p<0.01$.
[e] DAS given for 5 weeks post-carcinogen.

of esophageal cancer and its metabolism has been well-characterized to be mediated through cytochrome P450IIE1.[20,21] These findings are supported by recent evidence by Brady *et al.*[22] who found DAS to inhibit NMBA demethylase in the liver and selective suppression of P450IIE1 activity in microsomes. Of course it remains to be determined whether DAS and related compounds are themselves metabolized by the cytochrome systems effectively competing for carcinogen activation.

Current experiments in our laboratory are concentrating on special preparations of garlic for detection of chemopreventive effects. Aged garlic extracts have been examined for biological effects in a number of animal models.[10,24] Since these extracts are widely consumed it is important to observe whether they impart any tumor inhibiting effect and contrast such activities with known effects of purified organosulfur agents from garlic.

V. Summary

Experimental chemoprevention studies have lent themselves to a rapid exploration of garlic and associated members of the allium vegetables for substances that inhibit cancer development. At least two organosulfur compounds have been shown to suppress tumorigenesis at several organ sites. More needs to be learned about the metabolic fate of these naturally occurring sulfur-rich compounds, and perhaps, with this more will be known about their mechanism of tumor suppression. The pre-clinical development of these agents shows promise: they are natural substances found in food, their toxicity does not appear to be a limiting factor, and efficacy has been shown in independent tumor bioassays at multiple sites. A recent ecological study in China[24] and a case-control study in Italy[25] are suggestive of protection from gastrointestinal cancer when garlic and other alliums are a continuing part of the diet. Controlled chemoprevention trials in the high risk subject for cancer would seem to be a viable next step for these intriguing compounds so well-appreciated for their impact on nose and palate.

Acknowledgements

The authors wish to acknowledge the research support provided for these studies by American Institute for Cancer Research grant 89B25, a grant from the Wakunaga Pharmaceutical Company, Osaka, Japan, and the McCormick Company.

References

1. Block, E., The chemistry of garlic and onions, *Sci. Amer.*, 252, 114, 1985.

2. Fenwick, G.R. and Hanley, A.B., The genus *Allium*, *CRC. Crit. Rev. Food. Sci. Nutr.*, 23, 1, 1985.

3. Belman, S., Onion and garlic oils inhibit tumor promotion, *Carcinogenesis*, 4, 1063, 1983.

4. Perchellet, J.P., Perchellet, E.M., Abney, N.L., Zirnskin, J.A., and Belman, S., Effects of garlic and onion oils on glutathione peroxidase activity, the ratio of reduced/oxidized glutathione and ornithine decarboxylase induction in isolated mouse epidermal cells treated with tumor promotors, *Cancer Biochem. Biophys.*, 8, 299, 1986.

5. Belman, S., Sellakumar, A., Bosland, M.C., Savarese, K., and Estensen, R.D., Papilloma and carcinoma production in DMBA-initiated, onion oil-promoted mouse skin, *Nutr. Cancer*, 14, 141, 1990.

6. Sadhana, A.S., Rao, A.R., Kucheria, K., and Bijani, V., Inhibitory action of garlic oil on the initiation of benzo(a)pyrene-induced skin carcinogenesis in mice, *Cancer Lett.*, 40, 193, 1988.

7. Athar, M., Raza, H., Bickers, D.R., and Mukhtar, H., Inhibition of benzoyl peroxide-mediated tumor promotion in 7,12-dimethylbenz(a)anthracene initiated skin of sencar mice by antioxidants nordihydroguaiaretic acid and diallyl sulfide, *J. Invest. Dermatol.*, 94, 162, 1990.

8. Hussain, S.P., Jannu, L.N., and Rao, A.R., Chemopreventive action of garlic on methylcholanthrene-induced carcinogenesis, *Cancer Lett.*, 49, 175, 1990.

9. Hayes, M.A., Rushmore, T.H., and Goldberg, M.T., Inhibition of hepatocarcinogenic responses to 1,2-dimethylhydrazine by diallyl sulfide, a component of garlic oil, *Carcinogenesis*, 8, 1155, 1987.

10. Nakagawa, S., Kasuga, S., and Matsuura, H., Prevention of liver damage by aged garlic extract and its components in mice, *Phyto. Res.*, 1, 1, 1988.

11. Wargovich, M.J., Diallyl sulfide, a flavor component of garlic (*Allium sativum*) inhibits dimethylhydrazine-induced colon cancer, *Carcinogenesis*, 8, 487, 1987.

12. Wargovich, M.J., Woods, C., Eng, V.W.S., Stephens, L.C., and Gray, K.N., Chemoprevention of nitrosomethylbenzylamine induced esophageal cancer in rats by the thioether, diallyl sulfide, *Cancer Res.*, 48, 6872, 1988.

13. Thurnherr, N., Deschner, E.E., Stonehill, E.H., and Lipkin, M., Induction of adenocarcinomas of the colon in mice by weekly injections of 1,2-dimethylhydrazine, *Cancer Res.*, 33, 940, 1973.

14. Fiala, E.S., Investigations into the metabolism and mode of action of the colon carcinogens 1-2-dimethylhydrazine and azoxymethane, *Cancer*, 40, 2436, 1977.

15. Sumiyoshi, H. and Wargovich, M.J., Chemoprevention of 1,2-dimethylhydrazine-induced colon cancer in mice by naturally occurring organosulfur compounds, *Cancer Res.*, 50, 5084, 1990.

16. Imada, O., Toxicity aspects of garlic, in *Garlic in Biology and Medicine*, Lin, R., Ed., Nutrition International, Irvine, CA, in press.

17. Baer, A.R. and Wargovich, M.J., Role of ornithine decarboxylase in diallyl sulfide inhibition of colonic radiation injury in the mouse, *Cancer Res.*, 49, 5073, 1989.

18. Stinson, S.F., Squire, R.A., and Sporn, M.B., Pathology of esophageal neoplasms and associated proliferative lesions induced by N-methyl-N-benzylnitrosamine, *JNCI*, 61, 1471, 1978.

19. Hodgson, R.M., Wiessler, M., and Kleihues, P., Preferential methylation of target organ DNA by the oesophageal carcinogen, N-nitrosomethylbenzylamine, *Carcinogenesis*, 1, 861, 1980.

20. Li, N.H., Lu, S.H., Ji, C., Wang, M.Y., Cheng, S.J., and Jin, C.L., Formation of carcinogenic N-nitroso compound in corn bread inoculated with fungi, *Sci. Sin.*, 22, 471, 1979.

21. Barch, D.H., Kuemmerle, S., Hollenberg, P., and Lannacone, P., Esophageal microsomal metabolism of N-nitrosomethylbenzylamine in the zinc-deficient rat, *Cancer Res.*, 44, 5629, 1984.

22. Brady, J.F., Li, D., Ishizaki, H., and Yang, C.S., Effect of diallyl sulfide on rat liver microsomal nitrosamine metabolism and other monooxygenase activities, *Cancer Res.*, 48, 5937, 1988.

23. Unnikrishan, M.C., Soudamini, K.K., and Kuttan, R., Chemoprotection of garlic extract toward cyclophosphamide toxicity in mice, *Nutr. Cancer*, 13, 201, 1990.

24. You, W.C., Blot, W.J., Chang, Y.S., Ershow, A., Yang, Z.T., An, Q., Henderson, B.E., Fraumeni, J.F., and Wang, T.G., Allium vegetables and reduced risk of stomach cancer, *JNCI*, 81, 162, 1989.

25. Buiatti, E., Palli, D., Decarli, A., Amadori, D., Avellini, C., Bianchi, S., Biserni, R., Cipriani, F., Cocco, P., Giacosa, A., Marubini, E., Piutoni, R., Vindigni, C., Fraumeni, F., and Blot W., A case control study of gastric cancer and diet in Italy, *Int. J. Cancer*, 44, 611, 1989.

Chapter 7

Genotoxicity of Ni^{2+} in *Xenopus*: Search for the Molecular Mechanisms

F. William Sunderman, Jr., Gregory S. Makowski, Marilyn C. Plowman, and Sidney M. Hopfer

Table of Contents

I. Introduction

This chapter describes the initial steps in our search for the molecular mechanisms whereby Ni^{2+} causes genotoxicity, using embryos of the South African clawed toad, *Xenopus laevis*, as the experimental system. *Xenopus* embryos seem ideally suited for this investigation, since they are available in large numbers, are fertilized externally, develop rapidly, and are amenable to experimental interventions, such as microinjection. *Xenopus* embryos have been used in embryological research for over a century and have recently come under close scrutiny at the molecular level, stemming from the discovery that growth factors related to mammalian oncogenes are involved in cell-signalling processes that specify cell fate during *Xenopus* embryogenesis. Since the genotoxicity of nickel compounds has not previously been studied in *Xenopus*, several basic investigations were necessary in order to initiate this avenue of research.

II. Uptake of Ni^{2+} by *Xenopus* Embryos

The *first step* in this research program was to ascertain whether Ni^{2+} would enter *Xenopus* embryos spontaneously, or whether Ni^{2+} would need to be administered to the embryos by microinjection. The procedural details of this study have been reported.[1] Briefly, in each experiment, an adult *Xenopus* female was induced to ovulate by injections of gonadotropin. After the eggs were laid, they were promptly fertilized by exposure to fresh sperm suspension, prepared by mincing a testis excised from an adult *Xenopus* male. Batches of ~250 fertilized eggs were dejellied and suspended in a 1:10-dilution of modified Barth's saline solution ("0.1x-MBS"); samples of ~20 fertilized eggs were then transferred to Petri dishes for exposures to various concentrations of $^{63}NiCl_2$ dissolved in 0.1x-MBS solution. After exposures to $^{63}Ni^{2+}$ at 24°C for selected 0.5 h intervals during the period from 1 to 4.5 h post-fertilization, samples of 3 to 10 embryos were removed, rinsed three times with 0.1x-MBS solution, homogenized in distilled water, and assayed for ^{63}Ni by liquid scintillation counting. In experiments to measure ^{63}Ni binding to fertilization envelopes, groups of washed embryos were dissected with microforceps under a stereomicroscope; the envelopes were removed and placed directly into scintillation vials. In experiments to test the effect of fertilization on the uptake of ^{63}Ni, the eggs from a *Xenopus* female were divided between two Petri dishes: the eggs in one dish were fertilized, while the other eggs were left unfertilized. After dejellying, groups of fertilized and non-fertilized eggs were exposed for 0.5 h to specified concentrations of $^{63}Ni^{2+}$ and assayed for ^{63}Ni uptake.

As reported by Sunderman *et al.*,[1] these experiments showed that *Xenopus* embryos are readily permeable to $^{63}Ni^{2+}$ during early cleavage stages. When batches of embryos were exposed to $^{63}Ni^{2+}$ (0.3 or 3.0 μmol/L) from 1 to 1.5 h post-fertilization, ^{63}Ni uptake averaged 0.74 (SD ± 0.35) and 3.3 (SD ± 1.4) pmol/embryo, respectively. These mean values were 12 to 17 times the corresponding means for non-fertilized eggs ($p < 0.05$) (Figure 1). The integument that surrounds *Xenopus* eggs undergoes complex biochemical changes shortly after fertilization, converting the vitelline envelope to the fertilization envelope, releasing proteases from cortical granules, and activating transport channels for Ca^{2+}. The increased uptake of $^{63}Ni^{2+}$ by embryos, compared to non-fertilized eggs,

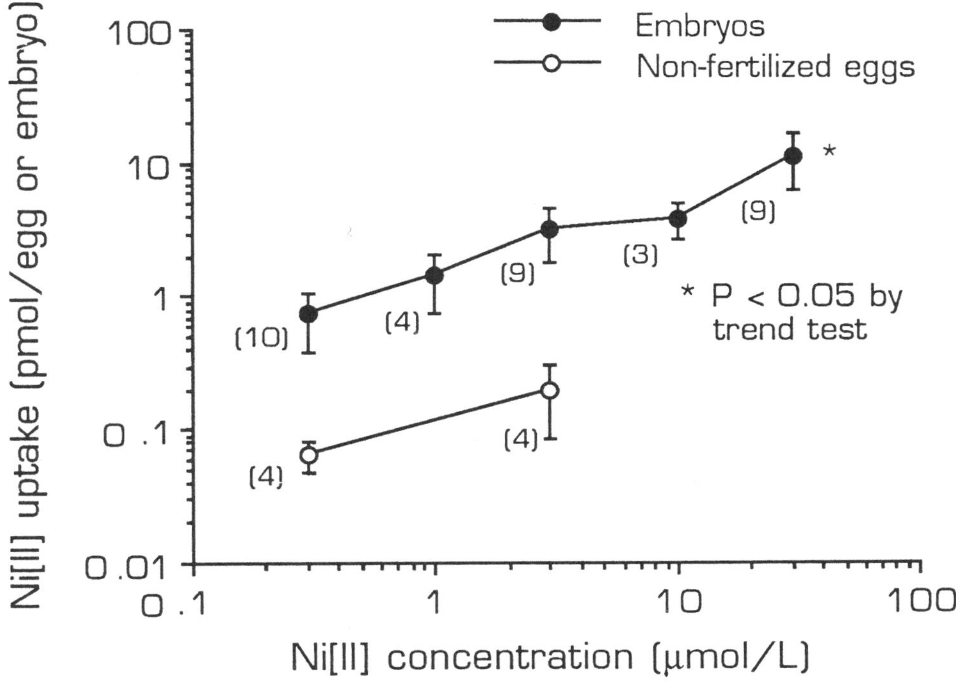

Figure 1. The uptake of ^{63}Ni in non-fertilized eggs (o) or embryos (•) exposed to specified concentrations of $^{63}Ni^{2+}$ from 1 to 1.5 h after collection or fertilization. The numbers of *Xenopus* females whose eggs or embryos were tested at each exposure level are given in parentheses; the error bars denote ± 1 SD; * = p <0.05 by trend test.[1]

suggests that the process of envelope conversion greatly enhances the integumentary permeability to $^{63}Ni^{2+}$, possibly via the activated Ca^{2+} channels.[1]

The ^{63}Ni was not simply adsorbed onto the surface of *Xenopus* embryos, since the fertilization envelopes, isolated by microdissection, contained only 5% of the corresponding ^{63}Ni content of the intact embryos. These measurements indicate that most of the ^{63}Ni traversed the fertilization envelope and entered one or more internal compartments. As shown in Figure 2, the uptake of ^{63}Ni by *Xenopus* embryos diminished progressively during 4 h post-fertilization. For example, when batches of embryos were exposed to $^{63}Ni^{2+}$ (0.3 or 3.0 μmol/L) from 4 to 4.5 h post-fertilization (*i.e.*, during the large cell blastula stage), ^{63}Ni uptake averaged 55% and 40%, respectively, of the corresponding values for embryos exposed from 1 to 1.5 h post-fertilization (*i.e.*, during the first cleavage stage, $p < 0.05$). The ^{63}Ni in *Xenopus* embryos was not completely or irreversibly bound to macromolecular constituents, since significant efflux of ^{63}Ni occurred after the $^{63}Ni^{2+}$-exposed embryos were returned to nickel-free medium.[1]

III. Teratogenicity of Ni^{2+} in *Xenopus* Embryos

As summarized in reviews on the embryotoxicity and teratogenicity of nickel compounds,[2-4] numerous studies have shown that administration of Ni^{2+} to rodents during early gestation causes embryotoxicity (*e.g.*, reduced litter size and

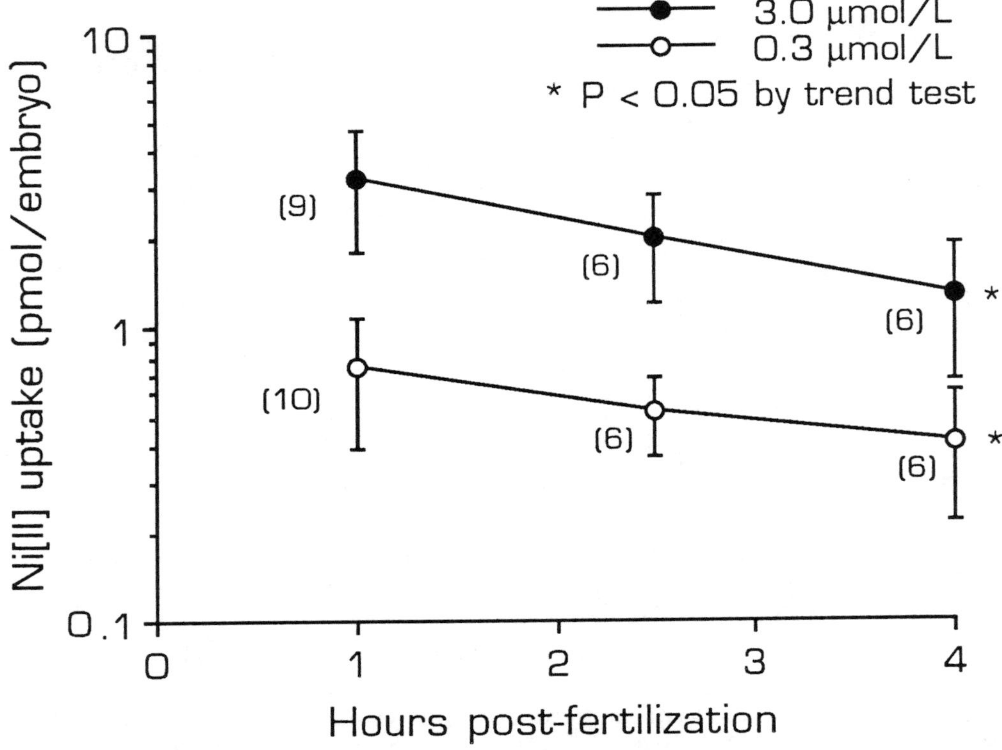

Figure 2. The uptake of ^{63}Ni in embryos exposed to $^{63}Ni^{2+}$ (3.0 µmol/L, •; or 0.3 µmol/L, o) for 0.5 h, beginning at the specified times post-fertilization. The numbers of *Xenopus* females whose embryos were tested at each interval are given in parentheses; the error bars denote ± 1 SD; * = $p < 0.05$ by trend test.[1]

enhanced neonatal mortality) and fetal malformations (*e.g.,* exencephaly, anophthalmia, cleft palate, skeletal anomalies, and cystic lungs). The *second step* in our research program was to determine whether or not Ni^{2+} causes such developmental toxicity in *Xenopus laevis.* This question was addressed by the FETAX (Frog Embryo Teratogenesis Assay; *Xenopus*) technique, which was developed by Dumont *et al.,*[5] standardized in Bantle's laboratory,[6-8] and validated as a screening test for teratogenic hazards from chemical agents.[9-12]

Our protocol for the FETAX assay has been described in detail,[13] and the assay results for Ni^{2+} have been reported by Hopfer *et al.*[14] In brief, groups of ~25 *Xenopus* embryos were incubated at 23°C for 4 days in FETAX media that contained graded concentrations of $NiCl_2$ (ranging from 0.1 µmol/L to 3 mmol/L); control groups were incubated in FETAX medium without added $NiCl_2$. The FETAX medium, an artificial pond water prepared from reagent-grade chemicals and distilled water, was replenished daily and was adjusted to pH 6.8, instead of the usual pH 7.8, in order to avoid precipitation of $Ni(OH)_2$. After exposure for 4 days (*i.e.* from 5 to 101 h post-fertilization, during which interval the embryos undergo cleavage, gastrulation, and organogenesis), the surviving embryos in each group were counted, fixed in formalin, and examined by microscopy to determine their developmental stages, malformations, and head-to-tail lengths.

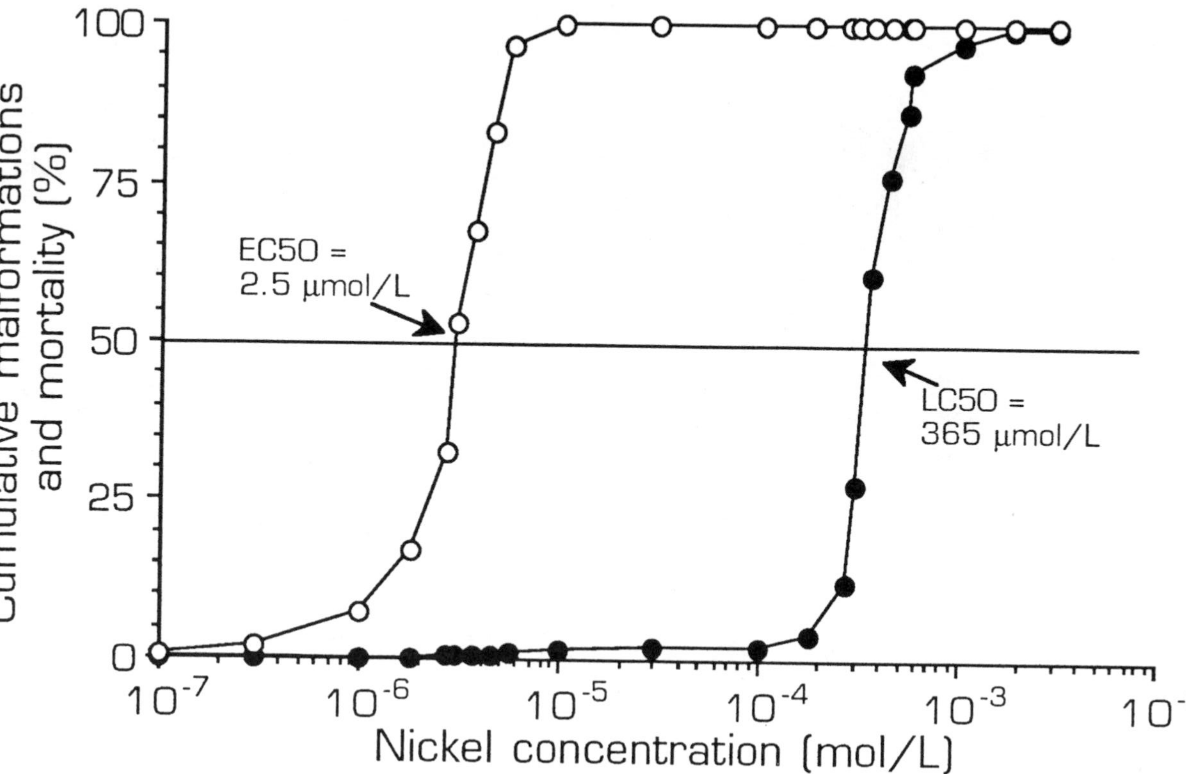

Figure 3. Cumulative incidence curves for malformations (o) and deaths (•) of *Xenopus* embryos exposed in the FETAX assay to 21 graded concentrations of Ni^{2+} during the period from 1 to 105 h post-fertilization.[14]

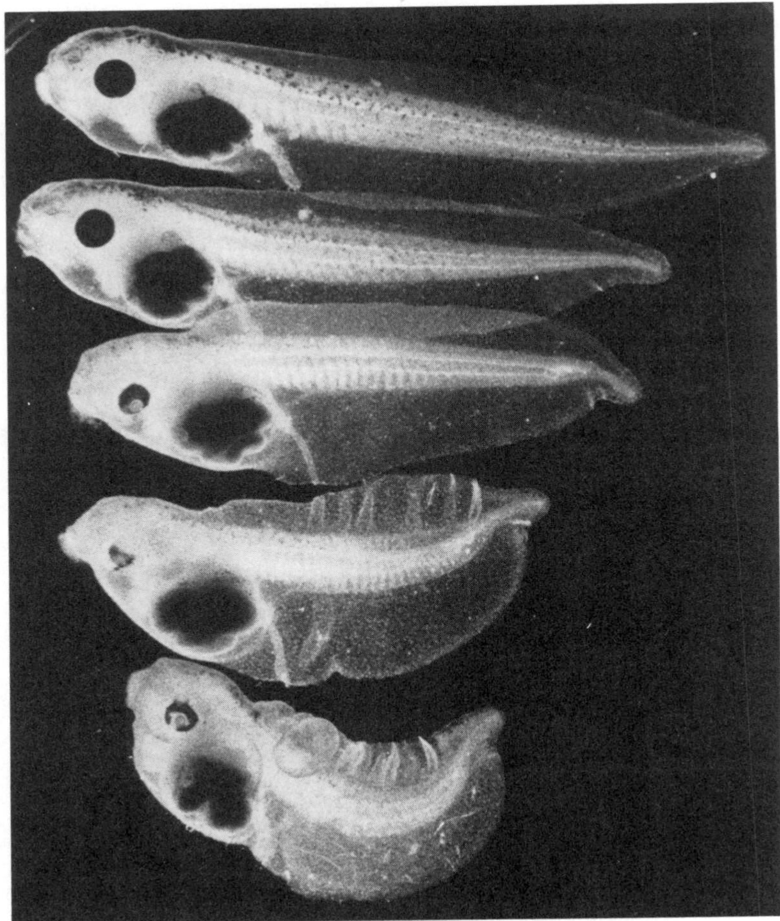

Figure 4. Photomicrograph of typical control and Ni^{2+}-exposed *Xenopus* tadpoles at 101 h post-fertilization, upon the completion of the FETAX assay. The tadpoles are viewed by dark-field illumination (unstained, 8x magnification). The tadpoles are stacked from top-to-bottom in order of increasing Ni^{2+} concentrations in the FETAX medium (*top:* control; *next-to-top:* 3 µmol/L; *middle:* 30 µmol/L; *next-to-bottom:* 100 µmol/L; *bottom:* 300 µmol/L). At 3 µmol/L, the tip of the tail is bent slightly downward, gut coiling is incomplete, pigmentation is diminished, and the dorsal fin extends higher than normal above the vertebrae. At 30 µmol/L, the tip of the tail is severely kinked downward, craniofacial anomalies are evident, gut coiling is impaired, the eyes are small and the lens is displaced, the dorsal and ventral fins extend broadly from the vertebrae, and pigmentation is diminished. At 100 µmol/L, stunted growth is obvious, anomalies of the head, face, and tail are marked, the eyes are small and mishapen, gut coiling is reduced, cardiomegaly is present, fin ruffling is prominent, and pigmentation is severely reduced. At 300 µmol/L, the embryo is extremely deformed and stunted, the tail bends upward, although the tip is kinked downward, midfacial hypoplasia is present with upward displacement of the nares, the eyes are malformed with open choroid fissure and scleral herniation, cardiomegaly and cardioptosis are noted, fin ruffling is severe, and dermal blisters or blebs are seen on the thorax and dorsal fin.[14]

The FETAX assay of Ni^{2+}, repeated seven times with similar results, showed that Ni^{2+} is a potent teratogen for *Xenopus,* inducing malformations of the eyes, skeleton, intestine, face, heart, and integument.[14] In control embryos, the survival at the end of the assay was consistently $\geq$ 95% and the incidence of malformations was $\leq 7\%$. In exposed embryos, the *Median Embryolethal Concentration* (LC_{50}) of Ni^{2+} was 365 (SE 9) μmol/L; the *Median Teratogenic Concentration* (EC_{50}) of Ni^{2+} was 2.5 (SE 0.1) μmol/L; and the *Teratogenic Index* (TI = LC_{50}/EC_{50}) was 147 (SE 5), which far exceeded the TI value of 1.5 that is considered the threshold level for positive teratogenicity in FETAX assays.[12] Exposure-response curves for malformations and mortality in Ni^{2+}-exposed embryos are shown in Figure 3. Control and Ni^{2+}-exposed embryos are illustrated in Figure 4.

Certain abnormalities, which were not classified as malformations, became more prominent with increasing Ni^{2+} concentrations, such as stunted growth, effusions or hemorrhages into coelomic cavities, and dermal hypopigmentation. The head-to-tail length of tadpoles was inversely correlated with the logarithm of the Ni^{2+} concentration ($r = 0.97$, $p < 0.001$, Figure 5). The *Minimum Concentration to Inhibit Growth* (MCIG) for Ni^{2+} in the FETAX assay was 5.6 μmol/L.[14]

In one experiment, four groups of *Xenopus* embryos were exposed to FETAX medium that contained Ni^{2+} (30 μmol/L) during specific 24 h periods post-fertilization; at other times, the embryos were kept in FETAX medium without added Ni^{2+}. When the assay ended at 101 h post-fertilization, the proportions of malformed embryos among the survivors in the respective groups were as follows: *Group A* (Ni^{2+}-exposure on day 1) = 32/123 (26%); *Group B* (Ni^{2+}-exposure on day 2) = 112/122 (92%); *Group C* (Ni^{2+}-exposure on day 3) = 117/117 (100%); and *Group D* (Ni^{2+}-exposure on day 4) = 24/117 (21%) ($p < 0.01$ by ANOVA). These results show that *Xenopus* embryos are most susceptible to Ni^{2+}-induced malformations on the second and third days of life, during the most active period of organogenesis. The pattern of malformations was affected by the timing of the Ni^{2+}-exposures, since facial, cardiac, and intestinal anomalies were more common in *Group C* than in *Group B* ($p < 0.05$), while ocular or skeletal anomalies were equally common in the two groups.[14]

IV. $^{63}Ni^{2+}$ Technique to Probe Western Blots for Ni^{2+}-Binding Proteins

The *third step* in our research program was to devise a sensitive technique to identify proteins that might be involved in the embryotoxic effects of Ni^{2+}. This project stemmed from our hypothesis that the Zn-finger domains of certain transcription factors, hormone receptors, oncogenes, and tumor-suppressor genes are potential molecular targets for metal ions.[15,16] Our hypothesis suggests that the substitution of foreign metal ions (*e.g.*, Ni^{2+}, Cd^{2+}) for Zn^{2+} in the finger-loop domains of such proteins could cause genotoxicity by affecting the conformation or stability of the DNA-binding structures. The foreign metal ions in finger-loop domains might generate oxygen free radicals close to specific gene loci, inducing DNA cleavage or DNA-protein cross-links. Furthermore, by substituting for Zn^{2+} in finger-loop domains of enzymes that repair DNA damage (e.g., poly(ADP-ribose)polymerase), the foreign metal ions might reduce the fidelity of DNA repair or produce sister chromatid exchanges. To pursue this avenue of investigation, a protein-blotting method was developed to detect $^{63}Ni^{2+}$-binding proteins in cell extracts.[17]

Aoki *et al.*[18,19] used $^{109}Cd^{2+}$ as a probe in a Western blotting procedure to detect metallothionein and other Cd^{2+}-binding proteins in tissue extracts. Schiff *et al.*[20,21] and Mazen *et al.*[22,23] employed such techniques to detect $^{65}Zn^{2+}$-binding

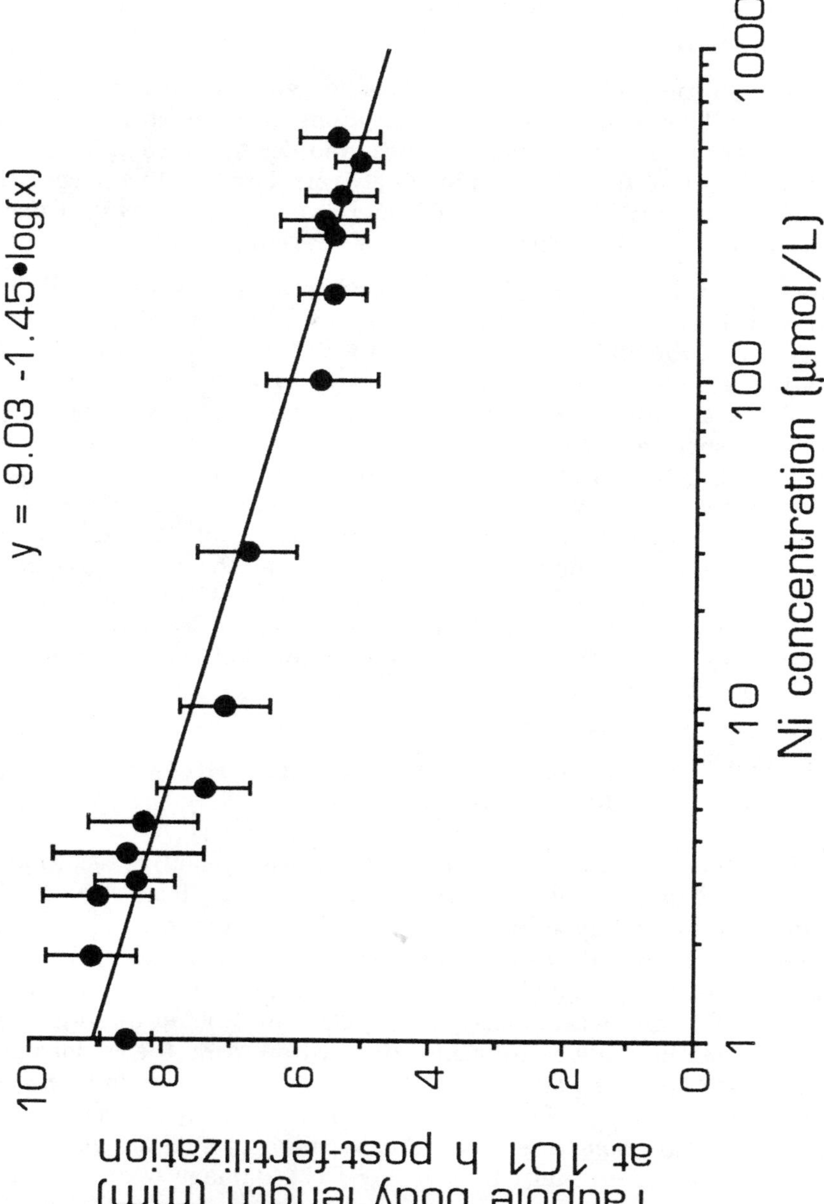

Figure 5. Head-to-tail lengths (mean ± SD) of *Xenopus* tadpoles exposed to Ni^{2+} in the **FETAX** assay. The least squares regression equation shows an inverse correlation of body length *vs.* the logarithm of the Ni^{2+} concentration ($r = 0.97$).[14]

to proteins with Zn-finger-like domains. An analogous procedure was devised in our laboratory to detect $^{63}Ni^{2+}$-binding proteins. The procedural details have been published.[17,24] Briefly, the procedure involves the following steps: (*a*) tissue extracts are boiled for 5 min in sample buffer that contains 10% glycerol, 1% sodium dodecylsulfate (SDS), and 5% 2-mercaptoethanol, prior to SDS-PAGE fractionation by the Laemmli procedure,[25] using slab gels that contain 9 to 12% polyacrylamide and 0.1% SDS; (*b*) the proteins are transferred to a nitrocellulose membrane by electroblotting according to Tobin *et al.*,[26] with addition of 0.015% SDS to the blotting buffer; (*c*) the membrane is rinsed in a buffer solution (pH 7.4, tris-HCl 100 mmol/L; NaCl, 50 mmol/L; $CaCl_2$, 5 mmol/L) to remove SDS and other contaminants from the electrophoresis and electroblotting steps; (*d*) the proteins are partially renatured by incubating the membrane at 25°C for 1 h in the same buffer, with added dithiothreitol (DTT, 0.5 mmol/L); (*e*) ^{63}Ni-binding proteins are labelled by incubating the membrane for 0.5 h in the same buffer, with freshly added $^{63}NiCl_2$ (5 µmol/L, 3.3 mCi/L), with DTT; (*f*) unbound $^{63}Ni^{2+}$ is removed by washing the membrane for 0.5 h in several rinses of the buffer, without DTT; (*g*) the membrane is dried overnight by pressing between blotting papers, (*h*) ^{63}Ni-binding proteins are visualized by autoradiography, using Eastman Kodak X-ray film and intensifying screens, with exposure at -70°C for 2 to 3 days; and (*i*) proteins on the membrane are stained with amido black.

The procedure for probing Western blots with $^{63}Ni^{2+}$ was optimized by experiments on jack bean urease, a nickel metalloprotein, carbonic anhydrase, a zinc metalloprotein, and rat kidney cytosol, which was previously shown to contain several ^{63}Ni-binding proteins.[27] To achieve optimal stringency and sensitivity, the following conditions were selected: (*a*) low radioprobe concentration (*i.e.*, 2 to 7 µmol ^{63}Ni/L), with high specific radioactivity (*e.g.*, 11 mCi ^{63}Ni/mg Ni); (*b*) tris-HCl buffer (100 mmol/L), within the pH range from 7.0 to 7.5, containing sufficient NaCl (50 to 100 mmol/L) and $CaCl_2$ or $MgCl_2$ (5 mmol/L) to prevent nonspecific binding of the radioprobe; and (*c*) incubation of the membrane in tris-HCl buffer that contains the salts plus a reducing agent (*i.e.*, DTT, 0.5 mmol/L) between the electroblotting and radioprobing steps.[17,24] Following the removal of SDS, the proteins undergo partial renaturation on the nitrocellulose membrane. Although the original three-dimensional protein structure is unlikely to be completely recovered, short polypeptide segments become sufficiently restored to permit metal binding to finger-loop domains and other high-affinity sites.[28]

V. $^{63}Ni^{2+}$-Binding to Zn-Finger Proteins in *Xenopus* Ovary Extracts

The structure and functions of Zn-finger proteins, a recently discovered class of DNA-binding proteins, have been reviewed in several recent articles.[15,16,29,30] The Zn-finger domains, usually 20 to 30 amino acids long, have pairs of cysteine or histidine residues, separated by 2 to 5 other amino acids, at each extremity. Tetrahedral coordination of Zn^{2+} to the thiol sulfur atoms of the cysteine residues and the imidazole nitrogen atoms of the histidine residues stabilizes the segment in a structure that fancifully resembles a finger. Site-specific binding of Zn-finger domains to double-stranded DNA is one of the mechanisms whereby proteins modulate gene expression. Transcription factor IIIA (TFIIIA) of *Xenopus* oocytes, the first Zn-finger protein to be identified and one of the most thoroughly studied of this class of regulatory proteins, contains a tandem array of 9 Zn-fingers.[31] The *fourth step* in this research program was to test our prediction that TFIIIA would be detected by probing Western blots of ovary extracts with $^{63}Ni^{2+}$ and other radiolabelled metal ions.

As summarized by Joho *et al.*,[32] previtellogenic oocytes in the ovaries of juvenile *Xenopus* females are laden with 7S ribonucleoprotein (RNP) particles that contain TFIIIA bound to ovary-specific 5S RNA in an equimolar ratio. The previtellogenic oocytes also contain abundant 42S RNP particles that represent a tetrameric assembly of subunits, each composed of ovary-specific 5S RNA, tRNA, and two major proteins (with approximate molecular weights of 43 and 48 kD) in molar ratio of 1:3:1:2. The p43 protein of the 42S RNP particles contains 9 putative Zn-finger domains. The 33% amino acid identity between TFIIIA and p43 consists mostly of the conserved amino acids that are characteristic of Zn-fingers. In addition to being a component of 7S RNP particles, TFIIIA promotes transcription of the 5S gene by binding specifically to the intragenic control region; Zn^{2+} is required for site-specific TFIIIA binding to both RNA and DNA. In contrast, p43 is solely a constituent of 42S RNP particles and evidently does not bind to the genes for 5S RNA or tRNA. The presence and possible role of Zn^{2+} in the putative finger-loop domains of p43 have not been established.[32]

Ovaries from juvenile *Xenopus* females were fractionated to obtain 7S and 42S RNP particles and to isolate TFIIIA. Proteins were probed with $^{63}Ni^{2+}$, $^{65}Zn^{2+}$ and $^{109}Cd^{2+}$ after separation by SDS-PAGE and blotting onto nitrocellulose membranes. The details and experimental results have been reported by Makowski *et al.*[24] Briefly, ovaries of juvenile *Xenopus* females were homogenized and centrifuged for 15 min at 16,500 x g at 4°C. The supernatant cytosol was fractionated by glycerol gradient centrifugation, according to Pelham and Brown.[33] The 7S RNP particles were harvested from the middle of the gradient and purified by DEAE-cellulose chromatography, according to Hanas *et al.*[34] The 42S RNP particles that sedimented in the pellet of the glycerol gradient were tested without further purification. In certain experiments, TFIIIA was isolated from 7S RNP particles by RNAase digestion and cleaved with CNBr. To probe Western blots with $^{65}Zn^{2+}$ and $^{109}Cd^{2+}$, the same technique was used as for $^{63}Ni^{2+}$, substituting $^{65}ZnCl_2$ (5 µmol/L, 0.5 mCi/L) or $^{109}CdCl_2$ (8 nmol/L, 125 µCi/L), and shortening the exposures to 1 to 2 days for ^{65}Zn, or 4 to 6 h for ^{109}Cd.

As shown in Figure 6, fractionations of *Xenopus* ovary cytosol by SDS-PAGE demonstrated three major protein bands with molecular weights of approximately 40, 43, and 48 kD (lane 4). The 40 kD protein was present in 7S RNP particles (lane 2) and the 43 and 48 kD proteins were present in 42S RNP particles, along with several minor proteins (lane 6). The 40 kD protein was identified as TFIIIA by immunoblotting with a specific anti-TFIIIA antibody, which reacted with TFIIIA at each step of its purification, but did not react with any other proteins in ovary extracts. Autoradiograms of Western blots probed with $^{63}Ni^{2+}$, $^{65}Zn^{2+}$, or $^{109}Cd^{2+}$ showed that the three radioligands bound strongly to TFIIIA and faintly to p43, wherever they were present (Figure 7).

Two proteins (68 kD and 74 kD) in ovary cytosol reacted with $^{63}Ni^{2+}$, but not with $^{65}Zn^{2+}$ or $^{109}Cd^{2+}$. These ^{63}Ni-binding proteins are isoforms of *Xenopus* albumin, as previously identified in homogenates of other *Xenopus* tissues.[17,35] When Western blots of purified TFIIIA and its CNBr-cleavage fragments were

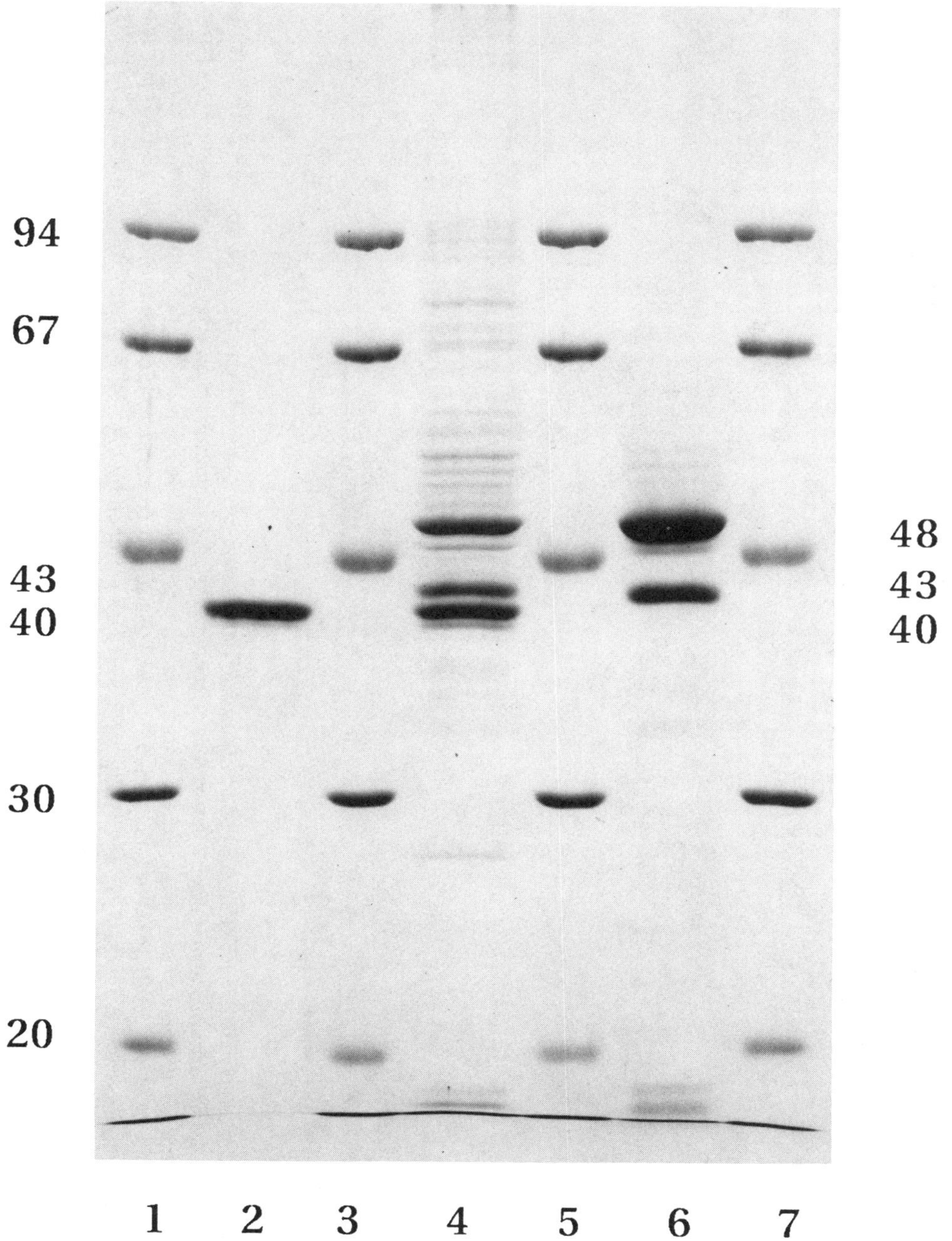

Figure 6. Comparison of proteins in *Xenopus* ovary cytosol and extracts of 7S and 42S RNP particles (SDS-PAGE, 10% gel, Coomassie blue stain). *Lanes 1, 3, 5 & 7:* mol. wt. markers (rabbit muscle phosphorylase B, 94 kD; bovine serum albumin, 67 kD; chicken ovalbumin, 43 kD; bovine RBC carbonic anhydrase, 30 kD; soybean trypsin inhibitor, 20 kD). *Lane 2:* 7S RNP particles obtained by DEAE-cellulose chromatography, showing a single 40 kD protein (TFIIIA). *Lane 4:* ovary cytosol, showing three major protein constituents (40, 43, & 48 kD). *Lane 6:* 42S RNP particles obtained by glycerol gradient centrifugation, showing two major protein constituents (43 & 48 kD).[24]

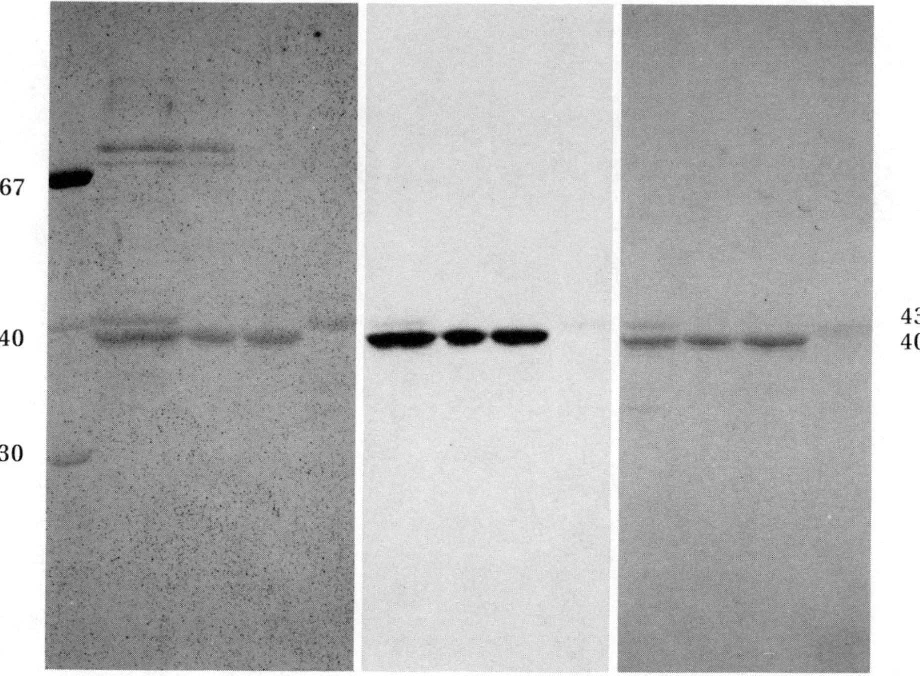

Figure 7. Binding of $^{63}Ni^{2+}$, $^{65}Zn^{2+}$ and $^{109}Cd^{2+}$ to TFIIIA and p43 in Western blots of ovary cytosol and extracts of 7S and 42S RNP particles (SDS-PAGE, 10% gel). *Left panel:* ^{63}Ni-autoradiogram after 3 day exposure; *center panel:* ^{65}Zn-autoradiogram after 2 day exposure; *right panel:* ^{109}Cd-autoradiogram after 4 h exposure. *Lane 1:* mol. wt. markers (same as Figure 6, plus horse liver alcohol dehydrogenase, 40 kD). *Lanes 2, 6, & 10:* ovary cytosol; *Lanes 3, 7, & 11:* 7S RNP particles obtained by glycerol gradient fractionation; *Lanes 4, 8, & 12:* 7S RNP particles purified by DEAE-cellulose chromatography; *Lanes 5, 9, & 13:* 42S RNP particles obtained by glycerol gradient fractionation. The $^{63}Ni^{2+}$ visualizes bovine albumin (67 kD), alcohol dehydrogenase (40 kD), and carbonic anhydrase (30 kD) in *Lane 1, Xenopus* isoalbumins (74 & 68 kD) in *Lanes 2 & 3,* TFIIIA in *Lanes 2, 3, & 4,* and p43 in *Lanes 2 & 5.* The $^{65}Zn^{2+}$ visualizes TFIIIA intensely in *Lanes 6, 7, & 8* and p43 weakly in *Lanes 6 & 9.* The $^{109}Cd^{2+}$ visualizes TFIIIA clearly in *Lanes 10, 11, & 12* and p43 weakly in *Lanes 10 & 13.*[24]

probed with $^{65}Zn^{2+}$, $^{63}Ni^{2+}$, or $^{109}Cd^{2+}$, the radioligands bound to the parent TFIIIA, the 22 kD middle fragment, and the 11 kD fragment (N-terminus), which all contain finger-loop domains, but *not* to the 13 kD fragment (C-terminus), which lacks finger-loop domains.[24] These observations suggest that the radioligands became bound to the finger-loop domains of TFIIIA.

VI. $^{63}Ni^{2+}$-Binding to Proteins in *Xenopus* Oocytes and Embryos

The blotting assay was used to prepare a developmental profile of ^{63}Ni-binding proteins in individual *Xenopus* eggs and embryos during early cleavage stages (Figure 8). The experiment has been reported by Lin *et al.*[17] The samples included an unfertilized egg, a fertilized egg, and embryos at the 2-cell, 4-cell, and 8-cell stages of development. The major ^{63}Ni-binding band in all samples was a 31 kD protein; faint ^{63}Ni-binding proteins of 40 and 43 kD were also detected in all samples. This experiment demonstrated the feasibility of probing for ^{63}Ni-binding proteins on Western blots of single *Xenopus* embryos. The 31 kD protein in *Xenopus* eggs and embryos, which binds ^{63}Ni avidly during early cleavage stages, is developmentally regulated, for it becomes much less prominent by the fourth day post-fertilization. Currently, a major focus of this research program is the isolation, characterization, and identification of the 31 kD ^{63}Ni-binding protein, which may play an important role in the uptake and embryotoxicity of Ni^{2+} in *Xenopus*.

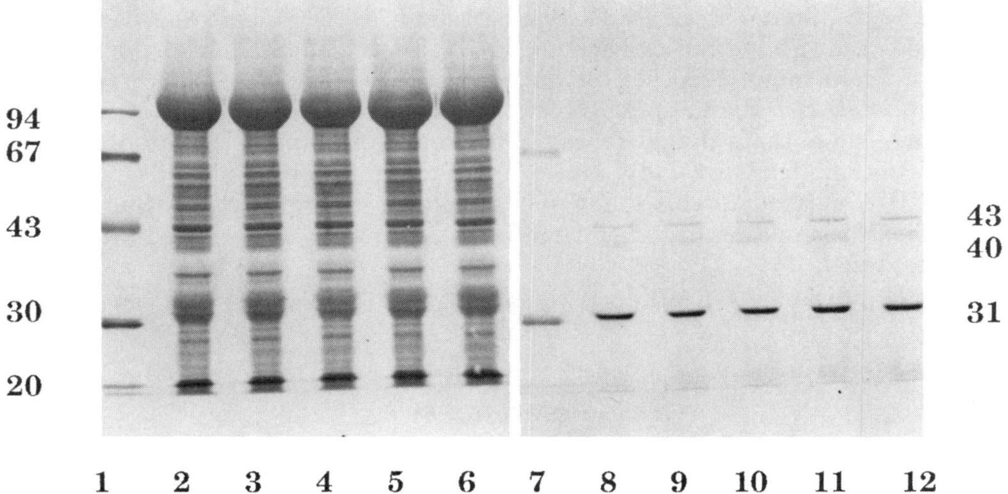

Figure 8. Blotting assay for $^{63}Ni^{2+}$-binding proteins in single *Xenopus* eggs and embryos. The left half shows the nitrocellulose membrane stained for proteins with amido black; the right half shows the ^{63}Ni-autoradiogram of the same membrane after 2 day exposure. *Lanes 1 & 7:* mol. wt. markers (see Figure 6); *Lanes 2 & 8:* unfertilized egg; *Lanes 3 & 9:* 1-cell embryo (fertilized egg); *Lanes 4 & 10:* 2-cell embryo (1.5 h post-fertilization); *Lanes 5 & 11:* 4-cell embryo (2 h); *Lanes 6 & 12:* 8-cell embryo (2.5 h). The major ^{63}Ni-binding band in all of the samples is a 31 kD protein; ^{63}Ni-binding to proteins of 40 and 43 kD is faintly visible in all samples.[17]

VII. Summary

New experimental models and analytical techniques have been developed in order to study the molecular mechanisms of Ni^{2+}-induced genotoxicity and teratogenicity. *Xenopus laevis* embryos were found to be readily permeable to $^{63}Ni^{2+}$ during early cleavage stages, providing a suitable species for investigations of Ni^{2+} uptake and embryotoxicity. Assays by the FETAX (Frog Embryo Teratogenesis Assay: *Xenopus)* procedure showed that Ni^{2+} is a potent teratogen for *Xenopus,* inducing malformations of the eyes, skeleton, intestine, face, heart, and integument. *Xenopus* embryos were shown to be most susceptible to the teratogenic effects of Ni^{2+} on the second and third days post-fertilization, during the most active period of organogenesis. A novel technique was devised to detect Ni-binding proteins, using $^{63}Ni^{2+}$ to probe Western blots. The usefulness of the technique was demonstrated by its ability to detect two Zn-finger proteins, TFIIIA (a constituent of 7S RNP particles) and p43 (a constituent of 42S RNP particles) in ovary extracts of juvenile *Xenopus* females. Proteins from individual *Xenopus* eggs and embryos were probed by the $^{63}Ni^{2+}$-blotting technique, revealing an intensely labelled Ni-binding protein (31 kD), which may be involved in the uptake and embryotoxicity of Ni^{2+} in *Xenopus.* Experiments are underway to isolate, characterize, and identify the 31 kD protein.

Acknowledgements

The authors are grateful for valuable advice and assistance from John A. Bantle, Ph.D., Bonnie Beck, Ph.D., Sean Brennan, Ph.D., Robert A. Finch, Ph.D., Shan-Mei Lin, Ph.D., Shozo Nomoto, Ph.D., Henry M. Smilowicz, Ph.D., and Kevin R. Sweeney, Ph.D. The authors acknowledge the expert technical assistance of Mr. Frank J. Mongillo, Ms. Jennifer Martin, and Ms. Odette Zaharia. The authors thank Robert G. Roeder, Ph.D., and Elizabeth Morefield, Ph.D., (Rockefeller University, New York) for the generous gift of monoclonal anti-TFIIIA antibody. This study was supported by grants to Dr. Sunderman from the National Institutes of Health, the March of Dimes, and Northeast Utilities, Inc.

References

1. Sunderman, F.W., Jr., Mongillo, F.J., Plowman, M.C., and Brennan, S.M., Uptake and release of $^{63}Ni^{2+}$ by *Xenopus* embryos during early cleavage stages, *Biol. Metals*, 2, 214, 1990.

2. Sunderman, F.W., Jr., Reid, M.C., Shen, S.K., and Kevorkian, C.B., Embryotoxicity and teratogenicity of nickel compounds, in *Reproductive and Developmental Toxicity of Metals*, Clarkson, T.W., Nordberg, G.F., and Sager, P.R., Eds., Plenum Press, New York, 1983, 399.

3. Mas, A., Holt, D., and Webb, M., The acute toxicity and teratogenicity of nickel in pregnant rats, *Toxicology*, 35, 47, 1985.

4. Leonard, A. and Jacquet, P., Embryotoxicity and genotoxicity of nickel, in *Nickel in the Human Environment*, Sunderman, F.W., Jr., Ed.-in-Chief, Oxford Univ. Press, Oxford, 1984, 277.

5. Dumont, J.N., Schultz, T.W., Buchanan, M., and Kao, G., Frog embryo teratogenesis assay-*Xenopus* (FETAX). A short-term assay applicable to complex environmental mixtures, in *Symposium on the Application of Short-term Bioassays in the Analysis of Complex Environmental Mixtures III*, Waters, M.D., Sandhu, S.S., Lewtas, J., Claxon, L., Chernoff, N., and Nesnow, S., Eds., Plenum Press, New York, 1983, 393.

6. Dawson, D.A. and Bantle, J.A., Development of a reconstituted water medium and preliminary validation of the frog embryo teratogenesis assay: *Xenopus* (FETAX), *J. Appl. Toxicol.*, 7, 237, 1987.

7. Fort, D.J., Dawson, D.A., and Bantle, J.A., Development of a metabolic activation system for the frog embryo teratogenesis assay: *Xenopus* (FETAX), *Teratogen. Carcinogen. Mutagen.*, 8, 251, 1988.

8. Fort, D.J. and Bantle, J.A., Use of frog embryo teratogenesis assay-*Xenopus* and an exogenous metabolic activation system to evaluate the developmental toxicity of diphenylhydantoin, *Fund. Appl. Toxicol.*, 14, 720, 1990.

9. Sabourin, T.D., Faulk, R.T., and Goss, L.B., The efficacy of three non-mammalian test systems in the identification of chemical teratogens, *J. Appl. Toxicol.*, 5, 225, 1985.

10. Dawson, D.A., Stebler, E.F., Burks, S.L., and Bantle, J.A., Evaluation of the developmental toxicity of metal-contaminated sediments using short-term fathead minnow and frog embryo-larval assays, *Environ. Toxicol. Chem.*, 7, 27, 1988.

11. Dawson, D.A., Fort, D.J., Smith, G.J., Newell, D.L., and Bantle, J.A., Evaluation of the developmental toxicity of nicotine and cotinine with frog embryo teratogenesis assay: *Xenopus*, *Teratogen. Carcinogen. Mutagen.*, 8, 329, 1988.

12. Dawson, D.A., Fort, D.J., Newell, D.L., and Bantle, J.A., Developmental toxicity testing with FETAX: evaluation of 5 compounds, *Drug Chem. Toxicol.*, 12, 67, 1989.

13. Hopfer, S.M., Plowman, M.C., and Sunderman, F.W., Jr., The FETAX test for teratogenicity of chemicals and environmental samples, in *Manual on Laboratory Diagnosis of Diseases of the Fetus, Neonate, and Childhood*, Sunderman, F.W., Ed., Institute for Clinical Science, Philadelphia, in press.

14. Hopfer, S.M., Plowman, M.C., Sweeney, K.R., Bantle, J.A., and Sunderman, F.W., Jr., Teratogenicity of Ni^{2+} in *Xenopus laevis*, assayed by the FETAX procedure, *Biol. Trace Elem. Res.*, in press.

15. Sunderman, F.W., Jr., Finger-loop domains and trace metals, in *Trace Elements in Clinical Medicine*, Tomita, H., Ed., Springer-Verlag, Tokyo, 1990, 291.

16. Sunderman, F.W., Jr., Regulation of gene expression by metals: Zinc finger-loop domains in transcription factors, hormone receptors, and proteins encoded by oncogenes, in *Metal Ions in Biology and Medicine*, Collery, P., Poirier, P.A., Manfait, M., and Etienne, J.C., Eds., John Libbey Eurotext, Paris, 1990, 549.

17. Lin, S.-M., Hopfer, S.M., Brennan, S.M., and Sunderman, F.W., Jr., Protein blotting method for detection of nickel-binding proteins, *Res. Commun. Chem. Pathol. Pharmacol.*, 65, 275, 1989.

18. Aoki, A., Kunimoto, M., Shibata, Y., and Suzuki, K.T., Detection of metallothionein on nitrocellulose membrane using Western blotting technique and its application to identification of cadmium-binding proteins, *Anal. Biochem.*, 157, 117, 1986.

19. Aoki, A. and Suzuki, K.T., Characterization of cadmium-binding proteins detected in rat liver by the Western blotting technique, *J. Biochem. Toxicol.*, 2, 67, 1977.

20. Schiff, L.A., Nibert, M.L., Co, M.S., Brown, E.G., and Fields, B.N., Distinct binding sites for zinc and double-stranded RNA in the reovirus outer capsid protein σ3, *Mol. Cell Biol.*, 8, 273, 1988.

21. Schiff, L.A., Nibert, M.L., and Fields, B.N., Characterization of a zinc blotting technique: Evidence that a retroviral gag protein binds zinc, *Proc. Natl. Acad. Sci. USA*, 85, 4195, 1988.

22. Mazen, A., Gradwohl, G., and de Murcia, G., Zinc-binding proteins detected by protein blotting, *Anal. Biochem.*, 172, 39, 1988.

23. Mazen, A., Menissier-de-Murcia, J., Molinete, M., Simonin, F., Gradwohl, G., Poirier, G., and de Murcia, G., Poly(ADP-ribose)polymerase: A novel finger protein, *Nucl. Acids Res.*, 17, 4689, 1989.

24. Makowski, G.S., Lin, S.M., Brennan, S.M., Smilowicz, H.M., Hopfer, S.M., and Sunderman, F.W., Jr., Detection of two Zn-finger proteins of *Xenopus laevis*, TFIIIA and p43, by probing Western blots of ovary cytosol with $^{65}Zn^{2+}$, $^{63}Ni^{2+}$, or $^{109}Cd^{2+}$, *Biol. Trace Elem. Res.*, in press.

25. Laemmli, U.K., Cleavage of structural proteins during the assembly of the head of bacteriophage T_4, *Nature*, 227, 680, 1970.

26. Towbin, H., Staehelin, T., and Gordon, J., Electrophoretic transfer of proteins from polyacrylamide gels to nitrocellulose sheets: Procedure and some applications, *Proc. Nat. Acad. Sci. USA*, 76, 4350, 1979.

27. Sunderman, F.W., Jr., Mangold, B.L., Wong, S.H.-Y., Reid, M.C., and Jansson, I., High-performance size-exclusion chromatography of ^{63}Ni-constituents in renal cytosol and microsomes from $^{63}NiCl_2$-treated rats, *Res. Commun. Chem. Pathol. Pharmacol.*, 39, 477, 1983.

28. Maruyama, K., MIkawa, T., and Ebashi, S., Detection of calcium binding proteins by ^{45}Ca autoradiography on nitrocellulose membrane after sodium dodecyl sulfate gel electrophoresis, *J. Biochem.*, 95, 511, 1984.

29. Berg, J.M., Zinc fingers and other metal binding domains: Elements for interactions between molecules, *J. Biol. Chem.*, 265, 6513, 1990.

30. Berg, J.M., Zinc finger domains: hypotheses and current knowledge, *Annu. Rev. Biophys. Chem.*, 19, 405, 1990.

31. Miller, J., McLachlan, A.D., and Klug, A., Repetitive zinc-binding domains in the protein transcription factor IIIA from *Xenopus* oocytes, *EMBO J.*, 4, 1609, 1985.

32. Joho, K.E., Darby, M.K., Crawford, E.T., and Brown, D.D., A finger protein structurally similar to TFIIIA that binds exclusively to 5S RNA in *Xenopus*, *Cell*, 61, 293, 1990.

33. Pelham, H.R.P., and Brown, D.D., A specific transcription factor that can bind either the 5S RNA gene or 5S RNA, *Proc. Natl. Acad. Sci. USA*, 77, 4170, 1980.

34. Hanas, J.S., Bogenhagen, D.F., and Wu, C.W., Cooperative model for the binding of *Xenopus* transcription factor A to the 5S RNA gene, *Proc. Natl. Acad. Sci. USA*, 80, 2142, 1983.

35. Graf, J.D. and Fischberg, M., Albumin evolution in polyploid species of the genus *Xenopus*, *Biochem. Genet.*, 24, 821, 1986.

Chapter 8

Rationale and Possible Mechanisms by Which Selenium Inhibits Mammary Cancer

John A. Milner

Table of Contents

I. Introduction

Considerable data point to the anticarcinogenic properties of selenium. Epidemiological studies show that higher selenium intake is associated with a reduction in tumors at various sites, including mammary tissue. Numerous studies also document the ability of dietary selenium to reduce the incidence and total number of tumors induced by a variety of carcinogens. Relatively high, but non-toxic, quantities of selenium are generally required to inhibit chemically induced tumors. The ability of selenium to alter the metabolism of some carcinogens, including the mammary carcinogen, 7,12-dimethylbenz(a)anthracene (DMBA), indicates that this trace element can be effective in inhibiting the initiation phase of carcinogenesis. Alterations in DMBA-DNA adducts resulting from dietary selenium supplementation were found to correlate with final tumor incidence and tumor number. Although the mechanism is unknown, several lines of evidence also point to the ability of selenium to effectively inhibit the promotion phase of carcinogenesis. Selenium supplements are also effective in depressing the incidence of virally induced mammary tumors. Likewise, clinical and laboratory studies reveal that selenium can inhibit the growth of some neoplastic cells, both *in vivo* and *in vitro*. The efficacy by which selenium inhibits chemically-induced, virally-induced and transplantable tumors makes it a unique dietary nutrient. Overall, considerable epidemiological and laboratory investigations support selenium as an effective anticarcinogenic agent.

II. Historical Background

Selenium is a trace element with an extremely provocative and controversial history. By the 1930's our knowledge of selenium was limited primarily to awareness about its toxicity.[1] In addition to concerns about its toxicity, safety controversies were sparked when Nelson *et al.*[2] reported that consumption of selenium led to an increased frequency of liver cell adenomas or low grade carcinomas in rats. While these data have been largely dismissed, the image of selenium as a highly toxic and possibly carcinogenic trace element remains even today.

Fortunately, by the late 50's and 60's increasing evidence was beginning to identify selenium as an essential nutrient in intermediary metabolism.[3-5] Evidence gradually accumulated that revealed that dietary selenium was effective in preventing an assortment of disorders including exudative diathesis in chicks, hepatosis dietetica in swine, unthriftness in cattle and white muscle disease in ruminants.[5] A metabolic function of this trace element was to remain elusive until the 70's; when it was shown to be an integral component of glutathione peroxidase, an enzyme involved in the catabolism of hydrogen and organic peroxides.[6,7] Most recently, prolonged inadequate intake of selenium in human beings has been reported to result in pain and tenderness in skeletal muscles and cardiac myopathy.[8-10] Although selenium is recognized as a component of several proteins in biological fluids and cells,[11-15] to date its requirement for glutathione peroxidase activity remains its only known biological function in mammals.

Although selenium has been proposed as an effective chemotherapeutic agent for almost 75 years,[16] it was not until 1949 when Clayton and Baumann[17] provided evidence that supplemental selenium protected rats from chemically induced carcinogenesis. Since that time substantial epidemiological and laboratory evidence have illustrated an inverse relationship between dietary selenium intake and cancer risk.

III. Human Findings

The geochemical environment in which food is produced can markedly influence the dietary selenium intake. Various indices of selenium status are known to correlate with the selenium content of locally grown plant crops. Shamberger and Frost[18] were among the first to report an inverse relationship between cancer mortality and selenium content of forage plants. Generally, epidemiological investigations have revealed an enhanced cancer mortality in geographic regions where the selenium content of the soil is low or deficient, compared to regions containing higher quantities of this trace element.[18-22] Age-corrected mortalities from cancer at 17 major sites in 27 countries correlated inversely with apparent dietary selenium intake.[20] Significant inverse correlations of cancer mortality of the breast, ovary, lung and leukemia with selenium intake have been observed. A similar inverse relationship between cancer at these sites and blood selenium concentrations of apparently healthy subjects located in the same geographic region were also detected.[21] The geographic occurrence of liver cancer in China is reported to relate inversely with the selenium content of locally available foods and the inhabitant's blood selenium concentration.[22] Thus, considerable epidemiological evidence points to an association of higher selenium intake with a reduction in cancer risk. This evidence does not imply that glutathione peroxidase activity is suboptimum or that selenium deficiency *per se* is a primary cause of increased cancer risk. Epidemiological studies implicate several identified, and possibly several unidentified, dietary factors which modify the risk of developing cancer. Selenium is one of relatively few dietary constituents that may, when consumed in greater quantities, significantly reduce cancer risk.

Several case-control studies have examined the hypothesis that lower selenium intakes and associated blood concentrations enhance cancer risk. Problems of generalized inadequate nutrient intake and secondary complications associated with the presence of cancer make the interpretation of some of these data difficult. However, more recent publications[23-27] have designed case-control studies that have largely avoided problems with confounding dietary inadequacy and thus are useful in examining the possible role of selenium as a modifier of cancer risk. Clark *et al.*[23] reported that low plasma selenium was associated with significant increases in the risk of nonmelanomous skin cancer. Likewise, a prospective case-control study by Salonen *et al.*[26] indicated low serum selenium concentrations were associated with increased cancer mortality. Willett *et al.*[27] detected a relative risk of 2.0 for cancer in subjects in the lowest versus highest quintiles of serum selenium concentration (<115 *vs.* 154 μg/ml). While these studies suggest an inverse relationship between selenium status and cancer risk, not all case-controlled studies have detected a relationship. Menkes *et al.*[25] did not detect a significant relationship of selenium status as a risk factor for lung cancer. Likewise, Peleg *et al.*[24] found that serum selenium did not differ from controls in a retrospective case-control study of 130 cancer cases matched for age, gender and race. The lack of consensus among these case-control studies implies that selenium is not a universal magic bullet against cancer. However, these data may also indicate that selenium may under certain circumstances, serve as a modifier of the risk of developing some types of cancers.

The selenium status of an individual may also influence the biological behavior of some neoplastic cells. In 1975, Broghamer *et al.*[28] reported that elevated blood selenium levels in cancer patients were associated with fewer recurrences, tumors that remained more localized and with a reduction in the number of metastases. These data suggest that selenium may modify the promotion and progression phases of carcinogenesis. However, in a subsequent retrospective study of patients with reticuloendothelial tumors no relationship between the aggressiveness of the tumor and selenium status was detected.[29] It remains unclear if selenium can modify the biological behavior of established tumors. However, the limited information available may simply indicate that all tumors are not equally affected by supplemental selenium. As discussed below the growth of some transplantable tumors, but not all, can be inhibited by supplemental selenium.

IV. Chemical Carcinogenesis

A variety of studies have established that dietary selenium supplementation can significantly inhibit the incidence of chemically induced tumors in animals (Table 1).[29-48] Chemically induced tumors in skin, liver, colon, pancreas and mammary tissue have been shown to be inhibited by dietary selenium supplementation. A reduction in the incidence and/or total tumor number in animals treated with diverse carcinogens including: 3′-methyl-4-dimethylaminoazobenzene, 7,12-dimethylbenz(a)anthracene (DMBA), benzo(a)pyrene, 2-acetylaminofluorene, 1,2-dimethylhydrazine (DMH), methylazoxymethanol acetate (MAM), aflatoxin B_1, methylbenzylnitrosamine and methylnitrosourea (MNU) have been shown to be inhibited by selenium supplementation. The ability of selenium to inhibit tumor formation resulting from such a wide variety of carcinogens and occurring in such a variety of tissues indicates a general mechanism rather than a tissue specific reaction.

A. Quantity and Form of Selenium

The quantity of selenium necessary to inhibit chemical carcinogenesis has varied from 0.5 to 6.0 µg/g of diet (Table 1). These quantities are considerably greater than the 0.05 to 0.1 µg/g of diet typically needed to optimize glutathione peroxidase activity. The need for relatively high, but not toxic, quantities of selenium to inhibit chemically induced cancer argues against an involvement of glutathione peroxidase. Both water and dietary supplements have been employed to examine the anticarcinogenic properties of selenium. Both routes of administration of selenium are generally effective in inhibiting tumors. However, the efficacy of selenium is known to depend upon the quantity of carcinogen administered, the quantity and form of selenium provided, as well as the content of other dietary constituents that are provided.

TABLE 1
Influence of Selenium on Chemically Induced Cancer

Selenium µg/g or ml	Tumor site	Carcinogen	Species	Reduction % controls	Reference
0.5	Breast	DMBA	Rat	8	30
1.0	Breast	DMBA	Rat	38	31
1.5	Breast	DMBA	Rat	21	30
2.0	Breast	DMBA	Mouse	48	32
2.5	Breast	DMBA	Rat	52	30
4.0	Breast	DMBA	Rat	52	33
6.0	Breast	DMBA	Mouse	62	34
2.5	Breast	AAF	Rat	31	35
4.0	Colon	DMH	Rat	54	36
2.0	Colon	AZM	Rat	15	37
2.0	Colon	AZM	Rat	7	38
4.0	Colon	AZM	Rat	42	36
1.0	Colon	BNA	Rat	45	39
1.0	Lung	BNA	Rat	100	39
2.0	Liver	DMAB	Rat	63	40
5.0	Liver	DMAB	Rat	50	41
2.5	Liver	AAF	Rat	59	35
4.0	Liver	AAF	Rat	50	42
1.0	Liver	AFB	Rat	80	43
1.0	Skin	DMBA	Mouse	38	44
1.0	Skin	BP	Mouse	45	44
5.0	Trachea	MNU	Hamster	-23	45
2.0	Sarcoma	BP	Mouse	65	47

Abbreviations used are DMBA = 7,12-dimethylbenz(a)anthracene; AAF = 2-acetylaminofluorene; DMH = 1,2-dimethylhydrazine; AZM = azoxymethanol; BNA = bis(2-oxopropyl)nitrosamine; DMAB = 3′-methyl-4-dimethylaminoazobenzene; AFB = aflatoxin B; and MNU = 1-methyl-1-nitrosourea.

The anticarcinogenic action of selenium does not appear to be mediated by its antioxidant function as a component of glutathione peroxidase. As indicated previously, quantities of selenium needed to inhibit chemically induced tumors generally exceed the requirement to optimize the activity of this enzyme. Conditions which increase free radical formation would be expected to increase the effectiveness of selenium if glutathione peroxidase were involved in the observed chemotherapeutic protection offered by this trace element. Ip[49] and Horvath and Ip[50] have examined the ability of vitamin E with or without selenium supplementation to modify the carcinogenicity of DMBA. In these studies, providing supplemental selenite above that found in the basal diet did not alter the activity of glutathione peroxidase in either liver or the mammary fat pad. Selenium supplementation at 2.5 µg/g was also ineffective in reducing the marked increase in lipid peroxidation resulting from dietary vitamin E deficiency. Although supplemental vitamin E was effective in preventing tissue peroxidation, it, unlike selenite, was ineffective in inhibiting DMBA induced tumor formation. Thus, these data provide strong evidence that the protective effects of selenium are not mediated through alterations in glutathione peroxidase or free radical metabolism. Nevertheless, providing adequate quantities of vitamin E may reduce the need for selenium to accommodate the challenges associated with oxidative stress and thereby facilitate selenium's anticarcinogenic properties.

Several forms of selenium are commercially available and have been used with varying efficacy in maintaining blood selenium and glutathione peroxidase activity. The ability of selenomethionine or other organic selenium compounds present in foods to inhibit the cancer process have not been extensively examined. Nevertheless, based upon the limited published data, seleno-amino acids appear to be less effective in inhibiting both the initiation and promotion phases of carcinogenesis than selenite supplements. Selenomethionine was found to be less effective in inhibiting the binding of DMBA to rat mammary cell DNA than was an equivalent quantity of selenite.[51] Likewise, selenite supplementation was more effective than selenomethionine in inhibiting the promotion phase of DMBA carcinogenesis.[48] Similarly, selenomethionine and selenocysteine have been found to be less effective in inhibiting the growth of tumor cells both *in vivo* and *in vitro* than equivalent quantities of selenium as sodium selenite.[52,53] It should be noted that the seleno-amino acids are generally effective in inhibiting tumor formation and development if provided in sufficient quantities. Since these selenocompounds are generally less toxic than some other forms of selenium their physiological significance should not be minimized. The reason for the reduced efficacy of selenomethionine possibly relates to the inability of methionine tRNA to discriminate the presence of selenium. Thus, a generalized incorporation of selenomethionine into cellular proteins likely reduces the effective concentration of selenium available to exert its anticarcinogenic property.

B. Selenium Deficiency and Chemical Carcinogenesis

Relatively few studies have examined the influence of selenium deficiency *per se* on the induction of chemically induced tumors. In those published reports the influence of selenium deficiency is inconclusive. Several studies have been unable to detect any alteration in tumor formation. The most extensively examined impact of selenium deficiency on chemical carcinogenesis has been with mammary tumor formation following treatment with 7,12-dimethylbenz(a)-anthracene.[31,46,49] Ip[31,49] provided strong evidence that the ability of selenium deficiency to increase the risk of tumor formation was dependent upon dietary lipid intake. These data suggest that selenium deficiency may alter the promotion phase of carcinogenesis. Unfortunately the impact of selenium deficiency on tumor induction with other carcinogen models has not been as well examined. Far too frequently, data relevant to this issue are not included in manuscripts or appropriate statistical evaluation of the data are not offered. Thus, the true impact of dietary selenium deficiency on chemically induced tumors must await further examination. If there is an influence of selenium deficiency on chemically induced tumors, it may well be on the promotion phase of carcinogenesis and therefore is likely influenced by other dietary constituents.

V. Selenium and the Initiation Phase of Carcinogenesis

The majority of studies examining selenium as an anticarcinogenic agent has used supplements throughout the experimental feeding period. Nevertheless, evidence for the ability of selenium to inhibit the initiation phase of carcinogenesis comes from several sources. The reduced ability of selenium to inhibit the incidence of cancer in animals treated with direct acting carcinogens compared to agents requiring metabolic activation provide some of the best evidence for an alteration in the initiation phase of carcinogenesis.[33,36]

Thompson *et al.*,[48] Ip[54] and Liu *et al.*[55] have provided evidence that dietary selenium supplementation can inhibit the initiation phase of DMBA carcinogenesis. Investigations by Liu *et al.*[55] showed that providing supplemental dietary selenium at 0.5 to 4.0 µg/g from two weeks prior to and two weeks following DMBA treatment led to a marked delay in the onset of mammary tumors and significantly reduced both tumor incidence and total tumor number compared to animals fed diets containing 0.1 µg Se/g (Figures 1 and 2). Comparison of rats fed supplemental selenium during the initiation and promotion phases revealed that much of the antitumorigenic effect of selenium could be attributed to changes in initiation.[55] The pronounced effect of selenite on the initiation phase of carcinogenesis in the studies of Liu *et al.*[55] likely were influenced by the low quantity of carcinogen administered. The percentage inhibition attributed to the initiation phase would be expected to decrease as the dose of DMBA is increased. Ip[54] has shown that the anticarcinogenic efficacy of selenium is diminished as the dose of the carcinogen is increased.

Considerable evidence points to the ability of selenium to alter the activation of procarcinogens.[51,55-60] Rasco *et al.*[57] provided evidence that selenium impedes activation and accelerates the detoxification of chemical carcinogens. Likewise, studies by Harbach and Swenberg[58] reported that addition of selenium to the drinking water of rats decreased hepatic DMH metabolism, as indicated by depressed expiration of azoxymethane. Studies in our laboratory show that dietary selenium supplementation can modify the metabolism of DMBA.[51,55,56,59] These studies reveal that selenium reduces those intermediates considered the most carcinogenic and mutagenic. Specifically, selenium inhibits the binding of DMBA to DNA and shifts the types of adducts that bind in both cultures of mouse embyro and mammary cells.[51,59] Concentrations of 0.5 µg Se/ml or more was effective in reducing the binding of DMBA to DNA. The reduction in binding was primarily due to a reduction in the occurrence of *anti* dihydrodiol epoxide adducts. The form of selenium added to the medium also influenced the percentage depression in DMBA-DNA binding. Selenodiglutathione and selenite were more effective in decreasing binding that selenomethionine or selenide. In subsequent studies, our laboratory has shown that mammary cells isolated from rats fed selenite at 2.0 µg/g have a reduced ability to activate DMBA to metabolites capable of binding to DMBA compared to rats fed diets containing 0.1 µg/g.[59] Approximately 7 days of feeding was necessary to significantly reduce the ability of mammary cells to metabolize DMBA to compounds capable of binding to DNA. Thus, dietary selenium can significantly influence the ability of target tissue to handle foreign and carcinogenic compounds.

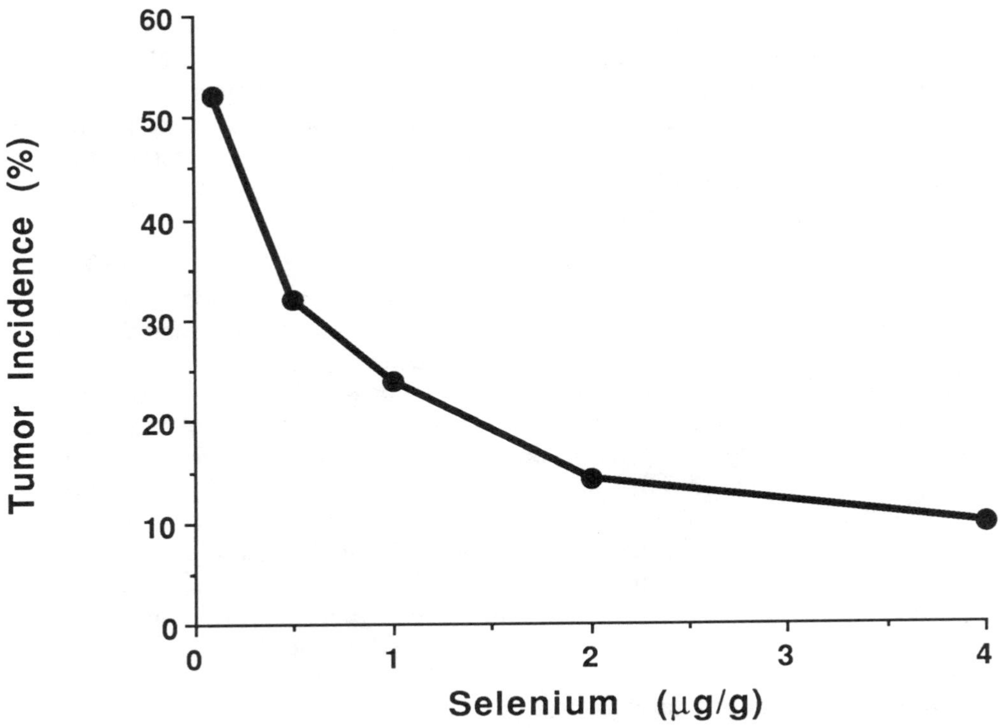

Figure 1. Influence of dietary selenium on mammary tumor incidence in rats treated with DMBA. Rats were fed the experimental diets two weeks before and two weeks after the administration of 1 mg DMBA. Selenium was added to the semipurified diet as sodium selenite. All rats were fed the basal diet (0.1 µg Se/g) two weeks after treatment with DMBA. Modified from ref. 55.

The effect of dietary selenite on the *in vivo* formation of DMBA adducts in rat mammary tissue has also been recently examined using a ^{32}P postlabelling technique.[60,61] Dietary supplemental selenite markedly decreased the binding of DMBA to mammary cell DNA (Table 2).[55] Likewise a marked reduction in *anti* dihydrodiol epoxide adducts was observed (Table 2). Increasing the dietary content of selenite resulted in a proportional decrease in binding of DMBA to DNA. A highly significant correlation (r=0.99) was found between DMBA-DNA binding and the incidence of DMBA induced mammary tumors. These studies clearly demonstrated that selenium is effective in modifying the initiation phase of carcinogenesis by altering carcinogen metabolism.

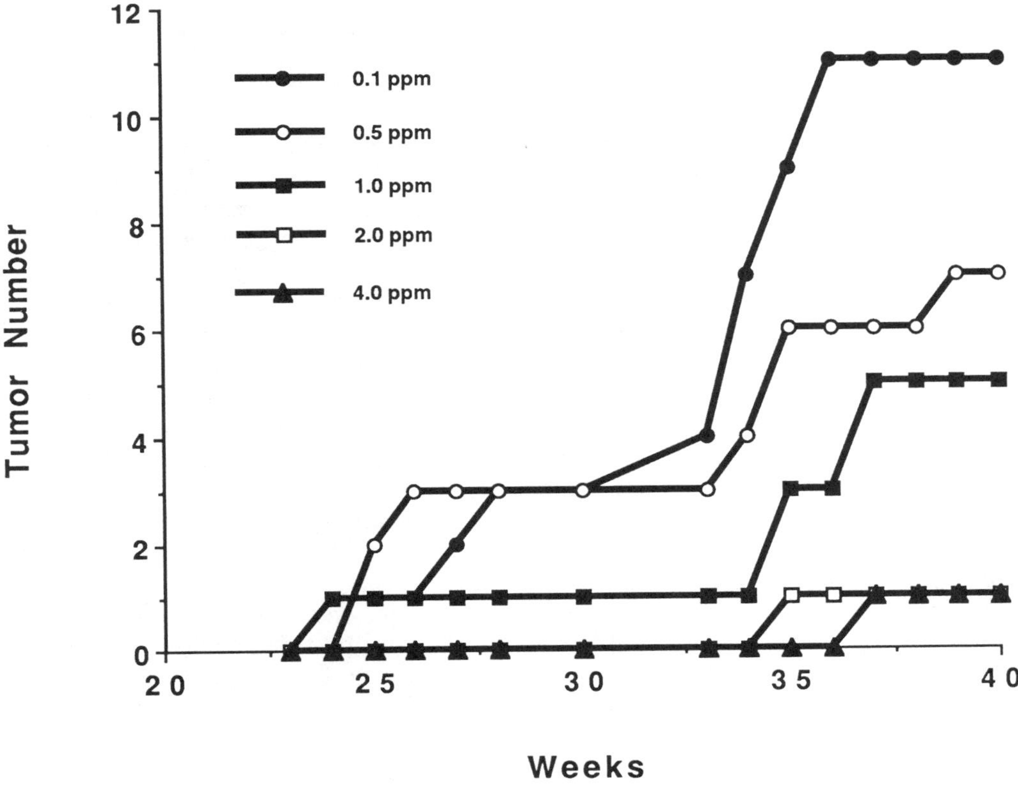

Figure 2. Influence of dietary selenium on palpable mammary tumors in rats treated with DMBA. Rats were fed the experimental diets two weeks before and two weeks after the administration of 1 mg DMBA. Selenium was added to the semipurified diet as sodium selenite. All rats were fed the basal diet (0.1 µg Se/g) two weeks after treatment with DMBA.

TABLE 2
Influence of Dietary Selenium on the *In Vivo* Formation of *Anti*-Dihydrodiol Epoxide-Deoxynucleotide Adducts and Total DMBA-DNA Binding

Se in diets (µg/g)	Adducts (nMol/Mol) *anti*-G adduct	Total adducts
0.1	23.9[a]	92.0[a]
0.5	17.3[b]	57.8[b]
1.0	8.4[c]	29.6[c]
2.0	8.2[c]	20.2[c,d]
4.0	6.2[d]	19.0[d]

Values are mean of 4 rats/treatment. Values with unlike superscripts differ at $p < 0.05$. Modified from ref. 55.

VI. Selenium and the Promotion Phase of Carcinogenesis

Inhibition of the initiation phase of carcinogenesis does not appear to totally explain the anticarcinogenicity of selenium. Banner *et al.*[62] found that selenium did not influence the acute alteration induced by 2-acetylaminofluorene or methylazoxymethanol and suggested that the anticarcinogenic properties of selenium were due to a mechanism other than an interference with carcinogen activation and interaction with cellular macromolecules. Furthermore, while the effect of selenium on the incidence of tumors resulting from treatment with direct acting carcinogens is less than observed with compounds requiring metabolic activation, there is nevertheless a significant reduction in total tumor number. Therefore, selenium likely inhibits both the initiation and promotion phases of carcinogenesis. The mechanism by which selenium alters the promotion phase of carcinogenesis is not well understood. Alterations in macromolecule biosynthesis, redox state, phosphorylation, hormonal status or alterations in immunity have been proposed to explain the ability of selenium to alter this phase of carcinogenesis. Additional information is needed to clarify the mechanism by which selenium alters the promotion phase. Several dietary constituents may alter the ability of selenium to inhibit this phase of carcinogenesis. Lipids are recognized as potent stimulators of the promotion phase of carcinogenesis. The efficiency of selenium to inhibit mammary tumorigenesis is known to be enhanced as the lipid content of the diet is increased.[31]

VII. Virally Induced Tumors and Selenium Intake

Another model frequently used in cancer research is the spontaneous or virally induced mammary tumor. Mouse mammary tumorigenesis is characterized by the presence of preneoplastic hyperplastic alveolar nodules that arise from normal mammary gland cell to develop mammary adenocarcinomas. Selenite supplements have been shown to dramatically reduce the incidence of mammary tumors in female virgin C_3H/St and BALB/cfC_3H mice.[63-65] The studies generally reveal that maximum reduction in tumor frequency occurs when supplemental selenium is provided through life.[63] However, data of Schrauzer *et al.*[63] suggest that some inhibition of mammary tumor development occurs when selenium supplements are begun during the later stages of life. The ability of selenium to inhibit this model of mammary cancer is known to depend upon the presence of other dietary constituents.[65] Dietary fat and protein appear to modify the ability of selenium to inhibit virally induced tumors.

VIII. Selenium and Transplantable Tumors

Studies with various transplantable tumors, including Murphy lymphosarcoma, Ehrlich ascites, L-1210, MCF-7 and MDA-MB 231, support the early hypothesis that selenium inhibits the growth of some neoplastic cells.[66-73] These data suggest selenium is able to inhibit the development of tumors originating at various sites. It is important to realize that the depression in the total number of tumors occurring in animals treated with chemical carcinogens may relate to a depression in the proliferation of the transformed cell. Thus, this model may reflect changes that occur during the promotion phase of carcinogenesis. As with other models of cancer, relatively high concentrations of selenium are required to inhibit tumor proliferation. Nevertheless there is some evidence that normal non-neoplastic cells are more resistant to the toxic effects of selenium than are neoplastic cells.[53]

The reason that some cells are particularly sensitive to the toxic effects of selenium is unknown. Available evidence suggests that cellular retention in not the primary factor accounting for differences in toxicity. Several studies suggest that selenium may inhibit cell proliferation by altering the biosynthesis of protein or other macromolecules. Studies[53,66] suggest that this effect may be mediated by an intermediate formed during selenium detoxification, such as selenodiglutathione. Selenodiglutathione has been shown to be more effective in inhibiting the growth of several tumor cells lines than is selenite.[53,72] Selenite is generally observed to be more effective than selenomethionine or selenide in inhibiting tumor growth.[52,53]

Intracellular changes induced by selenium supplementation may also account for the observed growth inhibition of some neoplastic cells. Morrison *et al.*[14] have observed that a 58 kD selenoprotein increases proportionally with the degree of growth inhibition caused by selenite. Alteration in the redox of the cell, including changes in oxidized and reduced glutathione, may also account for alterations in growth of neoplastic cells exposed to selenium.[74] Again alterations in hormonal status or immunity may be additional factors that may account for the efficacy of several forms of selenium to inhibit the growth of some neoplasms.

IX. Interactions Between Selenium and Other Dietary Constituents

A variety of studies show the interactive nature of selenium with other dietary constituents. The ability of selenium to interact with heavy metals is well established. Although there is relatively little information about such interactions in cancer models, one would expect heavy metals to decrease the ability of selenium to inhibit the cancer process. One of the most promising groups of candidates for chemoprevention is a combination of vitamin A and selenium. An additive effect of combined supplements of vitamin A and selenium in the inhibition of chemically induced mammary cancer has been observed.[75] Unfortunately, the presence of other dietary nutrients may have the opposite influence on the protection offered by selenium. Vitamin C appears to be one such nutrient. It has been reported to nullify the chemopreventive action of selenite. This effect is probably mediated through changing the redox state of selenium.[49] The ability of selenium to interact with sulfhydryls has sparked our laboratory to examine its interaction with garlic powder. Data of Liu *et al.*[76] revealed that a combination of garlic powder and selenium was more effective in inhibiting DMBA induced mammary cancer than either supplement provided singly.

X. Conclusion

Epidemiological and laboratory investigations reveal an inverse relationship between selenium intake and cancer risk. The ability of selenium to effectively inhibit the incidence of chemically and virally induced tumors and to depress the growth of some transplantable tumors, strongly supports the ability of this trace element to inhibit various stages of the cancer process. Some forms of selenium are clearly more effective than others in inhibiting the initiation and promotion phases of carcinogenesis. While the seleno-amino acids, selenomethionine and selenocystine, are less toxic they typically have a reduced ability to inhibit the proliferation of neoplastic cells or the binding of carcinogens to DNA compared to equivalent quantities of selenium as sodium selenite or selenodiglutathione. Additional studies are needed to determine whether a common link exists between the efficacy of selenium in inhibiting chemically-induced, virally-induced and transplantable tumor models of carcinogenesis. Such investigations should provide valuable insight into the form, dose and critical period in which providing supplemental selenium would be most effective in cancer inhibition.

References

1. Franke, K.W. and Painter, E.P., A study of the toxicity and selenium content of seliniteraus diets with statistical considerations, *Cereal Chem.*, 15, 1, 1938.

2. Nelson, A.A., Fitzhugh, O.G., and Calvery, H.O., Liver tumors following cirrhosis caused by selenium in rat, *Cancer Res.*, 3, 230, 1943.

3. Schwarz, K.A., Hitherto unrecognized factor against dietary necrotic liver degeneration in American Yeast (factor 3), *Proc. Soc. Exp. Biol. Med.*, 78, 852, 1951.

4. McCoy, K.E.M. and Weswig, P.H., Some selenium responses in the rat not related to vitamin E, *J. Nutr.*, 98, 383, 1969.

5. Underwood, E.J., *Trace Elements in Human and Animal Nutrition*, 4th ed., Academic Press, New York, 1977, 311.

6. Rotruck, J.T., Pope, A.L., Ganther, H.E., Swanson, A.B., Hafeman, D.G., and Hoekstra, W.G., Selenium: Biochemical role as a component of glutathione peroxidase, *Science*, 179, 588, 1973.

7. Ganther, H.E., Hafeman, D.G., Lawrence, R.A., Serfass, R.E., and Hoekstra, W.G., Selenium and glutathione peroxidase in health and disease: A review, in *Trace Elements in Human Health and Disease*, Vol. II, Pradad, A.S., Ed., Academic Press, New York, 1990, 165.

8. Van Rij, A.M., Thomson, C.D., McKenzie, J.M., and Robinson, M.F., Selenium deficiency in total parenteral nutrition, *Am. J. Clin. Nutr.*, 32, 2076, 1979.

9. Keshan Disease Research Group of the Chinese Academy of Sciences, Observations on the effect of selenium in prevention of Keshans disease, *Chinese Med. J.*, 92, 471, 1979.

10. Kein, C.L. and Ganther, H.E., Manifestations of chronic selenium deficiency in a child receiving total parenteral nutrition, *Am. J. Clin. Nutr.*, 37, 319, 1983.

11. Debski, B., Picciano, M.F., and Milner, J.A., Selenium content and distribution of human, cow and goat milk, *J. Nutr.*, 117, 1091, 1987.

12. Whanger, P.D., Pederson, N.D., and Weswig, P.H., Selenium proteins in ovine tissues II. Spectral properties of a 10,000 molecular weight selenium protein, *Biochem. Biophys. Res. Commun.*, 53, 1031, 1973.

13. Stadtman, T., Biological functions of selenium, *Trends in Biochem. Sci.*, 5, 203, 1980.

14. Morrison, D.G., Dishart, M.K., and Medina, D., Intracellular 58-kd selenoprotein levels correlate with inhibition of DNA synthesis in mammary epithelial cells, *Carcinogenesis*, 9, 1801, 1988.

15. Sunde, R.A., Molecular Biology of Selenoproteins, *Annual Rev. Nutr.*, 10, 451, 1990.

16. Walker, C.H. and Klein, E., "Selenium"—its therapeutic value—especially in cancer, *Am. Med.*, Aug., 628, 1915.

17. Clayton, C.C. and Bauman, C.A., Diet and azo dye tumors: Effect of diet during a period when the dye is not fed, *Cancer Res.*, 9, 575, 1949.

18. Shamberger, R.J. and Frost, D.V., Possible protective effect of selenium against human cancer, *Can. Med. Assn. J.*, 104, 82, 1969.

19. Shamberger, R.J., Relationship of selenium to cancer. I. Inhibitory effect of selenium on carcinogenesis, *J. Natl. Cancer Inst.*, 44, 931, 1970.

20. Schrauzer, G.N., White, D.A., and Schnieder, C.J., Cancer mortality correlation studies. III. Statistical association with dietary selenium intakes, *Bioinorg. Chem.*, 7, 23, 1977.

21. Schrauzer, G.N., White, D.A., and Schneider, C.J., Cancer mortality correlation studies. IV. Associations with dietary intakes and blood levels of certain trace elements, notable Se-antagonists, *Bioinorg. Chem.*, 7, 35, 1977.

22. Yu, S.Y., Chu, Y.J., Gong, X.L., Hou, C., Li, W.G., Gong, H.M., and Xie, J.R., Regional variation of cancer mortality incidence and its relation to selenium levels in China, *Biol. Trace Elem. Res.*, 7, 21, 1985.

23. Clark, L.C., Graham, G.F., Crounse, R.G., Grimson, R., Hulka, B., and Shy, C.M., Plasma selenium and skin neoplasma: A case-control study, *Nutr. Cancer*, 6, 13, 1984.

24. Peleg, I., Morris, S., and Hames, C.G., Is selenium a risk factor for cancer?, *Med. Oncol. Tumor Pharmacother.*, 2, 137, 1985.

25. Menkes, M.S., Comstock, G.W., Vuilleumier, J.P., Helsing, K.J., Rider, A.A., and Brookmeyer, R.P., Serum beta-carotene, vitamin A and E, selenium, and the risk of lung cancer, *N. Engl. J. Med.*, 315, 1250, 1986.

26. Salonen, J.T., Salonen, R., Lappetelainen, R., Maenpaa, P.H., Althan, G., and Puska, P., Risk of cancer in relation to serum concentrations of selenium and

vitamins A and E: Matched case-control analysis of prospective data, *Br. Med. J.*, 290, 417, 1985.

27. Willett, W.C. and Stampfer, M.J., Selenium and human cancer, *Acta Physiol. Toxicol.*, 59, 240, 1986.

28. Broghamer, W.L., Jr., McConnell, K.P., and Blotcky, A.L., Relationship between serum selenium levels and patients with carcinoma, *Cancer*, 37, 1384, 1976.

29. Broghamer, W.L., Jr., McConnell, K.P., Grimaldi, M., and Blotcky, A.L., Serum selenium and reticuloendothelial tumors, *Cancer*, 41, 1462, 1978.

30. Ip, C., Prophylaxis of mammary neoplasia by selenium supplementation in the initiation and promotion phases of chemical carcinogenesis, *Cancer Res.*, 41, 2683, 1981.

31. Ip, C. and Sinha, D., Anticarcinogenic effect of selenium in rats treated with dimethylbenz(a)anthracene and fed different levels and types of fat, *Carcinogenesis*, 2, 435, 1981.

32. Medina, D., Lane, H.W., and Tracey, C.M., Selenium and mouse mammary tumorigenesis: An investigation of possible mechanisms, *Cancer Res.*, 43, 2460s, 1983.

33. Thompson, J.J., Meeker, L.D., and Kokoska, S., Effect of an inorganic and organic form of dietary selenium on the promotion stage of mammary carcinogenesis in the rat, *Cancer Res.*, 44, 2803, 1984.

34. Medina, D. and Shepherd, F., Selenium-mediated inhibition of 7,12-dimethylbenz(a)anthracene-induced mouse mammary tumorigenesis, *Carcinogenesis*, 2, 451, 1981.

35. Harr, J.R., Exon, J.H., Whanger, P.D., and Weswig, P.H., Effect of dietary selenium on N-2-fluorenyl-acetamide (FFA)-induced cancer in vitamin supplemented selenium depleted rat, *Clin. Toxicol.*, 5, 187, 1972.

36. Jacobs, M.M., Jansson, B., and Griffin, A.C., Inhibitory effects of selenium on 1,2-dimethylhydrazine and methylazoxymethanol acetate induction of colon tumors, *Cancer Lett.*, 2, 133, 1977.

37. Jacobs, M.M., Selenium inhibition of 1,2-dimethylhydrazine-induced colon carcinogenesis, *Cancer Res.*, 43, 1646, 1983.

38. Nigro, N.D., Bull, A.W., Wilson, P.S., Souiller, B.K., and Alousi, M.A., Combined inhibitors of carcinogenesis: Effect on azoxymethane induced intestinal cancer in rats, *J. Natl. Cancer Inst.*, 69, 103, 1983.

39. Birt, D.F., Lawson, T.A., Julius, A.D., and Pour, P.M., Inhibition by dietary selenium on colon cancer induced in the rat by bis(2-oxopropyl)-nitrosamine, *Cancer Res.*, 42, 4455, 1982.

40. Daoud, A.H. and Griffin, A.C., Effect of retinoic acid, butylated hydroxytoluene, selenium and sorbic acid on azo-dye hepatocarcinogenesis, *Cancer Lett.*, 9, 299, 1980.

41. Clayt[illegible] [illegible]. and Baumann, C.A., Diet and azo dye tumors: Effect of diet during a pe[illegible] [illegible]ı the dye is not fed, *Cancer Res.*, 9, 575, 1949.

42. Marshall, M.V., Arnott, M.S., Jacobs, M.M., and Griffin, A.C., Selenium effects on the carcinogenicity and metabolism of 2-acetylaminofluorene, *Cancer Lett.*, 7, 331, 1979.

43. Grant, K.E., Conner, M.W., and Newberne, P.M., Effect of dietary sodium selenite upon lesions induced by repeated small doses of aflatoxin B_1, *Toxicol. Appl. Pharmacol.*, 41, 166, 1977.

44. Riley, J.F., Mast cells co-carcinogenesis and anticarcinogenesis in the skin of mice, *Experientia*, 24, 1237, 1968.

45. Thompson, H.J. and Becci, P.J., Effect of graded dietary levels of selenium on tracheal carcinomas induced by 1-methyl-1-nitrosourea, *Cancer Lett.*, 7, 215, 1979.

46. Ip, C. and Daniel, F.B., Effects of selenium on 7,12-dimethylbenz(a)anthracene-induced mammary carcinogenesis and DNA adduct formation, *Cancer Res.*, 45, 62, 1985.

47. Witting, C., Witting, U., and Krieg, V., The tumor protective effect of selenium in an experimental model, *J. Cancer Res. Clin. Oncol.*, 104, 109, 1982.

48. Thompson, H.J., Meeker, L.D., Becci, P.J., and Kokoska, S., Effect of short-term feeding of sodium selenite on 7,12-dimethylbenz(a)anthracene-induced mammary carcinogenesis in the rat, *Cancer Res.*, 42, 4954, 1982.

49. Ip, C., The chemopreventive role of selenium in carcinogenesis, in *Essential Nutrients in Carcinogenesis, Advances in Experimental Medicine and Biology*, Vol. 206, Poirier, L.A., Newberne, P.M., and Pariza, M.W., Eds., Plenum Press, New York, 1986, 431.

50. Horvath, P.M. and Ip, C., Synergistic effect of vitamin E and selenium in the chemoprevention of mammary carcinogenesis in rats, *Cancer Res.*, 43, 5335, 1983.

51. Milner, J.A., Pigot, M.A., and Dipple, A., Selective effects of sodium selenite on 7,12-dimethylbenz(a)anthracene-DNA binding in fetal mouse cell cultures, *Cancer Res.*, 45, 6347, 1985.

52. Greeder, G.A. and Milner, J.A., Factors influencing the inhibitory effect of selenium on mice inoculated with Ehrlich ascites tumor cells, *Science*, 209, 825, 1980.

53. Fico, M.E., Poirier, L.A., Watrach, A.M., Watrach, M.A., and Milner, J.A., Differential effects of selenium on normal and neoplastic mammary cells, *Cancer Res.*, 46, 3384, 1986.

54. Ip, C., Factors influencing the anticarcinogenic efficacy of selenium in dimethylbenz(a)anthracene induced mammary tumorigenesis in rats, *Cancer Res.*, 41, 2683, 1981.

55. Liu, J., Gilbert, K., Parker, H., and Haschek, W., Inhibition of 7,12-dimethylbenz(a)anthracene induced mammary tumors and DNA adducts by dietary selenite, Submitted.

56. Milner, J., Liu, J., Gilbert, K., Parker, H., and Haschek, W., Selenite inhibition of mammary tumors induced by 7,12-dimethylbenz(a)anthracene (DMBA), *FASEB J.*, 4, A1042, 1990.

57. Rasco, M.A., Jacobs, M.M., and Griffin, A.C., Effects of selenium on aryl hydrocarbon hydroxylase activity in cultured human lymphocytes, *Cancer Lett.*, 3, 295, 1977.

58. Harbah, P.R. and Swenberg, J.A., Effects of selenium on 1,2-dimethylhydrazine metabolism and DNA alkylation, *Carcinogenesis*, 2, 575, 1981.

59. Edaji, S., Bhattacharya, I.D., Voss, K., Singletary, K., and Milner, J.A., *In vitro* and *in vivo* effects of sodium selenite on 7,12-dimethylbenz(α)anthracene-DNA adducts formation in rat mammary epithelial cells, *Carcinogenesis*, 10, 823, 1989.

60. Reddy, M.V. and Randerath, K., Nuclease P1-mediated enhancement of sensitivity of ^{32}P-postlabeling test for structurally diverse DNA adducts, *Carcinogenesis*, 7, 1543, 1986.

61. Singletary, K.W., Parker, H., and Milner, J.A., Identification and *in vivo* formation of 32P-postlabled rat mammary DMBA-DNA adducts, *Carcinogenesis*, 11, 1959, 1990.

62. Banner, W.P., Tan, Q.H., and Zedeck, M.S., Selenium and the acute effects of the carcinogen 2-acetylaminofluorene and methylazoxymethanol acetate, *Cancer Res.*, 42, 2985, 1982.

63. Medina, D., Mechanisms of selenium inhibition of tumorigenesis, *J. Am. Coll. Toxicol.*, 5, 21, 1986.

64. Schrauzer, G.N., White, D.A., and Schneider, C.J., Inhibition of the genesis of spontaneous mammary tumors in C3H mice: Effects of selenium and of selenium-antagonistic elements and their possible role in human breast cancer, *Bioinorg. Chem.*, 6, 265, 1976.

65. Whanger, P., Schmitz, J.A., and Exon, J.H., Influence of diet on the effects of selenium in the genesis of mammary tumors, *Nutr. Cancer*, 3, 240, 1982.

66. Milner, J.A., Effect of selenium on virally induced and transplantable tumor models, *Fed. Proc.*, 44, 2568, 1985.

67. Ip, C., Ip, M.M., and Kim, U., Dietary selenium intake and growth of the MT-W9B transplantable rat mammary tumor, *Cancer Lett.*, 14, 101, 1981.

68. Medina, D. and Oborn, C.J., Differential effects of selenium on growth of mouse mammary cells in vitro, *Cancer Lett.*, 13, 333, 1981.

69. Milner, J.A. and Hsu, C.Y., Inhibitory effects of selenium on the growth of L1210 leukemic cells, *Cancer Res.*, 41, 1652, 1981.

70. Abdullaev, B., Gasanov, G.G., Ragimov, R.N., *et al.*, Selenium and tumor growth in experiments, *Dokl. Akad. Nauk. zerbaidzhanskoi S. S. R.*, 29, 18, 1973.

71. Mautner, H.G. and Jaffe, J.J., The activity of 6-selenopurine and related compounds against some experimental mouse tumors, *Cancer Res.*, 18, 294, 1958.

72. Poirier, K.A. and Milner, J.A., Factors influencing the antitumorigenic properties of selenium in mice, *J. Nutr.*, 113, 2147, 1984.

73. Vernie, L.N., Hamburg, C.J., and Bont, W.S., Inhibition of the growth of malignant mouse lymphoid cells by selenodiglutathione and selenodicystine, *Cancer Lett.*, 14, 303, 1981.

74. Le Boeuf, R.A. and Hoekstra, W.G., Changes in cellular glutathione levels: possible relation to selenium-mediated anti-carcinogenesis, *Fed. Proc.*, 44, 2563, 1985.

75. Thompson, H.J., Meeker, L.D., and Becci, P., Effect of combined selenium and retinyl acetate treatment on mammary carcinogenesis, *Cancer Res.*, 41, 1413, 1981.

76. Liu, J., Lin, R.I., and Milner, J.A., Inhibition of 7,12-dimethylbenz(a)anthracene (DMBA) induced mammary tumors and adducts by Garlic Powder, Submitted.

Chapter 9

Caloric Restriction and Cancer: Search for the Molecular Mechanisms

David Kritchevsky

Table of Contents

I. Introduction

The observation that restriction of food intake could inhibit tumor growth was made by Moreschi in 1909.[1] This area of tumor research has had a rather unusual history since. After a flurry of interest (which lasted about 15 years) in Moreschi's work, not much was heard about this aspect of cancer research until the work of Tannenbaum and of Baumann's group in the 1940's. Tannenbaum deserves special mention for his contributions to the area of diet and carcinogenesis. The interest ignited in the early 1940's flared for about a decade and then waned until it was revived in the early 1980's. Still there was enough interest and enough data for White[2] to be able to write a review of the field in 1961.

Caloric restriction can be achieved in several ways. The easiest approach involves simple underfeeding—the control animals are fed *ad libitum* and the test groups are fed less of the same diet. The problem in underfeeding is that it may lead to deficiencies of minerals, vitamins or even macronutrients if the *ad libitum* diet provides the minimum amount needed for nutritional adequacy. Later studies used diets containing chow plus cornstarch and skim milk powder. While an improvement it still gave no precise measure of which nutritional requirements were or were not being met. The first study using a precisely tailored semi-purified diet was that of Boutwell *et al.*[3] done in 1949. Use of a carefully devised semi-purified diet insures that both control and calorie-restricted animals will obtain the same amount of minerals, vitamins and protein. The area of caloric restriction and carcinogenesis has been reviewed in depth recently.[4-8] This chapter reviews historical and contemporary studies on caloric restriction and discusses potential mechanisms by which caloric restriction affects carcinogenesis.

II. Caloric Restriction and Carcinogenesis

A. Early Caloric Restriction Studies

Moreschi[1] showed in 1909 that underfeeding of mice inhibited growth of transplanted sarcomas (Table 1). A few years later Rous[9] showed that caloric restriction could also inhibit spontaneous tumorigenesis. The systematic study of underfeeding and carcinogenesis was begun by Tannenbaum in 1940.[10] He

TABLE 1
Underfeeding and Growth of Sarcoma 7 in Mice[a]

Group	Number	Feed intake (g/day)	Weight change (g)	Tumor weight (g)
A	8	ad lib	+1.8	7.6 ± 0.8
B	8	2.0	-2.4	5.2 ± 0.5
C	7	1.5	-1.9	3.6 ± 0.5
D	13	1.0	-4.2	1.3 ± 0.2

[a] After Moreschi, C., 1909 (ref. 1).

manipulated the diet so as to compare freely-fed mice with those whose weight was reduced by 25% or who were not permitted to gain weight while the controls were. In most cases this involved reducing the daily ration by 33-50%. The results of his initial study are presented in Table 2. In subsequent experiments Tannenbaum went to a form of semi-purified diet composed of chow, skim milk powder and cornstarch. Calories were reduced by deleting cornstarch. Using this diet he found that caloric restriction could inhibit growth of spontaneous mammary or lung tumors and induced epithelial tumors or sarcoma in ABC, DBA C57 Black or Swiss mice.[11] In the study of benzpyrene (BP)-induced skin tumors in male DBA mice, Tannenbaum[12] showed that by reducing mean intake from 9.6 to 8.9 cal/day, tumor incidence was reduced by 30%. Lavik and Baumann[13] compared effects of calories and fat on methylcholanthrene (MCA)-induced skin tumors in mice. Their data (Table 3) showed that calories, not amount of dietary fat, exerted the more significant effect. Thirty-four years later, in a summary of 82 published studies, Albanes [7] found that the collected data showed a similar relationship.

TABLE 2
Effect of Underfeeding on Tumorigenesis in Mice[a]

Tumor type (%)	Group	Tumor incidence
BP-induced skin	control	16
	underfed	4
BP-induced sarcoma	control	35
	underfed	22
Spontaneous mammary	control	40
	underfed	2

[a] After Tannenbaum, A., 1940 (ref. 10).

TABLE 3
Influence of Fat and Calories on MCA-Induced Skin Tumors in Mice[a]

Regimen		Tumor incidence
Fat	Calories	(%)
Low	Low	0
Low	High	54
High	Low	28
High	High	66

[a] After Lavik and Bowman, 1943 (ref. 13).

B. Contemporary Caloric Restriction Studies

We [14,15] examined the effects of 40% caloric restriction on 7,12-dimethylbenz(a) anthracene (DMBA)-induced mammary tumors in female Sprague-Dawley rats and of 1,2-dimethylhydrazine (DMH)-induced colon tumors in male F344 rats. The diets were designed to provide about 4% fat in the control diets and double that in the restricted ones. The data (Table 4) show that caloric restriction significantly reduces tumor incidence even when the diet contains more fat than the control. We also confirmed the observation of Carroll and Khor[16] that unsaturated fat is more co-carcinogenic than saturated fat. Boissoneault *et al.*[17] carried out a study involving calorie restriction of DMBA-treated rats. As the results show (Table 5) rats fed a high fat, calorie-restricted diet exhibited an 84% lower tumor incidence than rats fed a low fat diet *ad libitum*.

TABLE 4
Influence of Fat Type and 40% Caloric Restriction on Mammary and Colon Tumors in Rats[a]

Treatment	Fat[b]	% Fat	Incidence (%)
DMBA			
Ad libitum	CNO	3.9	58
Restricted	CNO	8.4	0
Ad libitum	CO	3.9	80
Restricted	CO	8.4	20
DMH			
Ad libitum	BO	3.9	85
Restricted	BO	8.4	35
Ad libitum	CO	3.9	100
Restricted	CO	8.4	53

[a] After Kritchevsky *et al.*, 1984 (ref. 14); and Klurfeld *et al.*, 1987 (ref. 15).

[b] CNO - Coconut Oil + 1% Corn Oil
CO - Corn Oil
BO - Butter Oil + 1% Corn Oil.

In an effort to determine the minimum level of caloric restriction which would be effective in inhibiting tumorigenesis we examined the effects of graded (10, 20, 30, 40%) caloric restriction on DMBA-induced mammary tumors in rats.[18] The results (Table 6) indicate that some effect is seen at 10% restriction, namely a 47% reduction in tumor burden and that a 33% reduction in tumor incidence becomes evident at 20% restriction. The effect of fat level was investigated in DMBA-treated rats whose caloric intake was reduced by 25% but whose actual daily fat intake was the same as that of the freely fed controls. Thus *ad libitum* or calorie restricted rats received exactly the same amount of fat daily. Even when the diets contained appreciable levels of fat,[19] caloric restriction inhibited tumor growth (Table 7).

TABLE 5
Effect of Calories and Fat on DMBA-Induced Mammary Tumors in Rats[a]

	Diets		
	High fat *ad libitum*	**High fat restricted**	**Low fat *ad libitum***
Corn oil (% of diet)	30	30	5
Fat intake (g/rat/day)	2.7	2.2	0.6
Tumor incidence (%)	73	7	43

[a] After Boissoneault *et al.*, 1986 (ref. 17).

TABLE 6
Influence of Graded Caloric Restriction on DMBA-Induced Mammary Tumors in Rats[a]

Regimen	Tumor incidence (%)	Tumor multiplicity	Tumor burden, g
Ad libitum	60	4.7 ± 1.3	10.1 ± 3.3
10% Restricted	60	3.0 ± 0.8	5.4 ± 3.0
20% Restricted	40	2.8 ± 0.7	4.7 ± 1.9
30% Restricted	35	1.3 ± 0.3	0.9 ± 0.8
40% Restricted	5	1.0	--
p	<0.005	NS	<0.05

[a] After Klurfeld *et al.*, 1989 (ref. 18).

The observation that caloric restriction inhibits tumor growth has now been made repeatedly. Restriction of calories has an effect when instituted late in life[20] or when exercised intermittently.[21] In the latter case, tumor incidence is highly correlated with feed-efficiency.

While caloric restriction generally inhibits spontaneous or induced tumorigenicity, Pollard and Luckert[22] found that caloric restriction inhibited the tumorigenicity of methylazoxymethanol, an indirect acting carcinogen, but not of methylnitrosourea which is a direct acting carcinogen. This observation suggests that caloric restriction may act as an energy requiring activation step.

TABLE 7
Effect of Fat Level and 25% Caloric Restriction on DMBA-Induced Mammary Tumors in Rats[a]

Regimen	Tumor incidence (%)	Tumor multiplicity	Tumor weight (g)	Burden (g)
Ad libitum				
5% Corn oil	65	1.9 ± 0.3	2.0 ± 0.7	4.2 ± 1.9
15% Corn oil	85	3.0 ± 0.6	2.3 ± 0.7	6.6 ± 2.7
20% Corn oil	80	4.1 ± 0.6	2.9 ± 0.5	11.8 ± 3.2
Restricted				
20% Corn oil	60	1.9 ± 0.4	0.8 ± 0.2	1.5 ± 0.5
26.7% Corn oil	30	1.5 ± 0.3	1.4 ± 1.0	2.3 ± 1.6
p	<0.005	<0.0001	<0.0001	<0.05

[a] After Klurfeld *et al.*, 1989 (ref. 19).

III. Possible Mechanisms for Inhibition of Tumorigenesis by Caloric Restriction

There are a number of hypothetical mechanisms by which caloric restriction could exert its inhibitory effect. These have been summarized by Ruggeri[8] (Table 8). Boutwell *et al.*[3] originally suggested that caloric restriction involved an activation of the pituitary-adrenocorticotropic axis as evidenced by reduced uterine and ovarian size and adrenal hypertrophy in female rats. Adrenalectomy has been shown to enhance DMBA-induced tumorigenicity in rats.[23] Cellular proliferation and mitotic activity have been shown to be reduced by rather severe

TABLE 8
Possible Mechanisms for Inhibition of Tumorigenesis by Caloric Restriction[a]

1. Elevated glucocorticoid levels leading to growth inhibition.
2. Reduced mitotic activity and cell proliferation.
3. Enhanced immune response.
4. Reduced nutrient available to preneoplastic cells.
5. Alterations in mammotropic hormones.
6. Alterations in peptide growth factors and receptors.
7. Repair of DNA damage.
8. Alterations in oncogene or protooncogene expression.

[a] After Ruggeri, B., 1990 (ref. 8).

food restriction.[24,25] Restriction of diet or calories eventually prolongs cell-mediated immunity.[26,27] Lagopoulos and Stalder[28] have suggested that limitation of nutrients available to preneoplastic cells could retard their progression. Ruggeri *et al.*[29] have found that tumors taken from rats subjected to caloric restriction show alterations in carbohydrate metabolism compared to tumors from *ad libitum*-fed rats. The observed changes suggest that the changes in carbohydrate metabolism of the tumor reflect the altered nutritional state of the host. Influence of caloric restriction on mammotropic hormones could play a role in its effects on breast cancer. Indeed, Sylvester and his associates[30] have reported that caloric restriction affects levels of circulating mammotropic hormones which, in turn, play a role in chemically induced mammary carcinogenesis. However, in view of the wide array of tumors which are affected by caloric restriction, effects on prolactin and estrogen may represent a special case.

Alteration in peptide growth factors offers an attractive hypothesis for the action of caloric restriction. Generally, the role of insulin[31] and its specific effects on tumor growth *in vitro*[32] and *in vivo*[33] are well documented. Caloric restriction has been shown to reduce plasma insulin levels in rats[18,19] but direct experimental proof of a relationship between food restriction, insulin levels and tumor growth remains to be shown. There are studies which suggest that caloric restriction may help the host to limit oxidative damage by increasing hepatic catalase[34] and lipid peroxidation.[35] Lymphocytes from calorie-restricted mice have an enhanced ability to repair damaged DNA.[36] Caloric restriction has also been shown to reduce oncogene expression.[37,38]

IV. Conclusion

Research on caloric restriction as it affects tumorigenicity has been through several reincarnations since Moreschi's initial work. In each renewal the observations persist but the methodology becomes increasingly refined. We now have at hand means of fine-tuning earlier studies and of testing a number of attractive hypotheses *vis-à-vis* mechanism(s) of action. Let us hope that the mechanism by which caloric restriction affects carcinogenesis will be delineated and that the knowledge is put to therapeutic use soon.

Acknowledgements

Supported, in part, by a Research Career Award (HL 00734) and a grant CA-43856-02 from the National Institutes of Health by grants-in-aid from the American Institute for Cancer Research and The Cancer Research Foundation and by funds from the Commonwealth of Pennsylvania.

References

1. Moreschi, C., Beziehungen Zwischen ernahrung und tumorwachstum, *Z. Immunitatsforsch*, 2, 651, 1909.

2. White, F.R., The relationship between underfeeding and tumor formation, transplantation, and growth in rats and mice, *Cancer Res.*, 21, 281, 1961.

3. Boutwell, R.K., Brush, M.K., and Rusch, H.P., Some physiological effects associated with chronic caloric restriction, *Am. J. Physiol.*, 154, 517, 1949.

4. Kritchevsky, D. and Klurfeld, D.M., Influence of caloric intake on experimental carcinogenesis: A review, *Adv. Exp. Med. Biol.*, 206, 55, 1986.

5. Pariza, M.W., Calorie restriction, *ad libitum* feeding and cancer, *Proc. Soc. Exp. Biol. Med.*, 183, 293, 1986.

6. Kritchevsky, D. and Klurfeld, D.M., Calorie effects on experimental mammary tumorigenesis, *Am. J. Clin. Nutr.*, 45, 236, 1987.

7. Albanes, D., Total calories, body weight and tumor incidence in mice, *Cancer Res.*, 47, 1987, 1987.

8. Ruggeri, B., The effects of caloric restriction on neoplasia and age-related degenerative processes, in *Human Nutrition*, Vol. 7, Alfin-Slater, R.B. and Kritchevsky, D., Eds., Plenum Press, New York, 1990, 187.

9. Rous, P., The influence of diet on transplanted and spontaneous tumors, *J. Exp. Med.*, 20, 433, 1914.

10. Tannenbaum, A., The initiation and growth of tumors. Introduction. I. Effects of underfeeding, *Am. J. Cancer*, 38, 335, 1940.

11. Tannenbaum, A., The genesis and growth of tumors. II. Effects of caloric restriction *per se*, *Cancer Res.*, 2, 460, 1942.

12. Tannenbaum, A., The dependence of tumor formation on the degree of caloric restriction, *Cancer Res.*, 5, 609, 1945.

13. Lavik, P.S. and Baumann, C.A., Further studies on tumor-promoting action of fat, *Cancer Res.*, 3, 749, 1943.

14. Kritchevsky, D., Weber, M.M., and Klurfeld, D.M., Dietary fat versus caloric content in initiation and promotion of 7,12-dimethylbenz(a)anthracene-induced mammary tumorigenesis in rats, *Cancer Res.*, 44, 3174, 1984.

15. Klurfeld, D.M., Weber, M.M., and Kritchevsky, D., Inhibition of chemically-induced mammary and colon tumor promotion by caloric restriction in rats fed increased dietary fat, *Cancer Res.*, 47, 2759, 1987.

16. Carroll, K.K. and Khor, K.T., Effect of level and type of dietary fat on incidence of mammary tumors induced in female Sprague-Dawley rats by 7,12-dimethylbenz(a)-anthracene, *Lipids*, 6, 415, 1970.

17. Boissonneault, G.A., Elson, C.E., and Pariza, M.W., Net energy effects of dietary fat on chemically-induced mammary carcinogenesis in F344 rats, *J. Natl. Cancer Inst.*, 76, 335, 1986.

18. Klurfeld, D.M., Welch, C.B., Davis, M.J., and Kritchevsky, D., Determination of degree of energy restriction necessary to reduce DMBA-induced mammary tumorigenesis in rats during the promotion phase, *J. Nutr.*, 119, 286, 1989.

19. Klurfeld, D.M., Welch, C.B., Lloyd, L.M., and Kritchevsky, D., Inhibition of DMBA-induced mammary tumorigenesis by caloric restriction in rats fed high fat diets, *Int. J. Cancer*, 43, 922, 1989.

20. Weindruch, R. and Walford, R.L., Dietary restriction in mice beginning at one year of age: Effect on life span and spontaneous cancer incidence, *Science*, 215, 1415, 1982.

21. Kritchevsky, D., Welch, C.B., and Klurfeld, D.M., Response of mammary tumors to caloric restriction for different periods of time during the promotion phase, *Nutr. Cancer*, 12, 259, 1989.

22. Pollard, M. and Luckert, P.H., Tumorigenic effect of direct- and indirect-acting carcinogens in rats on a restricted diet, *J. Natl. Cancer Inst.*, 74, 1347, 1985.

23. Carter, J.H., Carter, H.W., and Meade, J., Adrenal regulation of mammary tumorigenesis in female Sprague-Dawley rats: Incidence, latency and yield of mammary tumors, *Cancer Res.*, 48, 3801, 1988.

24. Koga, A. and Kimura, S., Influence of restricted diet on the cell renewal of the mouse small intestine, *J. Nutr. Sci. Vitaminol.*, 25, 265, 1979.

25. Koga, A. and Kimura, S., Influence of restricted diet on the cell cycle in the crypt of mouse small intestine, *J. Nutr. Sci. Vitaminol.*, 26, 33, 1980.

26. Jose, D.G. and Good, R.A., Quantitative effects of nutritional protein and calorie deficiency upon immune responses to tumors in mice, *Cancer Res.*, 33, 807, 1973.

27. Weindruch, R.H., Devens, B.H., Raff, H.V., and Walford, R.L., Influence of dietary restriction on aging and natural killer cell activity in mice, *J. Immunol.*, 130, 933, 1983.

28. Lagopoulos, L. and Stalder, R., The influence of food intake on the development of diethylnitrosamine-induced liver tumors in mice, *Carcinogenesis*, 8, 33, 1987.

29. Ruggeri, B.A., Klurfeld, D.M., and Kritchevsky, D., Biochemical alterations in 7,12-dimethylbenz(a)anthracene-induced mammary tumors from rats subjected to caloric restriction, *Biochim. Biophys. Acta*, 929, 239, 1987.

30. Sylvester, P.W., Aylsworth, C.F., and Meites, J., Relationship of hormones to inhibition of mammary tumor development by underfeeding during the "critical period" after carcinogen administration, *Cancer Res.*, 41, 1383, 1981.

31. Kahn, C.R., The molecular mechanism of insulin action, *Ann. Rev. Med.*, 36, 429, 1985.

32. Taub, R., Roy, A., Dieter, R., and Koontz, J., Insulin as a growth factor in rat hepatoma cells, *J. Biol. Chem.*, 262, 10893, 1987.

33. Hill, D.J. and Milner, R.D.G., Insulin as a growth factor, *Pediatric Res.*, 19, 879, 1985.

34. Koizumi, A., Weindruch, R., and Walford, R.L., Influence of dietary restriction and age on liver enzyme activities and lipid peroxidation in mice, *J. Nutr.*, 117, 361, 1987.

35. Chipalkatti, S., De, A.K., and Aiyar, A.S., Effect of diet restriction on some biochemical parameters related to aging in mice, *J. Nutr.*, 113, 944, 1983.

36. Weraarchakul, N. and Richardson, A., Effect of age and dietary restriction on DNA repair, *FASEB J.*, 2, A1209, 1988.

37. Khare, A., Mountz, J., Fischbach, M., Talal, N., and Fernandes, G., Effect of dietary lipids and calories on oncogene expression in autoimmune LPR mice, *Fed. Proc.*, 46, 441, 1987.

38. Fernandes, G., Khare, A., Langamere, S., Yu, B., Sandberg, L., and Fredericks, B., Effect of food restriction and aging on immune cell fatty acids, functions and oncogene expression in SPF Fischer 344 rats, *Fed. Proc.*, 46, 567, 1987.

Chapter 10

Choline, Methionine, Folate and Chemical Carcinogenesis

Adrianne E. Rogers, Steven H. Zeisel, and Rizwan Akhtar

Table of Contents

I. Introduction

A central role in chemical carcinogenesis of dietary methyl supply and of methyl metabolism is increasingly apparent. Methyl groups are supplied in the diet principally by methionine and choline, and normal methyl metabolism requires, in addition, the nutrients folate and vitamin B_{12}. The importance of dietary methyl supply in carcinogenesis was determined in studies designed to induce fatty liver and cirrhosis in rats used as models for the study of alcoholic liver disease in humans.[1,2] In these studies rats were fed diets deficient in choline and methionine and, in some experiments, deficient also in folate or vitamin B_{12}. A propensity of the deficient animals to develop liver tumors was noted.[2]

II. Overview: Methyl Deficiency and Cancer

Deficiencies of choline, methionine or folate are of widely varying importance in humans, with folate deficiency being by far the most important. Folate deficiency can arise in pregnancy (during which demand for folate is greatly increased), alcoholism, malabsorption, exposure to several therapeutic drugs and, notably, exposure to the antifolate cancer chemotherapeutic drugs such as methotrexate (MTX). With respect to cancer, alcoholism and MTX exposure are of particular interest. MTX is of interest because it is given with other cancer chemotherapeutic agents, some of which are known or thought to be carcinogenic,[3-6] and alcoholism because of its association with increased risk for certain cancer.[7,8] Choline and phosphatidylcholine (PtdCho) are widely available in foods, and the only circumstances in which deficiency might be expected to occur is in patients given total parenteral nutrition (TPN) and, perhaps, in pregnancy.[9] Methionine is a limiting amino acid in many plant proteins and in certain animal proteins, and deficiency may arise, along with deficiencies of other amino acids, in people who eat protein-deficient or strict vegetarian diets.

Dietary methyl-deficient rats given no known carcinogen exposure or given chemical carcinogens, such as aflatoxin B_1, one of several nitrosamines, or N-2-fluorenylacetamide, develop hepatocellular carcinoma earlier and in higher incidence than rats fed control, nutritionally complete diets, without or with carcinogen exposure.[10-14] The metabolic and molecular bases of this dietary effect on carcinogenesis have been, and are being, intensively investigated. It is important to note that the dietary methyl deficiencies that induce increased susceptibility to spontaneous or chemically induced carcinogenesis in rodents are marginal or borderline deficiencies and that severe deficiency is *not* required for the effect. Therefore, subclinical or borderline deficiencies in people may be a risk factor for cancer.

In people, associations between folate deficiency, either systemic or local, and dysplasia or carcinoma have been documented in the gastrointestinal tract, uterine cervix, respiratory tract and bone marrow.[15-19] The demonstrated or postulated etiology of the folate deficiency varies with the tissue site. Deficient intake or absorption is associated with the gastrointestinal malignancies or dysplasias; pregnancy or oral contraceptive agents are associated with cervical dysplasias or malignancies and genetic abnormalities of metabolism are associated with hematopoietic malignancy. Dietary folate deficiency or abnormal folate absorption and metabolism may be factors contributing to the increased risk of certain cancers in alcoholics.[7,8,15] Signs of folate deficiency can be demonstrated in a significant fraction of alcoholic populations.[20] In addition, evidence of choline deficiency can be detected in malnourished, alcoholic cirrhotic patients.[21]

III. Induction of Methyl Deficiency

Of particular interest are cancer patients treated with MTX and other chemotherapeutic drugs and, also, patients who may receive TPN in conjunction with their therapy. MTX-treated patients manifest markedly reduced plasma methionine, which indicates perturbation of methyl as well as folate metabolism by the drug.[22] The complex interactions of methylation pathways and phospholipid turnover are poorly understood. Among laboratory animals the metabolic defects induced by lipotrope deficiency are most marked in male weaning rats, although female rats and male mice are also susceptible to the deficiency and to its effects on carcinogenesis.[2,23,50] Reduction of the dietary supply of methyl groups is accomplished by: 1) lowering animal protein (usually casein) in the diet and replacing it with plant proteins (soybean, peanut) that are low in methionine, and 2) eliminating choline from the diet. In some cases folate also has been eliminated. Generally the diet is relatively high (15-20% by weight) in fat which increases the demand of the liver for methyl groups needed in lipoprotein synthesis and secretion. Failure of normal hepatic clearance of triglycerides leads to the fat accumulation in hepatocytes, i.e. fatty liver, which is the major morphologic characteristic of dietary methyl group deficiency and leads to the classification of methionine and choline as lipotropes. Since choline and methionine can substitute for each other in supplying methyl groups, diets must be deficient in both to induce deficiency.[23,24] Two excellent recent reviews of methionine and choline metabolism are available.[9,25] From studies in cultured normal or choline-deficient hepatocytes, it has been concluded that newly synthesized PtdCho was needed for very low density lipoprotein (VLDL) secretion and that significant utilization was not made of preexisting PtdCho.[26]

IV. Metabolic Effects of Methyl Group Deficiency

In considering dietary methyl group deficiency, investigators have tended to emphasize the role of deficiency of choline or methionine and to view folate as an accessory nutrient, although the interactions of the nutrients have been recognized since the initial studies were performed. The ability of choline and methionine to substitute for each other in prevention of liver damage has been amply demonstrated.[1,2,9,24,25] One cannot clearly separate the roles of choline and methionine in the intersecting biochemical pathways affected by dietary methyl group deficiency, and the ability of folate deficiency to enhance the effects of the deficiency is easily understood. The liver probably is more dependent on choline for critical biochemical pathways than most other tissues because of the demands made by lipoprotein secretion. It appears that PtdCho synthesis is the first priority for choline use in lipotrope-deficient liver.[9] In addition only liver has the capacity to regenerate methionine by homocysteine transmethylation from choline via betaine.[25] Other tissues can regenerate methionine only via folate- and vitamin B_{12}-mediated methylation of homocysteine. Choline can be generated in liver, mammary gland and other tissues by sequential methylation of phosphatidylethanolamine using methyl supplied by S-adenosylmethionine (Adomet).[9] This pathway accounts for 15–40% of PtdCho in liver but is, of course, severely compromised in methyl group-deficient rats since dietary methionine is inadequate.[9]

Dietary methyl group deficiency alters hepatic metabolism of folate; it decreases hepatic total folate by 31% without markedly altering folate distribution.[27] The liver is responsible for metabolism and, to some extent, storage of folates. It serves as a reservoir for other tissues as well as performing continuous synthesis and release of 5-methyltetrahydrofolate and other folate coenzymes.[28]

There are many cellular, metabolic and compositional effects of methyl-group deficiency in the liver (Table 1) and, probably, in other organs; the majority of studies have been performed in liver. Alterations of xenobiotic metabolism, nucleic acid methylation, membrane phospholipids, signal transduction pathways and increased hepatocyte turnover occur. These changes are likely contributors to enhanced carcinogenesis in the deficient liver. However, the many ramifications of perturbed methyl supply and metabolism (including, for example, alterations in folate pathways and in sulfhydryl metabolism because of the dual role of methionine) contribute to the complexity of identifying the key, characteristic change responsible for enhanced carcinogenesis in the liver.

TABLE 1

Biochemical and Cellular Abnormalities in Lipotrope-deficient Rodent Liver[a]

Triglyceride accumulation and decreased VLDL secretion

Decreased content of choline, S-adenosylmethionine, folate

Hyperplasia of hepatocytes

Increased lipid peroxidation

Reduced xenobiotic metabolism

Reduced nucleic acid and protein methylases

Undermethylation of DNA

Oncogene activation and hypomethylation (c-H-ras; c-myc)

Increased plasma membrane 1,2-sn-diacylglycerol (DAG)

Increased protein kinase C (PKC)

Increased activity of phospholipases A_2 and C

Increased prostaglandin E_2

[a] Compiled from references 1,2,9,10,13,23,26,27,34,56,59,60,61

An obvious site for methyl interaction with carcinogenesis is in control of cell division, which is regulated in part by methylation of nucleic acids. Methyl groups are needed also for synthesis and repair of DNA and other cell components. There is renewed interest in the role that cell division plays in the initiation, promotion and further development of cancer.[29,30] Many factors increase the rate of cell division in tissues. Lipotrope deficiency increases cell division in the hepatocytes, and it induces early development of hyperplastic, atypical foci within liver.[2,10,31] Additional factors that interact with cell division to determine tumor incidence and latency include carcinogen metabolism, which is altered in deficient rats, rate and extent of DNA damage and repair, which may be altered, and genetic and tissue-specific factors.[32]

V. Methyl Deficiency and Cancer

The earliest and most marked effect of dietary methyl group deficiency in enhancing chemical hepatocarcinogenesis was reported in aflatoxin B_1 (AFB_1)-treated rats.[2,31] Among potential mechanisms to explain the effect, in addition to hepatocyte hyperplasia, are alteration of AFB_1 metabolism,[10] formation and repair of AFB_1-DNA adducts,[33] and early hypomethylation of DNA[34] and of oncogenes.[13,35]

Chemical carcinogens can interfere with methyl group metabolism in animals fed complete diets. There have been observations of reduction of hepatic Adomet and early hypomethylation of oncogenes in rats fed a complete diet and given the hepatic carcinogen, diethylnitrosamine (DEN).[36] DEN also perturbs hepatic folate metabolism.[37] Another hepatic carcinogen, ethionine, seriously perturbs hepatic methyl metabolism.[38] Direct interactions of carcinogens with methyl metabolism are of great interest since they provide other evidence of the importance of methyl metabolism in carcinogenesis and may be important in tissues other than liver.

Metabolic and carcinogenic or co-carcinogenic effects of dietary methyl group deficiency have been much less extensively studied in organs other than liver. Deficient male rats have increased susceptibility to mammary gland carcinogenesis induced by procarbazine (PCZ)[39] and to pancreatic preneoplastic changes induced by l-azaserine.[40] They may have increased susceptibility to colon carcinogenesis induced by dimethylhyrdrazine and to esophageal carcinogenesis induced by DEN, but the findings with those carcinogens have not been entirely consistent.[10]

The mammary gland studies[39] are of particular interest. They were performed using procarbazine-hydrochloride (PCZ), a cancer chemotherapeutic agent used in treating Hodgkin's Disease and other tumors.[41] PCZ induces hematopoietic, mammary gland and Zymbal's gland tumors in rats and hematopoietic tumors and sarcomas in non-human primates.[42,43] It was chosen for study in methyl-deficient rats because of its leukemogenic properties, the hypothesis being that, since methyl group deficiency perturbs bone marrow metabolism and cell production, it may alter the neoplastic response of the marrow cells to PCZ. A second hypothesis examined in the same study was that MTX would enhance PCZ carcinogenesis because it blocks formation of folate coenzymes and, therefore, induces some of the same biochemical abnormalities as are induced by dietary methyl group deficiency.[44,45]

In these studies, an attempt was made to induce similar degrees of methyl deficiency, assessed by measurement of several biochemical parameters in liver, in deficient and in MTX-treated rats. The experiments were based on earlier studies[46,47] of dietary methyl group deficiency and MTX that had demonstrated the following:

1. Moderate deficiency tripled hepatic triglycerides and reduced hepatic choline concentration to 42% of normal, phosphocholine (PCho) concentration to 18% of normal, betaine concentration to 30% of normal and Adomet concentration to 57% of normal.

2. MTX, 0.1 mg/kg/d, did not reduce hepatic choline concentration but reduced PCho concentration to 48% of normal, betaine concentration to 55% of normal and Adomet concentration to 75% of normal.

3. The methyl group deficiency and MTX in combination gave results similar to results with the deficiency alone except that the increase in hepatic triglycerides (5 times normal) and the reduction of Adomet concentration (33% of normal) were much more marked.

VI. Roles of Methyl Metabolism in Liver and Mammary Gland Carcinogenesis

The extent to which disturbance of folate metabolism by MTX causes changes characteristic of methyl group deficiency depends, in part, upon the level of DNA synthesis in the target tissue. It has been emphasized recently that the effect of dihydrofolate reduction inhibitors (such as MTX) on tetrahydrofolate (THF)-dependent pathways (including methionine synthesis) may not be significant in cells not synthesizing thymidylate and DNA. Only in thymidylate synthesis is THF not regenerated.[45] This fact probably accounts for the greater reduction in Adomet and increase in triglycerides in deficient rats given MTX than in rats given either treatment alone, since the deficiency increases hepatocyte turnover. Reduction of-THF and 5-me-THF by MTX was enhanced in methyl-deficient rats.[27]

In the carcinogenesis study[39] weanling male, Sprague-Dawley rats were fed control (C) or methyl group-deficient (D) diet for 3 weeks and then given PCZ, 25 mg/kg, MTX, 0.2 mg/kg, the 2 drugs together or isotonic saline only by intraperitoneal injection, 2 or 3 days per week for 14 weeks. After 5 weeks of drug treatment a sample of rats was killed, and their livers were assayed for choline, PCho, and betaine. The PCZ-treated deficient rats had increased hepatic choline (17-fold increase) and doubled PCho. In rats fed control diet, PCZ again doubled PCho, but choline increased only 1.5 times. The addition of MTX to PCZ treatment in rats fed control diet enhanced the effect of PCZ, tripling hepatic choline content while still doubling PCho (Table 2).

In the rats treated for 14 weeks PCZ-induced mammary tumor incidence was increased 50–70% in deficient or MTX-treated rats compared to rats given control diet and PCZ only (Table 3). The cumulative probability for mammary tumor was significantly increased in deficient PCZ-treated rats, compared to rats fed control diet ($p = 0.05$), and was increased, but not significantly, by MTX. Tumor numbers were significantly increased in both deficient and MTX-treated rats

TABLE 2
Hepatic Choline and Phosphocholine in Male Procarbazine (PCZ)-Treated Rats[39]

Diet Group	PCZ	Hepatic[a] Choline	Hepatic[a] Phosphocholine
Control	-	0.7 ± 0.3	6.7 ± 1.8
	+	1.0 ± 0.6	14.7 ± 10.2
Deficient	-	0.2 ± 0.05	2.1 ± 0.7
	+	4.0 ± 2.4[b]	4.8 ± 2.0

[a] nmol/mg protein
[b] Significantly greater than deficient diet alone, $P < 0.01$

TABLE 3
Mammary Gland Tumors in Male and Female PCZ[a]-treated Sprague-Dawley Rats[39,50]

Diet	MTX[b]	Mammary gland tumors % Incidence		No./Rat	
		Males	Females	Males	Fe-males
Control	-	30	66	1.6	2.6
	+	49	70	1.7	3.2
Deficient	-	48	78	1.9	4.0

[a] Total dose: 790 mg/kg (males) and 300 mg/kg (females)
[b] Methotrexate, 0.2 mg/kg, in addition to PCZ

($p < 0.005$). Leukemia and lymphoma incidence were not affected by the deficiency or by MTX.[39]

Since MTX is one component of adjuvant drug regimens used to treat breast cancer,[48,49] its effect on mammary carcinogenesis is of great interest and was investigated further. In a second study, the same hypotheses were tested in female rats, with the addition that several levels of methyl deficiency were induced, and a diet that contained more choline and methionine than are required was tested also. Histopathologic examination of tumors is still in progress; the results for methyl deficiency using gross tumor data appear similar to the results in male rats. The differences between groups are smaller, presumably because females are less susceptible than males to the deficiency, but there is evidence that tumorigenesis is inversely related to dietary methyl supply when that supply is deficient to adequate.[50] In contrast to the result with male rats, MTX did not appear to alter PCZ carcinogenesis in female rats. It is not clear whether hypersupplementation with methionine and choline had an effect.

Another attempt to reduce carcinogenesis by hypersupplementation of diet with lipotropes has been reported recently. In that study mice were fed a nutritionally complete diet with or without added methionine and choline and given DEN. There was some reduction in liver tumors in association with choline hypersupplementation, but it was not significant. The authors suggested that it may have been, at least in part, the result of reduced weight gain in supplemented mice.[51]

PCZ forms methyl adducts with DNA via its methyldiazonium metabolite.[52-55] PCZ is activated by microsomal, xenobiotic-metabolizing enzymes with formation of methyl-DNA adducts in liver [52] and white blood cells.[54,55] The activiy of DNA methyltransferases is, presumably, of significance in determining the rate and extent of DNA repair. While changes in hepatic tRNA and protein methylases in methyl-deficient rats have been reported,[56] changes in DNA methyltransferase have not been reported.

Mammary gland epithelium concentrates choline and folate from the blood and secretes milk containing large amounts of folate bound to folate-binding proteins [28] and large amounts of choline.[57] The gland can also synthesize choline.[58] It seems likely that the gland would be sensitive to diet- or drug-induced perturbations of methyl metabolism.

The female rat gland is much more sensitive to PCZ carcinogenesis than the male gland (Table 3). Both showed a similar response enhancement of carcinogenesis with reduction in dietary methyl groups. It is important to obtain information on methyl metabolism in the gland itself and to examine the stages of mammary carcinogenesis under the experimental conditions used in the PCZ carcinogenesis studies. If the mammary gland, like the liver, shows interference by PCZ in choline metabolism, the results will be signifcant mechanistically.

References

1. Follis, R.H., Choline, in *Deficiency Disease,* Charles C. Thomas, Springfield, Illinois, 1958, 251.

2. Newberne, P.M., Lipotropic factors and oncogenesis, in *Essential Nutrients in Carcinogenesis*, Poirier, L.A., Newberne, P.M. and Pariza, M.W., Eds., Plenum Press, New York, 1986, 223.

3. Tucker, M.A., Coleman, C.N., Cox, R.S., Varghese, A., and Rosenberg, S.A., Risk of second cancers after treatment for Hodgkin's disease, *N. Engl. J. Med.,* 318, 76, 1988.

4. Kaldor, J.M., Nicholas, E.D., Pettersson, F., Clarke, E.A., Pedersen, D., Mehnert, W., Bell, J., Host, H., Prior, P., Karjalainen, S., Neal, F., Koch, M., Band, P., Choi, W., Pompe Kirn, V., Arslan, A., Zaren, B., Belch, A-R., Strom, H., Kittelmann, B., Fraser, P., and Stovall M., Leukemia following chemotherapy for ovarian cancer, *N. Engl J. Med,* 322, 1, 1990.

5. Kaldor, J.M., Day, N.E., Clarke, E.A., VanLeeuwen, F.E., Henry-Amar, M., Fiorentino, M.V., Bell, J., Pedersen, D., Band, P., Assouline, D., Koch, M., Choi, W., Prior, P., Blain, V., Langmark, F., Pompe Kirn, V., Neal, F., Peters, D., Pfeiffer, R., Karjalainen, S., Cuzick, J., Sutcliffe, S., Somers, R., Pellae-Cosset, B., Pappagallo, G.L, Fraser, P., Strom, H., and Stovall, M., Leukemia following Hodgkin's disease, *N. Engl. J. Med,* 322, 7, 1990.

6. Lavey, R.S., Eby, N.L., and Prosnitz, L.R., Impact on second malignancy risk of the combined use of radiation and chemotherapy for lymphomas, *Cancer,* 66, 80, 1990.

7. Rogers, A.E. and Conner, M.W. Alcohol and cancer, in *The Role of Essential Nutrients in Carcinogenesis,* Poirier, L., Newberne, P. and Pariza, M., Eds., Plenum Press, New York, 1987, 473.

8. Rogers, A.E. and Conner, M.W., Interrelationships of alcohol and cancer, in *Human Nutrition: A Comprehensive Treatise,* Alfin-Slater, R.B. and Kritchevsky, D., Eds., Plenum Press, New York, 1990.

9. Zeisel, S.H., Choline deficiency, *J. Nutr. Biochem.*, 1, 332, 1990.

10. Rogers, A.E. and Newberne, P.M., Lipotrope deficiency in experimental carcinogenesis, *Nutrition and Cancer,* 2, 104, 1980.

11. Rogers, A.E., Dietary effects on chemical carcinogenesis in the liver of rats, in *Rat Hepatic Neoplasia,* Newberne, P. and Butler, W.H., Eds., The MIT Press, Cambridge, Massachusetts and London, England, 1978,242.

12. Mikol, Y.G., Hoover, J.L., Creasia, D., and Poirier, L.A., Hepatocarcinogenesis in rats fed methyl-deficient amino acid-defined diets, *Carcinogenesis,* 4, 1619, 1983.

13. Chandar, N., Lombardi, B., and Locker, J., C-myc gene amplification during hepatocarcinogenesis by a choline-devoid diet, *Proc. Natl. Acad. Sci. USA,* 86, 2703, 1989.

14. Sawada, N., Poirier, L., Moran, S., Xu, Y.H., and Pitot, H.C., The effect of choline and methionine deficiencies on the number and volume percentage of altered hepatic foci in the presence or absence of diethylnitrosamine initiation in rat liver, *Carcinogenesis,* 11, 273, 1990.

15. Eto, J. and Krumdieck, C.L., Role of vitamin B_{12} and folate deficiencies in carcinogenesis, in *Essential Nutrients in Carcinogenesis,* Poirier, L.A., Newberne, P.M., and Pariza, M.W., Eds., Plenum Press, New York, 1986, 313.

16. Lashner, B.A., Heidenreich, P.A., Su, G.L, Kane, S.V., and Hanauer, S.B., The effect of folate supplementation on the incidence of dysplasia and cancer in chronic ulcerative colitis, *Gastroenterology,* 97, 255, 1989.

17. Branda, R.F., Moldow, C.F., and MacArthur, J.R., Folate-induced remission in aplastic anemia with familial defect of cellular folate uptake, *N. Engl. J. Med.,* 298, 469, 1978.

18. Butterworth, C.E., Hatch, K.D., Gore, H., Mueller, H., and Krumdieck, C.L., Improvement in cervical dysplasia associated with folic acid therapy in users of oral contraceptives, *Am. J. Clin. Nutr.,* 35, 73, 1982.

19. Rosenberg, I.H. and Mason, J.B., Folate, dysplasia, and cancer, *Gastroenterology,* 97, 502, 1989.

20. Gimsing, P., Melgaard, B., Andersen, K., Vilstrup, H., and Hippe, E., Vitamin B-12 and folate function in chronic alcoholic men with peripheral neuropathy and encephalopathy, *J. Nutr.,* 119, 416, 1989.

21. Chawla, R.K., Wolf, D.C, Kutner, M.H., and Bonkovsky, H.L., Choline may be an essential nutrient in malnourished patients with cirrhosis, *Gastroenterology,* 97, 1514, 1989.

22. Broxson, E.H., Stork, L.C., Allen, R.H., Stabler, S.P., and Kolhouse, J.F., Changes in plasma methionine and total homocysteine levels in patients receiving methotrexate infusions, *Cancer Research,* 49, 5879, 1989.

23. Rogers, A.E., Nutrition, in *The Laboratory Rat,* I., Baker, H.J., Lindsay, J.R. and Weisbroth, S.H., Eds., Academic Press, New York, 1979, chap. 6.

24. Newberne, P.M., Rogers, A.E., Bailey, C., and Young, V.R., The induction of liver cirrhosis in rats by purified amino acid diets, *Cancer Research,* 29, 230, 1969.

25. Finkelstein, J.D., Methionine metabolism in mammals, *J. Nutr. Biochem.,* 1, 228, 1990.

26. Vance, J.E., Lipoprotein assembly and secretion by hepatocytes, *Annu. Rev. Nutr.,* 10, 337, 1990.

27. Selhub, J., Soyum, E., Pomfret, E.A., and Zeisel, S.H., Effects of choline deficiency and methotrexate treatment upon liver folate content and distribution, in press, 1990.

28. Henderson, G.B., Folate-binding proteins, *Annu. Rev. Nutr.,* 103, 19, 1990.

29. Ames, B.N. and Gold, L.S., Too many rodent carcinogens: Mitogenesis increases mutagenesis, *Science,* 249, 970, 1990.

30. Cohen, S.M. and Ellwein, L.B., Cell proliferation in carcinogenesis, *Science,* 249, 1007, 1990.

31. Rogers, A.E. and Newberne, P.M., Aflatoxin B_1 carcinogenesis in lipotrope-deficient rats, *Cancer Res.,* 29, 1965, 1969.

32. Lutz, W.K., Dose-response relationship and low dose extrapolation in chemical carcinogenesis, *Carcinogenesis,* 11, 1243, 1990.

33. Schrager, T.F., Newberne, P.M., Pikul, A.H., and Groopman, J.D., Aflatoxin-DNA adduct formation in chronically dosed rats fed a choline-deficient diet, *Carcinogenesis,* 11, 177, 1990.

34. Wainfan, E., Dizik, M., Stender, M., and Christman, J.K., Rapid appearance of hypomethylated DNA in livers of rats fed cancer-promoting, methyl-deficient diets, *Cancer Res.*, 49, 4094, 1989.

35. Poirier, L.A., Zapisek, W.F., Cronin, G.M., and Lyn-Cook, B.D., Oncogene hypomethylation in the livers of rats led methyl-deficient, amino acid-defined diets, *Proc. Amer. Assoc. for Cancer Res.,* 31, 142, 1990.

36. Pascale, R., Daino, L., Simile, M., Ruggiu, M., Cozzolino, P., Satta, G., Vannini, G., Lai, P., and Feo, F., Lipotrope content, DNA methylation and protooncogene expression in rat liver during the early stages of tumor promotion, *Proc. Amer. Assoc. for Cancer Res.*, 31, 154, 1990.

37. Poirier, L.A. and Whitehead, V.U., Folate deficiency and formiminoglutamic acid excretion during chronic diethylnitrosamine administration to rats, *Cancer Res.*, 33, 383, 1973.

38. Hoover, K.L, Hyde, C.L., Wenk, M.L, and Poirier, L.A., Ethionine carcinogenesis in CD-1, BALB/c and C3H mice, *Carcinogenesis*, 7, 1143, 1986.

39. Rogers, A.E., Akhtar, R., and Zeisel, S.H., Procarbazine carcinogenicity in methotrexate-treated or lipotrope-deficient male rats, *Carcinogenesis*, 11, in press, 1990.

40. Andry, C.D., Kupchik, H.Z., and Rogers, A.E., L-azaserine induced preneoplasia in the rat pancreas. A morphometric study of dietary manipulation (lipotrope deficiency) and ultrastructural differentiation, *Toxicologic Pathol.*, 18, 10, 1990.

41. Wiernik, P.H., Chemotherapy of hodgkins disease, in *Cancer Principles and Practice of Onocology*, 2nd ed., De Vita, V.T., Hellman, S., and Rosenberg, J.A., Eds., J.B. Lippincott Company, Philadelphia, update, 1988, 1.

42. IARC, *IARC Monographs* on the Evaluation of the carcinogenic risk of chemicals to humans: Some antineoplastic and immunosuppressive agents, vol. 26, 1981.

43. Adamson, R.H. and Sieber, S.M., Studies on the oncogenicity of procarbazine and other compounds in nonhuman primates, in *Malignant Lymphomas*, Vol. 3, Rosenberg, S. and Kaplan, H., Eds., Academic Press, San Diego, 1982, 239.

44. IARC, *IARC Monographs* on the Evaluation of carcinogenic risk, Suppl. 7, vol. 241, 1988.

45. Schweitzer, B.I., Dicker, A.P., and Bertino, J.R., Dihydrofolate reductase as a therapeutic target, *FASEB J.*, 4, 2441, 1990.

46. Pomfret, E.A., daCosta, K.A., and Zeisel, S.H., Effects of choline deficiency and methotrexate treatment upon rat liver, *J. Nutr. Biochem.*, 1, 505, 1990.

47. Zeisel, S.H., Zola, T., daCosta, K.A., and Pomfret, E.A., Effect of choline deficiency on S-adenosylmethionine and methionine concentrations in rat liver, *Biochem. J.*, 259, 725, 1989.

48. Fisher, B., Redmond, C., Dimitrov, N.V., Bowman, D., Legault-Poisson, S., Wickerham, D.L., Wolmark, N., Fisher, E.R., Margolese, R., Sutherland, C., Glass, A., Foster, R., Caplan, R., and others, A randomized clinical trial evaluating sequential methotrexate and fluorouracil in the treatment of patients with node-negative breast cancer who have estrogen-receptor-negative tumors, *N. Engl. J. Med.*, 320, 473, 1989.

49. Ludwig Breast Cancer Study Group, Combination adjuvant chemotherapy for node-positive breast cancer, *New Engl. J. Med*, 319, 677, 1988.

50. Akhtar, R. and Rogers, A.E., Modulation of procarbazine-induced mammary carcinogenesis in female rats by dietary lipotropes, in *Vitamins and Minerals in the*

Prevention and Treatment of Cancer, Jacobs, M.M., Ed., CRC Press, Inc., Boca Raton, FL, 1991.

51. Fullerton, F.R., Hoover, K, Mikol, Y.B., Creasia, D.A., and Poirier, L.A., The inhibition by methionine and choline of liver carcinoma formation in male C3H mice dose with diethylnitrosamine and fed phenobarbital, *Carcinogenesis*, 11, 1301, 1990.

52. Wiestler, O.D., Kleihues, P., Rice, J.M., Ivankovic, S., DNA methylation in maternal, fetal and neonatal rat tissues following perinatal administration of procarbazine, *J. Cancer Res. Clin. Oncol.*, 108, 56, 1984.

53. Erikson, J.M., Tweedie, D.J., Ducore, J.M., and Prough, R.A., Cytotoxicity and DNA damage caused by the azoxy metabolites of procarbazine in L1210 tumor cells, *Cancer Res.*, 49, 127, 1989.

54. Swaffar, D.S., Harker, W.G., Pomerantz, S., Nelson, C., and Yost, G.S., In vitro bioactivation of procarbazine to cytotoxic species in human leukemia cells, *Proc. Amer. Assoc. for Cancer Res.*, 31, 384, 1990.

55. Souliotis, V.L., Kaila, S., Boussiotis, V.A., Pangalis, G.A., and Kyrtopoulos, S.A., Accumulation of O^6-methylguanine in human blood leukocyte DNA during exposure to procarbazine and its relationships with dose and repair, *Cancer Res.*, 50, 2759, 1990.

56. Wainfan, E., Kilkenny, M., and Dizik, M., Comparison of methyltransferase activities of pair-fed rats given adequate or methyl-deficient diets, *Carcinogenesis*, 9, 861, 1988.

57. Chao, C., Pomfret, E.A., and Zeisel, S.H., Uptake of choline by rat mammary-gland epithelial cells, *Biochem. J.*, 254, 33, 1988.

58. Yang, E.K., Blusztajn, J.K., Pomfret, E.A., and Zeisel, S.H., Rat and human mammary tissue can synthesize choline moiety via the methylation of phosphatidylethanolamine, *Biochem. J.*, 256, 821, 1988.

59. Blusztain, J.K. and Zeisel, S.H., 1,2-sn-Diacylglycerol accumulates in choline-deficient liver: A possible mechanism of hepatic carcinogenesis via alteration in protein kinase C activity, *FEBS Letters*, 243, 267, 1989.

60. Singh, U., Yokota, K., Gupta, C., and Shinozuka, H., Choline deficiency activates phospholipases A_2 and C in rat liver without affect the activity of protein kinase C, *J. Nutr. Biochem.*, 1, 434, 1990.

Chapter 11

Effects of Folic Acid Deficiency on Tumor Cell Biology

Richard F. Branda

Table of Contents

I. Introduction

Folic acid is a vitamin which is found most abundantly in green leafy vegetables, liver, navy beans, nuts and whole wheat products.[1] Medical interest in this substance derived from an observation in 1931 that extracts of yeast or liver effectively treated tropical macrocytic anemia.[2] The structure of folic acid was elucidated a decade later.[2] The medicinal form of the vitamin, folic acid, consists of an oxidized pteridine ring, p-aminobenzoic acid and glutamic acid moieties. Naturally occurring coenzyme forms of the vitamin typically are reduced at the pteridine ring and contain multiple glutamic acid residues.[3]

Dietary insufficiency or decreased intestinal absorption of folate compounds eventually leads to a deficiency syndrome which clinically is most evident in the bone marrow, but all dividing cells are affected. The hallmark of the disease is megaloblastic changes in bone marrow precursor cells. The cells are large with a characteristic delay in nuclear compared to cytoplasmic maturation. There is evidence of ineffective erythropoiesis, in that the bone marrow is hypercellular but the reticulocyte count is low, and there are varying degrees of pancytopenia. Cytologic abnormalities resembling megaloblastosis can be identified in epithelial cells from the uterine cervix, mouth, stomach and intestine.[4]

Surveys have found evidence of poor folic acid nutrition in several population groups.[5,6] Pregnant women, adolescents, alcoholic subjects and individuals from lower socio-economic groups are particularly susceptible.[5,6] Abnormally low blood folate levels also have been reported in cancer patients. For example, Magnus described low serum folate levels in 85% of a series of patients with metastatic cancer, and Somayaji and colleagues found that serum folate was low in 11 of 18 patients.[7,8] This deficiency may occur because of decreased dietary intake and increased utilization of the vitamin by rapidly dividing tumor cells.[8] While replacement therapy with folic acid is usually indicated when deficiency is detected, treatment of folic acid deficiency in cancer patients is controversial because of concerns about possible promotion of tumor growth.

This uncertainty about the potential risks and benefits of folic acid administration to cancer patients spans nearly half a century. Initial reports in the early 1940's describing the use of newly purified folate compounds to treat tumors were optimistic. Leuchtenberger and colleagues found that an oxidized folate triglutamate inhibited the growth of sarcoma 180 and breast cancers in mice.[10] In 1947, Farber *et al.* reported that the same pteroyltriglutamic acid, when administered to patients with a variety of advanced malignant diseases, produced beneficial effects, including improved energy, appetite and sense of well being.[11] However, a year later Farber noted that children with leukemia who received folic acid conjugates (pteroylglutamic acid and pteroyldiglutamic acid) suffered an "acceleration phenomenon."[12] This observation led to the development and clinical testing of folic acid antagonists as chemotherapeutic agents.[12]

Subsequent studies in rodents indicated that nutritional deficiency of folic acid retarded the growth of ascitic lymphocytic neoplasms in mice and Walker carcinosarcoma 256 in rats.[13,14] Interpretation of these experiments is confounded by the fact that the animals on the folate deficient diets progressively lost weight, while the control animals gained and then maintained their weight. Since caloric restriction or treatments which prevent weight gain also impair tumor growth,[14] the restriction of tumor cell progression observed in these experiments may not have been due to folate deficiency alone. Attempts to extend this possible anti-tumor effect of nutritional folate deficiency to humans with cancer were disappointing. Gailani and colleagues found that they were able to reduce blood, liver and tumor levels of folic acid in patients with advanced malignancy with a folate deficient diet. Unfortunately, no antitumor effect was noted.[15]

Following Farber's seminal observations with folate antagonists in acute leukemia, numerous investigators have studied the effects of these drugs on the intermediary metabolism of folate compounds and on tumor cell biology. The impact of nutritionally induced folate deficiency on these processes has received much less attention. While there are many similarities between the effects of folate antagonists and nutritional folate deficiency on cellular metabolism, they are not congruent. For example, methotrexate treatment raises levels of dihydrofolate polyglutamates and inhibits AICAR, thereby blocking purine metabolism, an effect not seen with nutritional folate deficiency.[16] Further supporting the idea that folate antagonists and nutritional deficiency have differing effects on tumor cells are our observations that even the most stringent conditions of folate deficiency resulted in only an approximately 90% loss of viability in Chinese Hamster Ovary (CHO) cells,[17] while methotrexate treatment produced essentially total kill of either CHO or B16 melanoma cells at concentrations greater than 0.1 μM (unpublished data). In view of these differences, this review will focus primarily on the effects of nutritional folate deficiency on tumor cell biology.

II. Effects of Nutritional Folate Deficiency on Some Aspects of Tumor Cell Biology

A. Proliferation

Optimal Friend erythroleukemia cell replication occurs when adequate levels of exogenous folate monoglutamate and intracellular folate polyglutamates are available.[18] Supplementation with additional folate above these levels does not shorten the cell doubling time.[18] In the setting of low or absent exogenous folate, proliferation is accompanied by a progressive halving of intracellular folate levels. Eventually the folate supply is diluted among the progeny, folate deficiency develops, and tumor cell doubling time lengthens.[18] The number of potential duplications is proportional to the intracellular polyglutamyl folate levels.[18]

Murine B16 melanoma cells cultured in low-folate medium (0.26 ng/ml) proliferate at the same rate as cells in folate replete medium for 3 days (Figure 1). At that time, deoxyuridine suppression of exogenous thymidine incorporation, a measure of intracellular folate activity, becomes abnormal.[19] Continued culture in low folate medium completely inhibits cellular proliferation (Figure 2). If, however, these folate deficient cells are transferred to folate-containing medium, replication resumes at approximately the same rate as in melanoma cells which have never been folate deficient (Figure 2). This observation suggests that reversal of folate deficiency does not accelerate the growth of tumor cells. It merely permits growth-arrested cells to recommence replication. This interpretation was confirmed by an *in vivo* experiment. Murine melanoma cells were incubated for 3 days in either low-folate or complete medium. The cells were

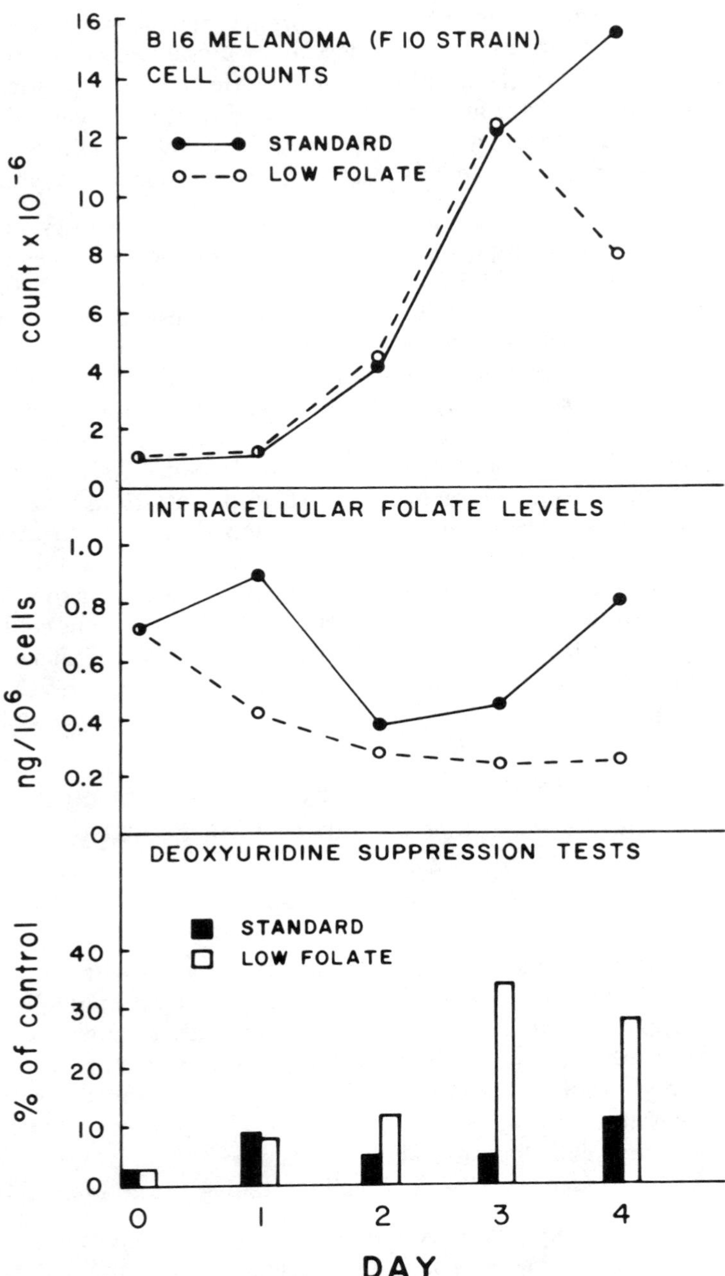

Figure 1. Changes in intracellular folate levels and activity during incubation of murine melanoma cells in low-folate medium and the same medium supplemented with folic acid (standard medium).

Top panel. Melanoma cells grown in low-folate medium (open circles) replicate at the same rate as control cells (closed circles) during the first 3 days in culture.

Middle panel. Intracellular folate levels, assayed by the *Lactobacillus casei* method, drop steadily in tumor cells incubated in low-folate medium during the first 3 days.

Bottom panel. The deoxyuridine suppression test, a measure in folate coenzyme activity, becomes abnormal after 3 days of growth in low-folate medium.

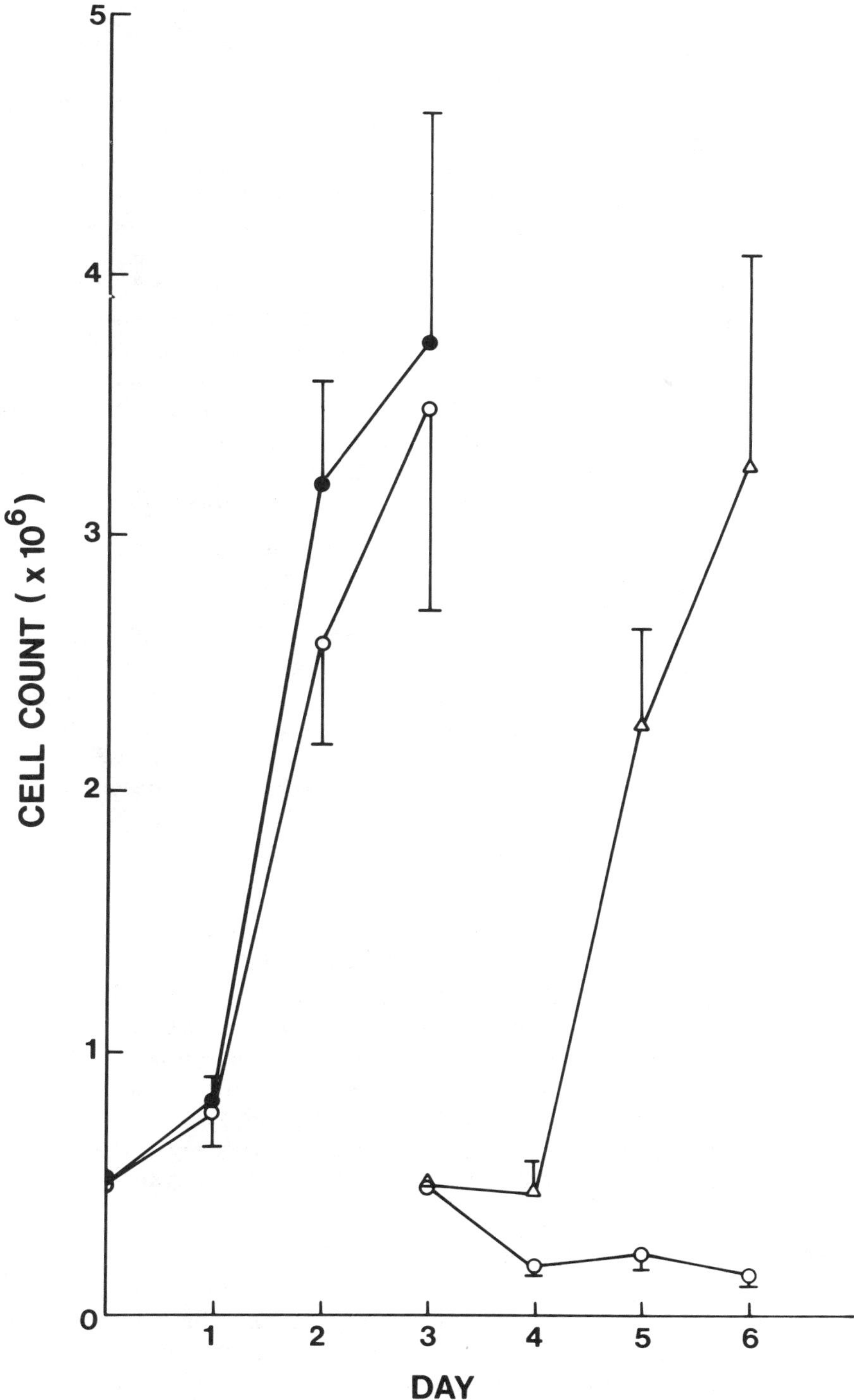

Figure 2. Effect of incubation in low-folate medium on melanoma cell proliferation. Murine B16 (F10 strain) melanoma cells were cultured in folate containing medium (closed circles) or low-folate medium (open circles). After 3 days, cells from the low-folate medium were split and inoculated into either the same medium or into folate-replete medium (triangles). Points, mean of at least 6 determinations; bars, SEM.

then injected subcutaneously into normal mice. Growth rates were comparable for both types of cells.[19]

Similar results were obtained with CHO cells. In this experimental system, incubation of tumor cells for 3 days in low-folate medium lowers intracellular folate levels approximately tenfold.[17] At this time there is a modest decrease in replication rate and a lower saturation density compared to folate-replete cells. If, however, the cells are maintained in low-folate medium, population cell growth is markedly inhibited. Transfer of these cells to folate-containing medium, or medium supplemented with both hypoxanthine and thymidine, is accompanied by a resumption of proliferation at the same rate as cells which were never folate deficient. Hypoxanthine or thymidine added singly did not improve the poor growth of folate-deficient cells. This observation suggests that the anti-proliferative effect of nutritional folate deficiency is mediated through impairment of both purine and pyrimidine synthesis. Although the restrictive effects of folate deficiency on proliferation were initially reversible, prolonged inhibition eventually was accompanied by a decline in cell viability.[17]

Taken together, these observations with tumor cells suggest that an adequate supply of both exogenous and endogenous folate compounds is necessary for optimal tumor cell proliferation. Reduced availability of folates eventually restricts replication. Initially this restriction is reversible, but if folate deprivation is prolonged and severe, loss of cell viability results. However, the degree of cell killing is not as extensive as that which occurs with folate antagonists. If folate deficiency is corrected, and cell growth resumes, it is at approximately the same rate as in tumor cells which were never deprived of folate. No "acceleration phenomenon" was seen in these experimental systems.

B. Cell Size

Tumor cell size increases coincident with the development of folate deficiency. In murine melanoma cells, intracellular folate levels, as determined by the *Lactobacillus casei* assay, drops progressively and folate activity, when measured with the deoxyuridine suppression test, becomes abnormal after 3 days of culture (Figure 1).[19] In 7 experiments, the mean size of melanoma cells in low-folate medium increased from 9041 ± 1245 fl (mean ± SD) on day 2.5 of culture, to 13,419 ± 864 fl on day 3.5, and to 15,790 ± 906 fl by day 4.5. In contrast, tumor cells in folate-containing medium maintained approximately the same size in culture during this period: 8364 ± 1237 fl; 9718 ± 799 fl; and 8389 ± 956 fl, respectively.[20]

The effect of nutritional folate deficiency on cell size also was studied in CHO cells (Figure 3). Again, control cell populations maintained a nearly constant mean cell volume throughout the culture period. Tumor cells in low-folate medium increased progressively in size, to approximately double the volume of cells in folate-supplemented medium, until growth arrest occurred.[17] Addition of both thymidine and hypoxanthine permitted maintenance of normal cell size. However, addition of these nucleosides singly had dramatically different effects. Cells provided thymidine supplementation of low-folate medium retained a normal mean cell volume. However, addition of hypoxanthine to this medium resulted in cells which were more than 3 times larger than cells in medium containing folate or both hypoxanthine and thymidine (Figure 3).[17]

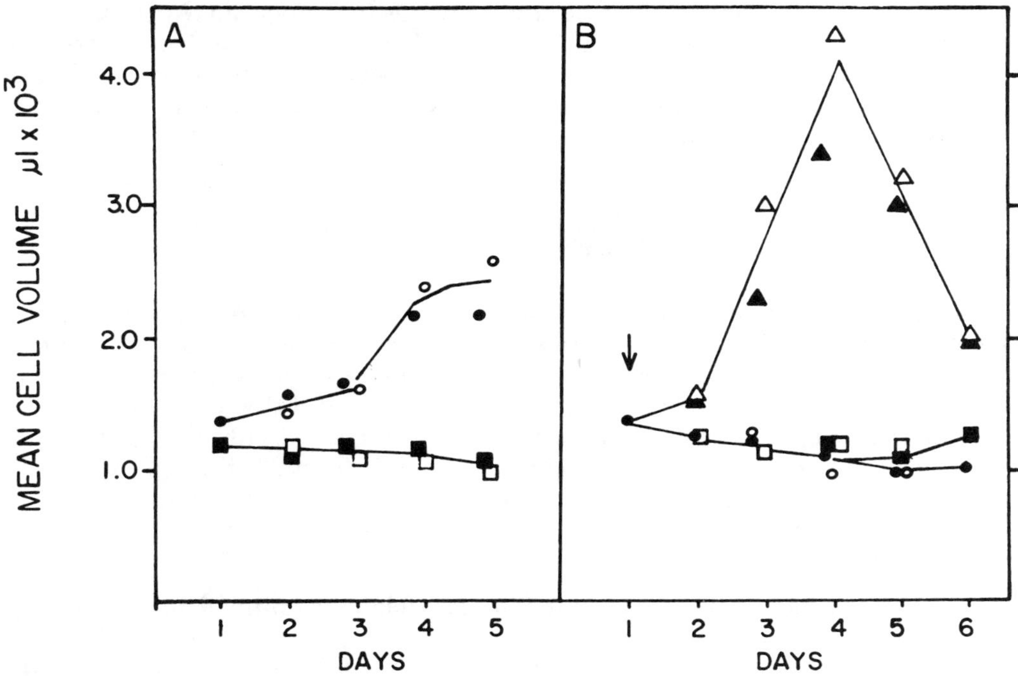

Figure 3. Mean cell volume of replated cultures.
A. CHO cells maintained in complete medium (boxes) or low-folate medium (circles).
B. Low-folate cultures, supplemented with 30 µM hypoxanthine (triangles), 3 µM thymidine (circles), or both precursors (squares).
The precursors were added to the cultures 24 hrs after seeding of the cells (arrow). The data plotted are averaged values from duplicate samples of each of two separate experiments (open and closed symbols).

These measurable changes in CHO cell size were accompanied by morphologic alterations. The cells in folate deficient medium were noticeably larger than cells in folate-supplemented medium. Addition of thymidine was associated with an elongated, spindle-shaped morphology, while cells grown in hypoxanthine-supplemented medium had a well spread cell shape and ruffled membrane surface.[17] Thus, thymidine supplementation ameliorated the effects of folate deficiency on cell size and morphology, while the addition of hypoxanthine exaggerated these alterations.

C. Cell Cycle Traverse

Measurement of DNA content in bone marrow cells from patients with megaloblastic anemias delineated an arrest of DNA synthesis and prolongation of the S and G2 phases of the cell cycle.[21] In addition, DNA synthesis continued beyond the point in cellular maturation (myelocyte stage) at which it normally terminates. Interestingly, the abnormalities occurred in only a proportion of cells. There were always some cells which passed normally through mitosis.[21] This observation is consistent with studies of the effects of folate deficiency on cellular proliferation and viability in tumor cells, which indicated that the deleterious sequelae were not ubiquitous.[17]

Murine melanoma cells incubated in low-folate medium demonstrated a progressive increase in the number of cells in S phase as folate deficiency developed, when studied by flow cytometry. After 3 days of incubation, approximately 25% of melanoma cells in low-folate medium had an accumulation of DNA synthesis in S phase, compared to approximately 10% of cells in folate-containing medium.[19] This accumulation became more striking on days 4 and 5 of culture.[19,20] If these folate deficient cells were transferred to folate-containing medium on day 3, they were able to resume DNA synthesis. One day later, their cell cycle distribution was essentially identical to tumor cells which had remained in complete medium. If, however, folate supplementation was delayed until day 5, the cells were unable to recover.[19] Cellular proliferation was impaired, and most cells were dead within 72 hours.

The effects of nutritional folate deficiency were studied in more detail in CHO cells. Confirming the findings with human bone marrow cells and murine melanoma cells, CHO cells showed an increase in the percentage of S phase cells coincident with the onset of folate deficiency (Figure 4). These folate deficient cells manifested an increased DNA and cellular protein content per cell during the period of S phase delay.[17] Persistent deficiency led to a delay in movement through S phase to cell division and population growth arrest.[17] These folate depleted cells could be rescued completely after 3 days of culture by adding folate or both thymidine and hypoxanthine to the medium. However, if the cells were maintained for a longer period of time under conditions of folate deprivation, DNA and protein contents and cell size increased, and viability declined. Thus, a transient delay in S phase progression was followed by irreversible changes in cellular proliferation.[17]

Addition of nucleosides singly to CHO cells in folate deficient medium resulted in strikingly different cell cycle distributions (Figure 4). Thymidine supplementation initially was associated with an essentially normal DNA distribu-

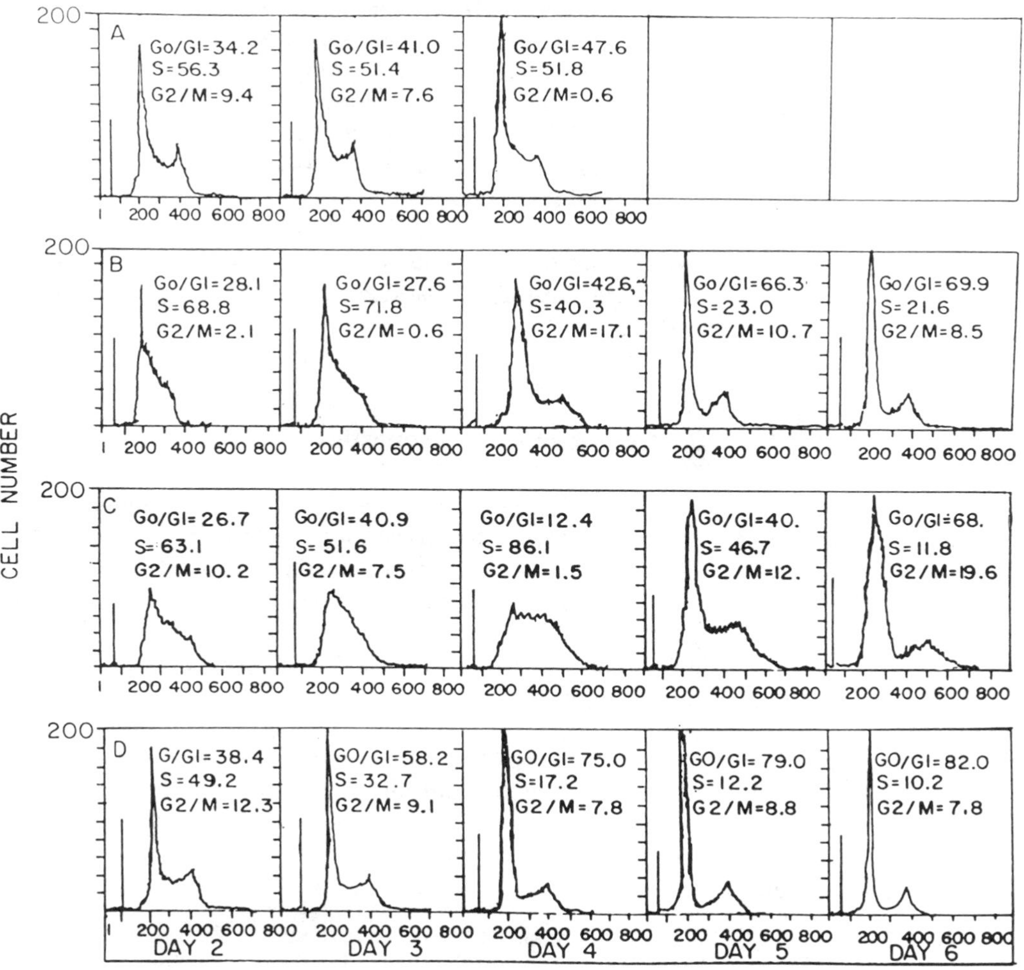

Figure 4. Red fluorescence histograms of the daily cellular DNA content of replated cultures grown in complete medium (A), or low-folate medium alone (B) or supplemented with 30 µM hypoxanthine (C) or 3 µM thymidine (D). The cell cycle distribution is presented for each population as quantitated by flow cytometry. Chick red blood cells were used as an internal standard and are represented as the first, sharp peak at about 50 fluorescence units. Data are from a single sample of a typical experiment.

tion, but more prolonged incubation in this folate and purine deficient medium produced a G0/G1 arrest. The relative DNA content of these cells was normal, while the cellular protein content was reduced.[17] These pyrimidine supplemented cells were best able to maintain viability.[17] In contrast, hypoxanthine supplementation of folate deficient cultures caused a remarkable increase in the number of cells in S phase, approaching 85% of the population. Eventually these cells re-established a near normal histogram, but this was associated with population growth arrest and greatly reduced viability.[17] These kinetic changes were accompanied by relative increases in cellular DNA and protein content.[17] Thus, in this experimental system pyrimidine supplementation tends to ameliorate, while purine addition exacerbates the abnormalities of cell cycle traverse and viability induced by folate deficiency.

D. Cell Membrane Properties

The onset of folate deficiency in tumor cells is accompanied by changes in the adhesive properties of the cells. Growth of murine melanoma cells in low-folate medium for longer than 2.5 days resulted in tumor cells which adhered more rapidly and in higher percentages to plastic or plastic dishes coated with laminin or fibronectin.[20] Although mean cell volume nearly doubled during a 4.5 day experimental period, the increase in adherence was not proportional. Cell doubling time likewise did not appear to correlate with adhesion, since folate deficient cells in both exponential and plateau phases of growth adhered more avidly than control cells. Consistent with this conclusion, there was no apparent relationship between the extent of accumulation of cells in S phase and the degree of adhesion. Therefore the changes in adhesive properties induced by folate deficiency probably are not mediated by changes in cell size, proliferative capacity or cell cycle distribution.

The adherence of CHO cells to the substratum was assayed with a trypsinization procedure.[17] Folate deficient cells required longer exposure periods or higher concentrations of trypsin to produce complete detachment from culture plates, compared to control cells in folate-supplemented medium. Nucleosides added singly modulated this membrane effect. The addition of hypoxanthine to folate deficient medium resulted in CHO cells which were very loosely adherent to the wells and were more easily detached than the control cells. In contrast, tumor cells grown in medium supplemented with thymidine were more tightly adherent than folate deficient cells, and less than half detached after prolonged incubation with standard (0.06%) concentrations of trypsin.[17]

The mechanism by which nutritional folate deficiency influences the membrane properties of tumor cells is unclear at present. Patients with severe megaloblastic anemia due to deficiencies of either folic acid or vitamin B12 have been reported to manifest decreased red cell filterability and an abnormal erythrocyte membrane pattern.[22,23] Dietary deficiency of folic acid in rats was associated with disorganization of cellular membranes and disruption of subcellular structures, particularly the mitochondria and rough endoplasmic reticulum.[24] The increased membrane adhesion observed in folate deficient tumor cells thus may reflect changes in membrane structure.

E. Chromosomes

1. **Karyotypic Abnormalities**. Cytogenetic analyses of bone marrow cells and peripheral blood lymphocytes from patients with megaloblastic anemia due to either vitamin B12 or folate deficiency have found that chromosomal abnormalities are frequent and diverse. In general, the extent of chromosomal aberrations and the severity of the megaloblastic changes are proportional.[25] Chromosome breakage is prominent. Gaps or breaks involving one or more chromatids and chromosomes, acentric fragments and dicentric forms occur in up to a third of metaphases.[21,25-27] Numerical chromosomal abnormalities and translocations are uncommon.[21,27] A second frequently encountered finding is thin, elongated chromosomes resulting from decreased contraction or despiralization.[21,25,27] In one series, despiralization of chromosomes was present in 40-70% of bone marrow metaphases and in 25-55% of lymphocyte metaphases from megaloblastic anemia patients.[27] A third type of chromosomal abnormality reported in these patients is centromere spreading, with centromeric constrictions of exaggerated size.[21,25,27] The centromere regions are widely spread, resulting in chromatid breaks.[27] All of these chromosomal abnormalities in bone marrow cells appeared to resolve promptly with vitamin replacement[21,25,27] but persisted in peripheral blood lymphocytes for as long as 12 months after hematological remission.[27]

Chromosomal changes in CHO cells induced by folate deficiency resembled those found in cells from patients with megaloblastic anemia. Approximately 20% of mitoses from folate deficient cells had chromosomal damage, compared to about 3% in control cells.[28] Nearly half of the aberrations were gaps, breaks and fragments of the chromatid type. Triradial and quadriradial exchanges and ring chromosomes were found commonly. Sixty percent of abnormal mitoses contained decondensed or allocyclic chromosomes.[28] These were either decondensed regions of individual chromosomes or of whole chromosomes. Most were typical of G2 chromosomes, but some decondensed chromosomes had G1 or S morphology.[28]

2. **Fragile Sites**. Chromosome gaps or breaks at specific sites can be induced by culture conditions used to prepare samples for cytogenetic analysis. The best characterized of these is a heritable fragile site at the end of the long arm of the X chromosome at Xq28. This chromosomal abnormality is associated with X-linked mental retardation and distinctive physical anomalies grouped together in the Fragile X Syndrome.[29,30] In 1979, Sutherland noted that incubation of cells from affected individuals in medium deficient in folic acid and thymidine increased expression of the fragile site.[31] Further studies in his laboratory and by others showed that the addition of methotrexate or fluorodeoxyuridine (a thymidylate synthetase inhibitor) to folate-containing medium also increased expression, while supplementation of low-folate medium with folinic acid or the thymidine analog bromodeoxyuridine suppressed expression of the fragile site.[31-33]

Most, but not all, heritable fragile sites are folate sensitive.[34] Deprivation of folic acid and thymidine can also enhance expression of "spontaneous" chromosome breaks, called by Yunis and Soreng constitutive fragile sites.[34] They reported that nearly half of heriditary and constitutive fragile sites map at or close to breakpoints found in human malignancies.[34] They suggested that a high expression of fragile sites may predispose to certain types of malignancies.[34] The results of subsequent studies have been conflicting. Some have supported an association between fragile sites and cancer chromosome breakpoints, while others have not.[35] Recent studies indicate that fragile site breakage caused by folate deficiency can lead to stable chromosome rearrangements.[36] Hecht and colleagues found that incubation of amniocytes in folate deficient medium was associated with an increased frequency of numerical and structural chromosome abnormalities. Breakage occurred at folate-sensitive fragile sites and led to nondisjunction and chromosome rearrangements.[36] While early cytogenetic analyses of cells from megaloblastic anemia patients indicated that the karyotypic changes were completely reversible with vitamin replacement, these studies by Hecht suggest that more subtle, stable abnormalities may persist. The potential contribution of chromosome rearrangements at fragile sites to the development of malignancies is unclear at present.

In the course of investigating folate metabolism in a kindred affected by the Fragile X syndrome, we found that the *in vitro* expression of the fragile site was strikingly reduced by treatment of the patients for one month with oral folic acid.[37] This finding is of potential clinical interest, since an inverse relationship between expression of the fragile site and IQ has been reported.[38] It also suggests that, if folate-sensitive fragile sites contribute to chromosomal rearrangements, the frequency of these abnormalities might be reduced by dietary supplementation with folic acid.

3. **Sister chromatid exchanges (SCE).** Interchanges of DNA, as measured by the rate of SCE, are more likely to occur in bone marrow cells and peripheral blood lymphocytes from patients with megaloblastic anemia.[39] Culture of lymphocytes from normal individuals in low-folate medium is associated with higher levels of SCEs.[37,40,41] While the nature of the DNA lesion which causes SCEs is not known, these interchanges are a sensitive indicator of mutagenesis. As was the case with the expression of fragile site Xq28, administration of oral folate for one month to patients was associated with a reduction in the frequency of SCEs. Therefore *in vivo* folate therapy can ameliorate two *in vitro* indices of chromosome damage.

4. **Double-stranded DNA breaks.** Nondenaturing elution of DNA from filters with time is a measure of DNA breaks. Elution rate is correlated with the number of double-stranded breaks. Incubation of human skin fibroblasts,[37] murine melanoma cells[19] or CHO cells (unpublished data) in folate deficient medium was associated with a more rapid rate of elution, indicating more strand breaks compared to cells in folate-supplemented medium. The effect became more pronounced with increasing severity of folate deficiency (Figure 5).[19]

5. **Nucleotide pool changes.** Direct evidence that DNA synthesis is impaired in folate deficient cells was provided by measurements showing that the migration of the DNA replication fork and the joining of Okazaki fragments are delayed. DNA molecules do not replicate continuously from one end to the other. They are subdivided into segments which have an origin and a terminus. The replicating fork is the point at which the two parental strands separate.[42] Within the replicating segments, synthesis occurs in short pieces approximately 50 to 150 nucleotides long called Okazaki fragments. These segments are joined together by removal of the RNA primer and gap-filling by further DNA synthesis.[42]

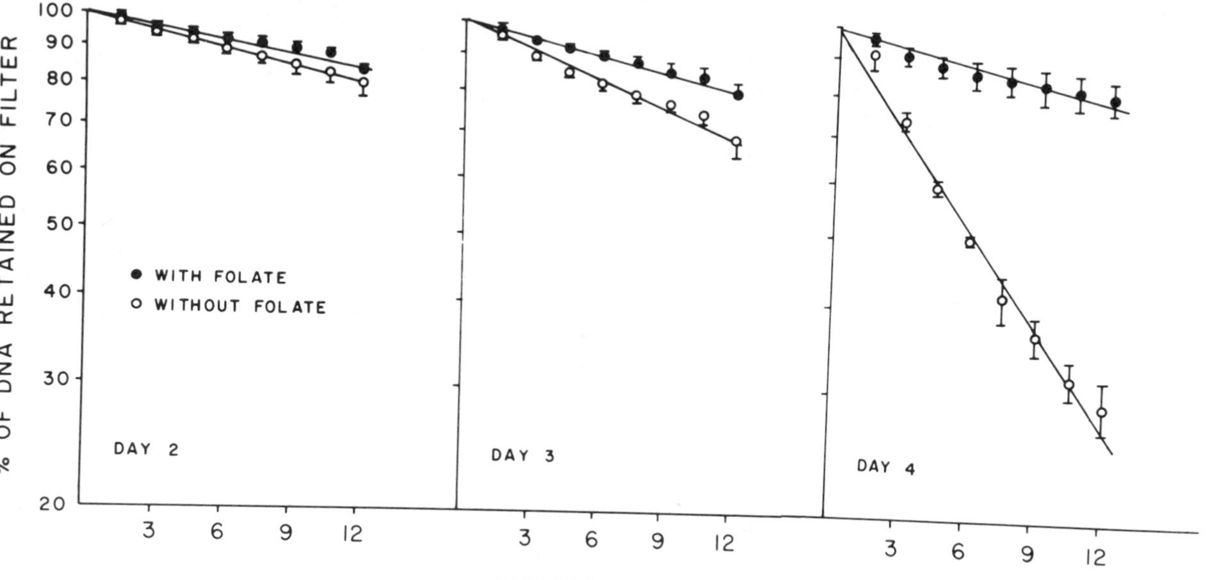

Figure 5. DNA strand breaks detected by alkaline filter elution in melanoma cells (F10 strain). Cells were cultured in folate-containing (closed circles) or low-folate (open circles) medium for the indicated number of days. Then cells were deposited on a filter and lysed, and the DNA eluted. At the indicated number of hours of elution, retention of radiolabeled DNA was determined. Points, mean of quadruplicate determinations; bars, SEM.

Mitogen-stimulated lymphocytes from patients with megaloblastic anemia due to folic acid or vitamin B12 deficiency were found to have retarded conversion of pulse-labeled DNA to full-sized DNA strands.[43] Replication fork rate was 40 to 92% of the rate in control cells.[44] The block in DNA maturation was not a permanent one, since continued incubation eventually resulted in full-sized strands. The investigators suggested that folate and vitamin B12 deficiencies primarily decreased "gap-filling" DNA synthesis, and that these incompletely replicated chromosomes were more likely to suffer breakage during mitosis.[42,43]

Since the folate coenzyme 5,10 methylene tetrahydrofolate is necessary for *de novo* thymidylate synthesis, it has been suggested that folate deficiency leads to a reduced availability of this nucleotide for DNA synthesis.[42] Studies with methotrexate demonstrated unbalanced deoxyribonucleotide synthesis in mitogen stimulated lymphocytes, with decreases in the dTTP pool and elevation of the dATP pool.[45] Other laboratories reported a substantial increase in the concentration of dUTP and a drop in dTTP in methotrexate treated lymphoid cells. It was suggested that cyclic incorporation and removal of dUMP during gap repair resulted in degradation of DNA and double strand breaks.[46]

Although a similar mechanism has been postulated to occur in folate deficiency, measurements of nucleotide pools in megaloblastic anemias have not found reduced amounts of dTTP.[47,48] There may, however, be functional compartmentalization of deoxyribonucleotide pools.[49] Because deoxynucleoside triphosphate pools are very small (it has been calculated that the pools can maintain DNA synthesis for only 30 seconds to 5 minutes), compartmentalization could quickly limit availability of dTTP for DNA replication.[50]

Deoxynucleotide pool imbalances might explain many of the chromosomal changes associated with folic acid deficiency. Thymine nucleotide deprivation in mammalian cells causes chromosome breaks and shattering, chromatid gaps, breaks and exchanges, chromosome aberrations including rings, dicentrics and quadriradial forms, and loss of viability.[51] Likewise, purine deoxynucleotide triphosphate excess or deprivation leads to DNA strand breakage, chromosome breaks and aberrations.[51] Alteration of nucleotide levels affects fragile site expression. Inhibition of thymidylate synthesis, depletion of dCTP, or elevation of uridine levels enhances expression of the rare folate-sensitive sites.[52] Common fragile sites, which are probably present in all individuals, are expressed more frequently in the setting of thymidylate stress or increased uridine levels.[52] Finally, nucleotide pool imbalances are mutagenic and increase the sensitivity of cells to mutagenic agents.[50]

Because of these reported interactions of folic acid deficiency, nucleotide pool imbalances and chromosomal damage, we became interested in studying these effects more directly. CHO cells were incubated in low-folate medium alone or this medium supplemented with hypoxanthine or thymidine singly. In this experimental system the addition of hypoxanthine greatly reduced the frequency of damaged mitoses and of decondensed chromosomes.[28] Thymidine supplementation affected neither the frequency nor the type of chromosomal damage. Thus purine, rather than pyrimidine, lack appears to have more influence on the chromosomal instability induced by nutritional folate deficiency. This finding was rather surprising, in that hypoxanthine supplementation tended to exaggerate, while thymidine addition ameliorated, the effects of folate deficiency on cellular phenotype and viability.[17] These diverse effects of folate deficiency and nucleoside supplementation on CHO cells are summarized semi-quantitatively in Table 1.

TABLE 1
Changes in CHO Cell Characteristics Following Growth in Low-Folate Medium Alone or the Same Medium Supplemented with Thymidine (+ dT) or Hypoxanthine (+ Hx)[a]

	Control	Low Folate	+dT	+Hx
Restricted growth	0	++	++	++
Cell size	+	++	+	++++
Adherence	++	+++	++++	+
S phase arrest	0	++	0	++++
Viability	++++	++	+++	+
Protein content	++	+++	+	++++
Chromosome damage	+	++++	++++	++

[a] Control cells were incubated in low-folate medium with added folic acid. Changes were graded semi-quantitatively on a scale of 0 to 4+.

These observations suggest that at least some types of chromosomal defects induced by nutritional folate deficiency are differentially sensitive to perturbations of nucleotide pools. This may be of clinical relevance because tumor and progenitor cells vary in their capacity to utilize *de novo* and salvage pathways for nucleosides. Thus, undifferentiated tumor cells and early hematopoietic cells appear to rely on salvage of pyrimidine nucleotides and *de novo* synthesis of purines, while cellular differentiation is characterized by increased *de novo* synthesis of pyrimidines and salvage of "higher" purines.[53] Cells which are folate deficient, with resultant impairment of *de novo* nucleotide synthesis, would salvage purines or pyrimidines to a different extent depending upon their stage of differentiation. This could lead to further imbalances of nucleotide pools and perhaps contribute to the type of chromosome damage found in our cultures. We postulate, therefore, that folate deficiency may represent a specialized case of the more general phenomenon of chromosomal instability induced by nucleotide pool imbalances.

III. Effects of Nutritional Folate Deficiency on Metastatic Potential

One of the most devastating characteristics of a malignancy is its ability to spread, since most patients succumb as a result of metastases to distant organs. Current evidence suggests that only a minority of the cells in a primary tumor express the constellation of phenotypic traits required to complete the many steps in the metastatic process.[54] These include: detachment from the primary mass; penetration into lymphatics or blood vessels; transport and interaction with host platelets, lymphocytes and other blood elements; arrest in a capillary bed; adherence to endothelium and extracellular matrix; extravasation; proliferation;

and vascularization.[54] Folic acid deficiency alters tumor cell properties which may be relevant to one or more of these steps.

To test the possibility that nutritional folate deficiency influences metastatic potential, murine B16 melanoma cell strains of high (F10) and low (F1) metastatic potential were grown in specially formulated folate-deficient Eagle's medium.[19] After 3 days in culture, these cells consistently developed characteristics of folate deficiency: restricted proliferation, increased size, S phase arrest, and impaired deoxyuridine suppression.[19]

These folate deficient and control melanoma cells were injected into the tail veins of normal host mice. Pigmented metastases were scored after 10 to 14 days. Cells from the high metastatic potential F10 line produced an average of 90 pulmonary metastases but no hepatic metastases (Figure 6). In contrast, folate deficient cells produced an average of 394 pulmonary metastases, a highly significant difference. Although the number of liver metastases was low, 9 of 11 animals injected with folate deficient cells had at least one metastasis, and this difference from control cells was also statistically significant.

Similar results were obtained with the low metastatic potential F1 line. In this case, control cells produced an average of 14 metastases in the lungs, and none in the liver, while injection of folate deficient cells resulted in an average of 42 metastases per animal. Seven of 12 animals had liver metastases as well (Figure 7).

In 13 experiments performed over a 3 year period, folate-deficient cells consistently initiated more pulmonary metastases in normal mice than melanoma cells grown in folate-supplemented medium.[19]

The mechanism or mechanisms by which nutritional folate deficiency enhances tumor cell metastatic potential is unclear at present. Deficiency of this vitamin is associated with changes in chromosomal stability, cell size, cell cycle distribution and membrane adherence properties which have been shown to influence metastasis formation. For example, increased genetic instability promotes the generation of tumor cells with the capacity to metastasize by fostering diversity. Survival of the few tumor cells that develop into a metastasis is due to unique properties of the surviving cells in response to host selection pressures. Recent studies suggest that metastatic capacity correlates with a higher rate of generation of metastatic variants.[55] Moreover, pretreatment of murine melanoma cells with ultraviolet light or chemotherapeutic agents enhances metastatic potential.[56,57] By analogy, folate deficiency might similarly promote tumor diversity and increase the possibility of developing cells with the ability to form metastases by enhancing chromosomal instability.

Evidence for genetic instability was sought in the murine melanoma cells in two ways: karyotypic analysis and alkaline filter elution. No major changes in mean chromosome number were found in this highly aneuploid cell line following induction of folate deficiency.[19] Other laboratories similarly found no relationship between metastatic potential and the generation of metacentric marker chromosomes, suggesting that more subtle changes may be responsible for alteration of metastatic capacity.[58] In contrast, increased DNA strand breaks were readily identified in folate deficient melanoma cells, and the onset of these breaks appeared to correlate with the enhancement of metastasis formation (Figure 5).[19] While this temporal association does not prove a causal relation-

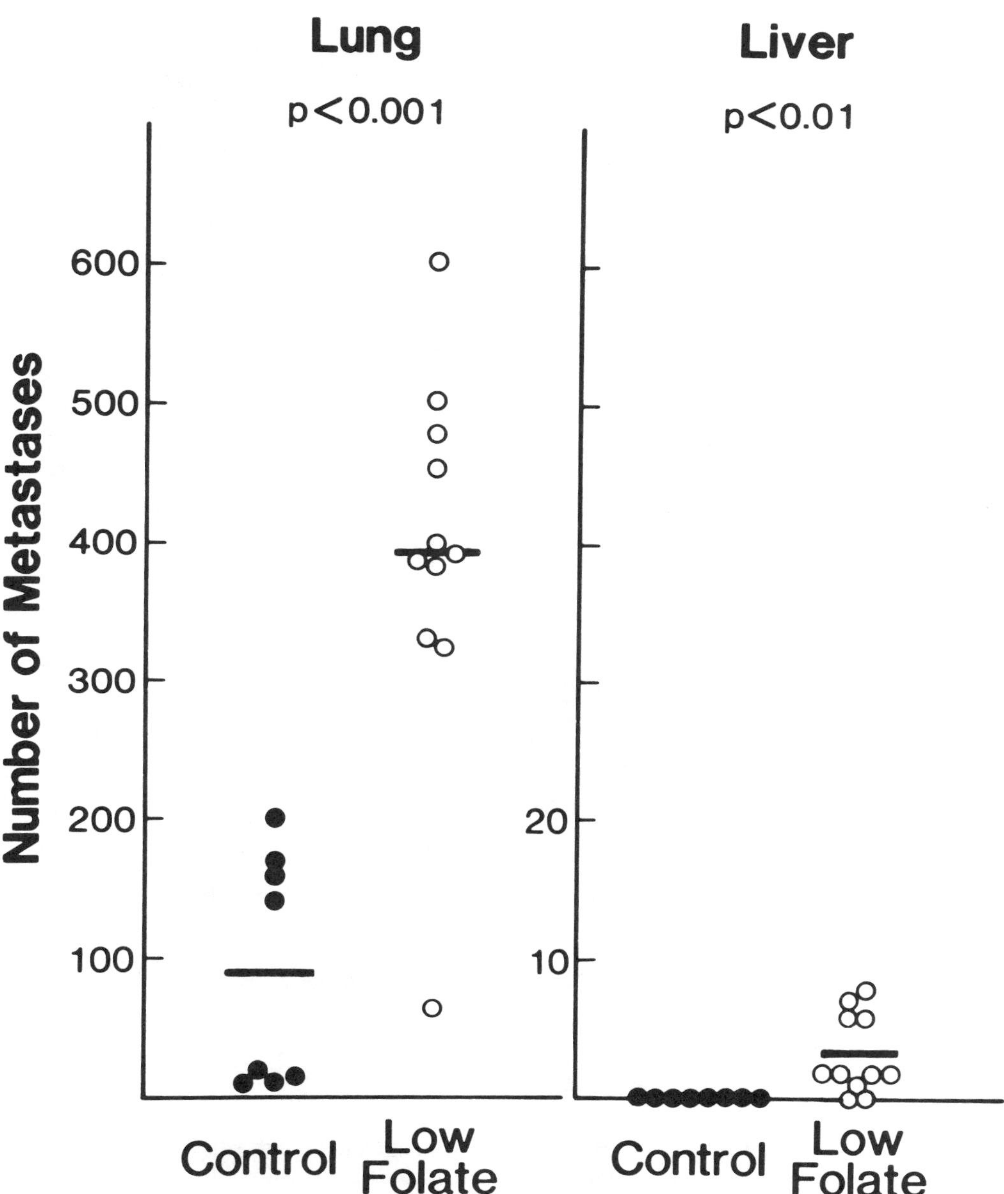

Figure 6. Number of pigmented metastases formed by murine B16 melanoma cells (F10 strain) in the lung (left panel) or liver (right panel) of mice after intravenous injection. Tumor cells were incubated for 3 days in low-folate (open circles) medium or the same medium supplemented with folic acid (closed circles).

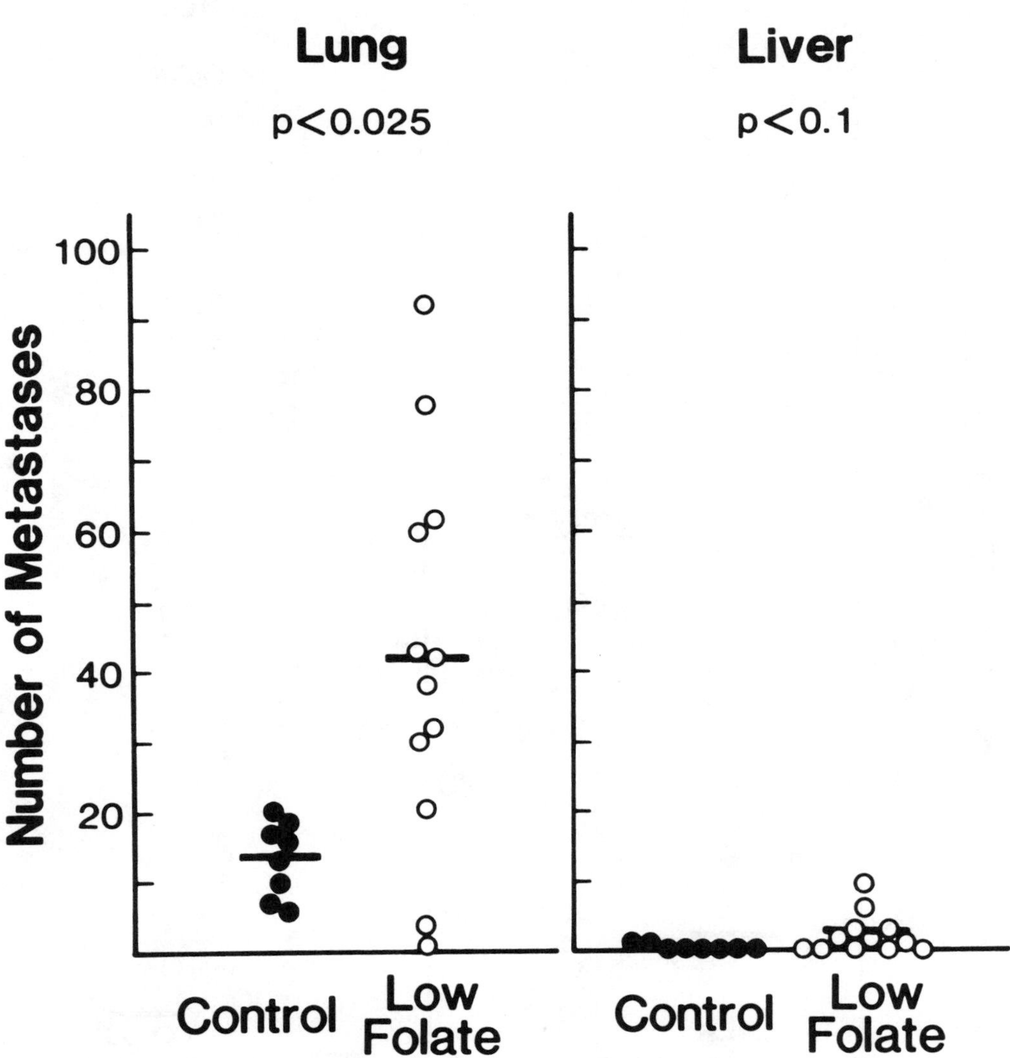

Figure 7. Number of metastases formed by F1 strain melanoma cells following growth for 3 days in low-folate (open circles) or folate-containing (closed circles) medium.

ship, it supports the idea that folate induced chromosomal instability may contribute to the potentiation of metastatic capacity.

Lung colony-forming ability in the FSA 1233 cell system is cell cycle and cell size dependent. Large cells and cells in S phase established the greatest number of colonies.[59] Since folate deficiency produces an increase in mean cell volume and an accumulation of cells in the S phase of the cell cycle, the possible influence of these changes on murine melanoma metastasis formation was investigated. In contrast to the studies cited above, in this experimental system larger cell size did not appear to be an important factor in metastasis formation. Although mean cell volume increased progressively with prolonged culture in folate deficient medium, there was not a parallel increase in metastatic potential, and the correlation between mean cell volume and metastasis formation was weak.[19] To test this possibility more directly, folate deficient murine melanoma cells were labeled with radioactive iododeoxyuridine and injected into the tail veins of normal C57/Bl6 mice. These cells were larger and had lower intracellular folate activity, as measured by the deoxyuridine suppression test, compared to control cells. In three experiments, there was no consistent evidence of significantly increased trapping of folate deficient cells compared to control cells in the lungs, kidney, spleen or liver (Table 2).

TABLE 2
Arrest of [^{125}I]deoxyuridine-Radiolabeled Tumor Cells in the Organs of C57BL Mice[a]

	WITH FOLATE Experiment #				WITHOUT FOLATE Experiment #			
Organ	**1**	**2**	**3**	**mean**	**1**	**2**	**3**	**mean**
15 minutes								
Lung	89	66	95	83	91	65	59	72
Kidney	0	0.1	0.2	0.1	0	0.2	0.1	0.1
Spleen	0	0.2	0.2	0.1	0	0.2	0.1	0.1
Liver	2	0.9	1.5	1.5	1	3	0.6	1.5
2 hours								
Lung	32	45	49	42	42	39	56	46
Kidney	0	0.2	0.2	0.1	0	0.2	0.1	0.1
Spleen	0	0.2	0.4	0.2	0	0.2	0.2	0.1
Liver	1	0.8	0.8	0.9	2	2.7	0.9	1.9
24 hours								
Lung	2	0.9	14	5.6	3	1.4	4	2.8
Kidney	0	0.2	0.2	0.1	0	0.1	0.1	0.1
Spleen	0	0.2	0.2	0.1	0	0.2	0.1	0.1
Liver	0	0.3	0.5	0.4	0	0.2	0.2	0.1

[a] Mice were given injections of approximately 5 x 10^4 viable B16 melanoma cells i.v. via the tail vein. Data are expressed as a percentage of radioactivity retained at various times after injection into four or five mice per sample.

The observation that folate deficient murine melanoma cells adhere more rapidly and completely to laminin or fibronectin coated plates suggests that this increased adhesion to extracellular matrix components may contribute to the greater metastatic potential of these cells.[20] Tumor invasion following hematogenous dissemination probably involves attachment via cell surface receptors to components of the basement membrane such as laminin and of the stroma such as fibronectin.[60] The adhesive and metastatic behavior of B16 cells can be modulated by exposure to these adhesion proteins; *in vitro* exposure to laminin increased metastatic potential, while fibronectin tended to reduce laminin binding and metastasis formation.[61] In many, but not all cases, increased membrane adhesion correlates with increased metastatic potential.[62,63] Therefore it is plausible to suggest that the increased adhesiveness associated with nutritional folate deficiency may contribute to the enhanced metastatic potential of these cells.

Another membrane property which is thought to influence metastatic potential is thrombin generation. Tumor cell membranes provide a surface for prothrombinase generation.[64] Prothrombinase is a complex of an active protease (Factor Xa) with a non-enzymatic cofactor (Factor Va) bound to a membrane surface in the presence of calcium. Without a suitable membrane surface, the ability of prothrombinase to convert prothrombin to thrombin is greatly impaired.[65] Therefore an appropriate membrane surface is necessary for fibrin deposition. Fibrin, in turn, may protect tumor cells from elimination by NK or other cytotoxic cells.[66,67] We found that folate deficient cells generally produced a higher rate of thrombin generation than folate replete cells. However, when the data were adjusted for cell number, these differences disappeared.[20] We conclude that folate deficiency does not alter the capacity of the cell membrane to facilitate prothrombinase complex formation. These observations also suggest that the effects of folate deficiency on membranes is relatively specific.

Thus, folate deficiency influences at least two known determinants of metastatic potential, namely genetic stability and membrane adhesion. These two mechanisms are not mutually exclusive because of postulated interconnections between cell structure, DNA stability and metastatic potential.[68]

IV. Summary

Tumor cells which are deprived of exogenous folates maintain near-normal doubling times while dividing their endogenous folate compounds among daughter cells.[69] When polyglutamyl folate levels drop below a critical level (approximately 1-1.5 μM), folate coenzymes are no longer available for nucleic acid and protein synthesis, resulting in major changes of cellular phenotype, kinetics and genotype.[17-19,69] Population cell growth is markedly inhibited. If folate is restored, replication resumes at approximately the same rate as in tumor cells which were never folate deficient. Prolonged folate deficiency causes a decline of reproductive viability. However, the response to folate deprivation is heterogeneous, and a sizable subpopulation of cells, at least 10%, survive even severe folate deficiency. The onset of reduced participation of folate compounds in pyrimidine metabolism, as measured by the deoxyuridine suppression test, coincides with an increase of mean cell volume, accumulation of DNA synthesis in the S phase of the cell cycle, elevated cellular protein levels and increased membrane adherence to substratum. Karyotypic analysis of these folate deficient tumor cells reveals numerous chromosomal abnormalities, including gaps, breaks, ring chromosomes, triradial and quadriradial exchanges, and decondensed chromosomes. The number of double strand DNA breaks, as detected by alkaline filter elution, increases with progressive folate deficiency. These effects of nutritional folate deficiency on tumor cells can be prevented by providing a source of both purines and pyrimidines.

Supplementation of tumor cells with single nucleosides differentially modifies the manifestations of folate deficiency. Addition of thymidine reduces cell size toward normal, releases S phase arrest, decreases cellular protein levels, increases membrane adherence, and improves viability, but it does not alter the frequency or distribution of chromosomal abnormalities. In contrast, hypoxanthine supplementation increases cell size and S phase arrest, elevates protein levels, decreases membrane adherence, lowers viability, and reduces the frequency of damaged mitoses and decondensed chromosomes. Neither nucleoside alone restores proliferation.

Because folate deficiency affects several important characteristics of tumor cells, inadequate levels of this vitamin may contribute to the progression of malignancies. Studies in mice indicate that folate deficient B16 melanoma cells produce more metastases than folate replete control cells. While the exact mechanism responsible for this enhanced metastatic capacity has not been elucidated, the effect appears to be mediated, at least in part, by the increased genetic instability and membrane adherence of folate deficient cells, rather than by the associated changes in cell size and cell cycle traverse. These experiments indicate that folate deficiency may be an important dietary factor influencing the spread of cancer. Since metastasis formation is a primary determinant of cancer morbidity and mortality, the consequences of folate deficiency require more careful consideration in patients with malignancies.

Acknowledgements

This work was supported by grants from the American Institute for Cancer Research and from the National Cancer Institute (CA 41843).

References

1. Hafen, B.Q., Ed., *Nutrition and Health: New Concepts and Issues*, Morton Publishing Co., Englewood, Colorado, 1985, 67.

2. Blakely, R.L., *The Biochemistry of Folic Acid and Related Pteridines*, North-Holland, Amsterdam-Holland, 1969, Chap. 1.

3. Herbert, V., Drugs effective in megaloblastic anemias, in *The Pharmacological Basis of Therapeutics*, 5th ed., Goodman, L.S. and Gilman, A., Eds., MacMillan, New York, 1975, Chap. 64.

4. Babior, B.M., The megaloblastic anemias, in *Hematology*, 4th ed., Williams, W.J., Beutler, E., Erslev, A.J., and Lichtman, M.A., Eds., McGraw-Hill, New York, 1990, Chap. 47.

5. Sauberlich, H.E., Detection of folic acid deficiency in populations, in *Folic Acid: Biochemistry and Physiology in Relation to the Human Nutrition Requirement*, National Academy of Science, Washington, D.C., 1977, Chap. 20.

6. Blakely, R.L., *The Biochemistry of Folic Acid and Related Pteridines*, North-Holland, Amsterdam-Holland, 1969, Chap. 12.

7. Magnus, E.M., Folate activity in serum and red cells of patients with cancer, *Cancer Res.*, 27, 490, 1967.

8. Somayaji, B.N., Nelson, R.S., and McGregor, R.F., Small intestinal function in malignant neoplasia, *Cancer*, 29, 1215, 1972.

9. Chanarin, I., Investigation and management of megaloblastic anaemia, *Clinics in Haematol.*, 5, 747, 1976.

10. Leuchtenberger, C. and Leuchtenberger, R., Growth-regulating effects of naturally occurring metabolites of folate and ascorbate on malignant cells, in *Nutritional Factors in the Induction and Maintenance of Malignancy*, Butterworth, C.E. and Hutchinson, M.L., Eds., Academic Press, New York, 1983, Chap. 9.

11. Farber, S., Cutler, E.C., Hawkins, J.W., Harrison, J.H., Peirce, E.C., and Lenz, G.G., The action of pteroylglutamic conjugates on man, *Science*, 106, 619, 1947.

12. Farber, S., Diamond, L.K., Mercer, R.D., Sylvester, R.F., and Wolff, J.A., Temporary remissions in acute leukemia in children produced by folic acid antagonist, 4-aminopteroyl-glutamic acid (aminopterin), *N. Engl. J. Med.*, 238, 787, 1948.

13. Potter, M. and Briggs, G.M., Inhibition of growth of amethopterin-sensitive and amethopterin-resistant pairs of lymphocytic neoplasms by dietary folic-acid deficiency in mice, *J. Natl. Cancer Inst.*, 28, 341, 1962.

14. Rosen, F. and Nichol, C.A., Inhibition of the growth of an amethopterin-refractory tumor by dietary restriction of folic acid, *Cancer Res.*, 22, 495, 1962.

15. Gailani, S.D., Carey, R.W., Holland, J.F., and O'Malley, J.A., Studies of folate deficiency in patients with neoplastic diseases, *Cancer Res.*, 30, 327, 1970.

16. Allegra, C.J., Huang, K., Yeh, G.C., Drake, J.C., and Baram, J., Evidence for direct inhibition of de novo purine synthesis in human MCF-7 breast cells as a principal mode of metabolic inhibition of methotrexate, *J. Biol. Chem.*, 262, 13520, 1987.

17. Borman, L.S. and Branda, R.F., Nutritional folate deficiency in Chinese Hamster Ovary Cells I. Characterization of the pleiotropic response and its modulation by nucleic acid precursors, *J. Cell. Physiol.*, 140, 335, 1989.

18. Steinberg, S.E., Fonda, S., Campbell, C.L., and Hillman, R.S., Folate utilization in Friend erythroleukemia cells, *J. Cell. Physiol.*, 114, 252, 1983.

19. Branda, R.F., McCormack, J.J., Perlmutter, C.A., Mathews, L.A., and Robison, S.H., Effects of folate deficiency on the metastatic potential of murine melanoma cells, *Cancer Res.*, 48, 4529, 1988.

20. Branda, R.F. and Tracy, P.B., Effects of Nutritional folate deficiency on the adhesive properties of murine melanoma cells, *Cancer Lett.*, in press.

21. Menzies, R.C., Crossen, P.E., Fitzgerald, P.H., and Gunz, F.W., Cytogenetic and cytochemical studies on marrow cells in B12 and folate deficiency, *Blood*, 28, 581, 1966.

22. Ballas, S.K., Saidi, P., and Constantino, M., Reduced erythrocytic deformability in megaloblastic anemia, *Am. J. Clin. Pathol.*, 66, 953, 1976.

23. Ballas, S.K., Abnormal erythrocyte membrane protein pattern in severe megaloblastic anemia, *J. Clin. Invest.*, 61, 1097, 1978.

24. Bremert, J.C., Dreosti, I.E., and Tulsi, R.S., A teratogenic interaction between dietary deficiencies of zinc and folic acid in rats: an electron microscope study, *Nutrition Res.*, 9, 105, 1989.

25. Heath, C.W., Cytogenetic observations in vitamin B12 an folate deficiency, *Blood*, 27, 800, 1966.

26. Kiossoglou, K.A., Mitus, W.J., and Dameshek, W., Chromosomal aberrations in pernicious anemia, *Blood*, 25, 662, 1965.

27. Das, K.C., Mohanty, D., and Garewal, G., Cytogenetics in nutritional megaloblastic anaemia: prolonged persistence of chromosomal abnormalities in lymphocytes after remission, *Acta Haemat.*, 76, 146, 1986.

28. Libbus, B.L., Borman, L.S., Ventrone, C.H., and Branda, R.F., Nutritional folate-deficiency in Chinese Hamster Ovary Cells: chromosomal abnormalities associated with perturbations in nucleic acid precursors, *Cancer Genet. Cytogenet.*, 46, 231, 1990.

29. Jacobs, P.A., Glover, T.W., Mayer, M., Fox, P., Gerrard, J.W., Dunn, H.G., and Herbst, D.S., X-linked mental retardation: a study of 7 families, *Am. J. Med. Genet.*, 7, 471, 1980.

30. Jennings, M., Hall, J.G., and Hoehn, H., Significance of phenotypic and chromosomal abnormalities in X-linked mental retardation (Martin-Bell or Renpenning syndrome), *Am. J. Med. Genet.*, 7, 417, 1980.

31. Sutherland, G.R., Heritable fragile sites on human chromosomes I. Factors affecting expression in lymphocyte culture, *Am. J. Hum. Genet.*, 31, 125, 1979.

32. Glover, T.W., FUdR induction of the X chromosome fragile site: evidence for the mechanism of folic acid and thymidine inhibition, *Am. J. Hum. Genet.*, 33, 234, 1981.

33. Sutherland, G.R., Fragile chromosomes, in *Nutritional Factors in the Induction and Maintenance of Malignancy*, Butterworth, C.E. and Hutchinson, M.L., Eds., Academic Press, New York, 1983, 63.

34. Yunis, J.J. and Soreng, A.L., Constitutive fragile sites and cancer, *Science*, 226, 1199, 1984.

35. Le Beau, M.M., Chromosomal fragile sites and cancer-specific breakpoints—a moderating viewpoint, *Cancer Genet. Cytogenet.*, 31, 55, 1988.

36. Hecht, F., Defendi, G.L., Bixenman, H.A., and Hecht, B.K., Human aneuploidy and folic acid deficiency, in *Aneuploidy, Part B: Induction and Test Systems*, Alan R. Liss, Inc., New York, 1988, 159.

37. Branda, R.F., Arthur, D.C., Woods, W.G., Danzl, T.J., and King, R.A., Folate metabolism and chromosomal stability in the Fragile X syndrome, *Am. J. Med.*, 77,602, 1984.

38. Chudley, A.E., Knoll, J., Gerrard, J.W., Shepel, L., McGahey, E., and Anderson, J., Fragile (X) X-linked mental retardation 1: relationship between age and intelligence and the frequency of expression of fragile (X) (q28), *Am. J. Med. Genet.*, 14, 699, 1983.

39. Knuutila, S., Helminen, E., Vuopio, P., and De La Chapelle, A., Increased sister chromatid exchange in megaloblastic anaemia—studies on bone marrow cells and lymphocytes, *Hereditas*, 89, 175, 1978.

40. Arthur, D.C., Danzl, T.J., and Branda, R.F., Cytogenetic studies of a family with a hereditary defect of cellular folate uptake and high incidence of hematologic disease, in *Nutritional Factors in the Induction and Maintenance of Malignancy*, Butterworth, C.E. and Hutchinson, M.L., Eds., Academic Press, New York, 1983, 101.

41. Tawn, E.J. and Earl, R., The influence of culture media on chromosome aberration levels, sister chromatid exchange frequencies, and the rate of cell proliferation: comparison of Iscove's low folate medium with Eagle's MEM, *J. Med. Genet.*, 25, 419, 1988.

42. Hoffbrand, A.V., Ganeshaguru, K., Hooton, J.W.L., and Tripp, E., Megaloblastic anaemia: initiation of DNA synthesis in excess of DNA chain elongation as the undelying mechanism, *Clinics Haem.*, 5,727, 1976.

43. Wickremasinghe, R.G. and Hoffbrand, A.V., Defective DNA synthesis in megaloblastic anaemia, *Biochem. Biophys. Acta*, 563, 46, 1979.

44. Wickremasinghe, R.G. and Hoffbrand, A.V., Reduced rate of DNA replication fork movement in megaloblastic anemia, *J. Clin. Invest.*, 65, 26, 1980.

45. Hoffbrand, A.V. and Tripp, E., Unbalanced deoxyribonucleotide synthesis caused by methotrexate, *Brit. Med. J.*, 2, 140, 1972.

46. Goulian, M., Bleile, B., and Tseng, B.Y., Methotrexate-induced misincorporation of uracil into DNA, *Proc. Natl. Acad. Sci. USA*, 77,1956, 1980.

47. Hoffbrand, A.V., Ganeshaguru, K., Lavoie, A., Tattersall, M.H.N., and Tripp, E., Thymidylate concentration in megaloblastic anemia, *Nature*, 248, 602, 1974.

48. Iwata, N., Omine, M., Yamauchi, H., and Maekawa, T., Characteristic abnormality of deoxyribonucleoside triphosphate metabolism in megaloblastic anemia, *Blood*, 60, 918, 1982.

49. Taheri, M.R., Wickremasinghe, R.G., and Hoffbrand, A.V., Alternative metabolic fates of thymine nucleotides in human cells, *Biochem. J.*, 194, 451, 1981.

50. Meuth, M., The genetic consequences of nucleotide precursor pool imbalance in mammalian cells, *Mutation Res.*, 126, 107, 1984.

51. Kunz, B.A., Genetic effects of deoxyribonucleotide pool imbalances, *Environ. Mutagen.*, 4, 695, 1982.

52. Sutherland, G.R., The role of nucleotides in human fragile site expression, *Mutation Res.*, 200, 207, 1988.

53. Shaw, T., The role of blood platelets in nucleoside metabolism: regulation of megakaryocyte development and platelet production, *Mutation Res.*, 200, 67, 1988.

54. Fidler, I.J., Tumor heterogeneity and the biology of cancer invasion and metastasis, *Cancer Res.*, 38, 2651, 1978.

55. Hill, R.P., Chambers, A.F., Ling, V., and Harris, J.F., Dynamic heterogeneity: rapid generation of metastatic variants in mouse B16 melanoma cells, *Science*, 224, 998, 1984.

56. Fisher, M.S. and Cifone, M.A., Enhanced metastatic potential of murine fibrosarcoma treated *in vitro* with ultraviolet radiation, *Cancer Res.*, 41, 3018, 1981.

57. McMillan, T.J. and Hart, I.R., Enhanced experimental metastatic capacity of a murine melanoma following pre-treatment with anticancer drugs, *Clin. Exp. Metastasis*, 4, 285, 1986.

58. Kendal, W.S., Wang, R-Y., Hsu, T.C., and Frost, P., Rate of generation of major karyotypic abnormalities in relationship to the metastatic potential of B16 murine melanoma, *Cancer Res.*, 47, 3835, 1987.

59. Suzuki, N., Frapart, M., Grdina, D.J., Meistrich, M.L., and Withers, H.R., Cell cycle dependency of metastatic lung colony formation, *Cancer Res.*, 37, 3690, 1977.

60. Liotta, L.A., Tumor invasion and metastases—role of the extracellular matrix: Rhoads Memorial Award Lecture, *Cancer Res.*, 46, 1, 1986.

61. Terranova, V.P., Williams, J.E., Liotta, L.A., and Martin, G.R., Modulation of the metastatic activity of melanoma cells by laminin and fibronectin, *Science*, 226, 982, 1984.

62. Maslow, D.E., Tabulation of results on the heterogeneity of cellular characteristics among cells from B16 mouse melanoma cell lines with different colonization potentials, *Invasion Met.*, 9, 182, 1989.

63. Zoller, M. and Matzku, S., Changes in adhesive properties of tumor cells do not necessarily influence metastasizing capacity, *Clin. Expl. Metastasis*, 7, 227, 1989.

64. Tracy, P.B., Eide, C.C., and Mann, K.G., Human prothrombinase complex assembly and function in isolated peripheral blood cell populations, *J. Biol. Chem.*, 260, 2119, 1985.

65. Nesheim, M.E., Taswell, J.B., and Mann, K.G., The contribution of bovine Factor V and Factor Va to the activity of prothrombinase, *J. Biol. Chem.*, 254, 10952, 1979.

66. Gilbert, L.C. and Gordon, S.G., Relationship between cellular procoagulant activity and metastatic capacity of B16 mouse melanoma variants, *Cancer Res.*, 43, 536, 1983.

67. Gorelik, E., Augmentation of the antimetastatic effect of anticoagulant drugs by immunostimulation in mice, *Cancer Res.*, 47, 809, 1987.

68. Pienta, K.J., Partin, A.W., and Coffey, D.S., Cancer as a disease of DNA organization and dynamic cell structure, *Cancer Res.*, 49, 2525, 1989.

69. Steinberg, S.E., Fonda, S., Campbell, C.L., and Hillman, R.S., Cellular abnormalities of folate deficiency, *Brit. J. Haematol.*, 54, 605, 1983.

Chapter 12

Recent Studies on the Neoplasia and Abnormal Cellular Differentiation in Methyl Insufficiency

Lionel A. Poirier

Table of Contents

I. Introduction

The induction of liver cancer by the dietary deficiencies of the methyl donors, methionine and choline, has been amply demonstrated in rodents.[1-5] Our own contributions to this area consisted in the observations that: 1) amino acid-defined methionine- and choline-deficient diets induced liver cancer in rats and mice;[1] 2) such diets also produced a hypomethylating environment in the livers of rats as determined by decreased ratios of S-adenosylmethionine/S-adenosylhomocysteine (SAM/SAH);[6] and 3) decreased 5-methyldeoxycytidine contents in hepatic DNA.[1] The changes wrought in hepatic SAM bioavailability and in DNA methylation by dietary methyl deprivation have also been produced by chronic hepatocarcinogen administration.[1] During the course of these studies, it was discovered that the chronic administration of severely deficient diets to rats resulted in the transdifferentiation of pancreatic acinar cells to hepatocyte-like cells in rats.[7] This finding led us to examine the possible role of specific gene methylation in hepatocarcinogenesis by methyl deprivation. In a series of ongoing studies, it was shown that the chronic administration of the methyl-deficient diets to rats led to hepatic hypomethylation of specific oncogenes during the early and late stages of hepatocarcinogenesis, as well as in the tumors produced.[8-10] Although the mechanistic significance of such hypomethylation remains to be determined, it is evident that the administration of methyl-deficient diets to rodents results both in a hypomethylating environment *in vivo*, as well as in hypomethylated macromolecules in the target tissue.

Of critical importance to this area of research is the extent to which physiological methyl insufficiency contributes to the carcinogenic process. As is shown in Figure 1, there are two major sources of methyl groups *in vivo*: the preformed and the *de novo*. The preformed sources consist of dietary methionine and choline; the *de novo* consists of methionine which is synthesized from 1-carbon fragments in the folate pool transferred to homocysteine via the cobalamin-dependent enzyme methionine synthase. A second pathway of methionine biosynthesis is mediated by the enzyme, betaine homocysteine methyltransferase, but this pathway mainly conserves pre-existing methyl groups derived from choline. It is worth noting that this enzyme is active principally in the liver and that human liver contains less than does rodent liver.[11,12]

II. Paradox

In light of the carcinogenic and cocarcinogenic activities of dietary methyl deprivation towards the liver, one would expect that deficiencies of vitamin B_{12} and folate, responsible for the *de novo* biosynthesis of methyl groups, would similarly enhance the activities of carcinogens *in vivo*. Yet, such is not the case (for reviews, *cf.* ref. 9,13). When adequately investigated, dietary deficiencies of vitamin B_{12} and of folic acid have tended to inhibit carcinogenesis, particularly in the liver.[9,13] It is thought that the tumor-suppressive effects of deficiencies of vitamin B_{12} and folic acid are related to their inhibition of DNA biosynthesis through the inhibition of thymidylate synthetase (Figure 1).[13-15] Indeed, the macrocytic and megaloblastic anemias associated with deficiencies of this vitamin have been attributed to this enzymatic defect.[14,15]

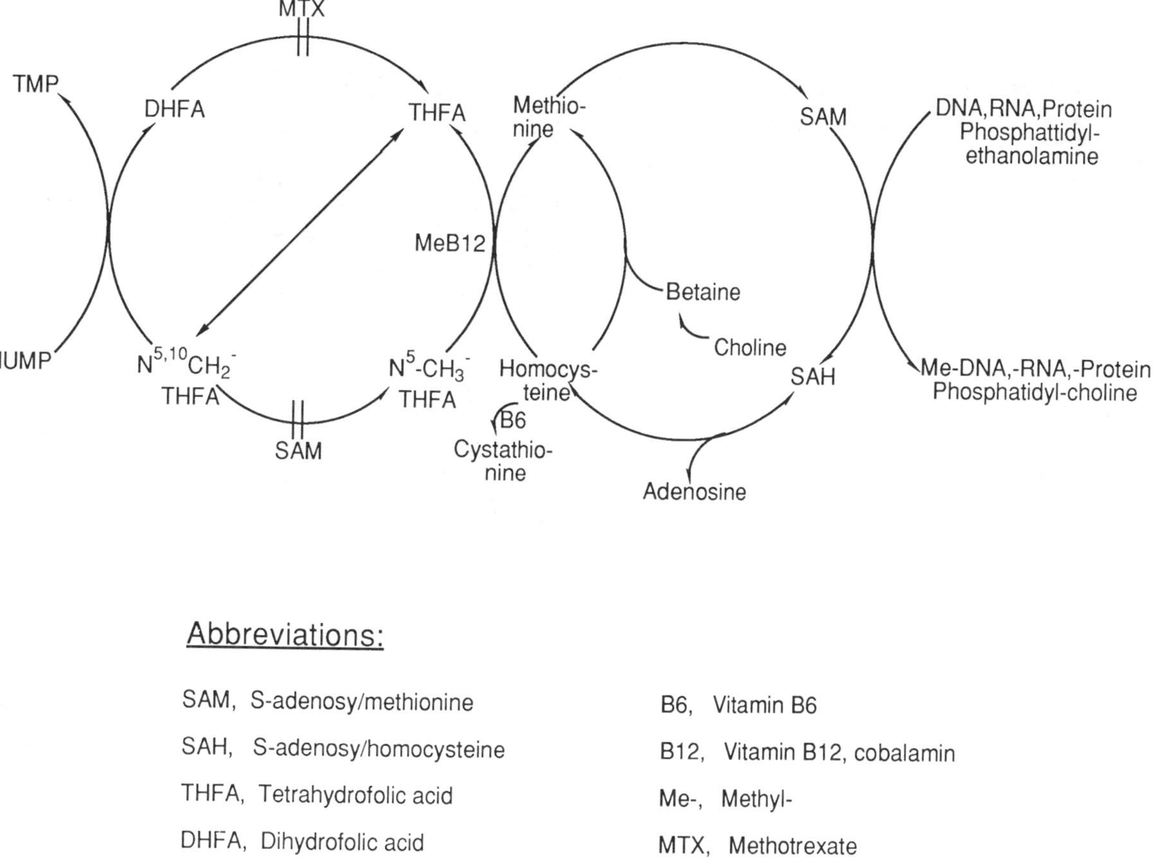

Figure 1. The regulation and transfer of one-carbon units in the metabolism of nucleic acids, proteins, amino acids and phospholipids.

Yet, there is evidence to show that folate and vitamin B_{12} deficiencies may play a role in enhancing carcinogenesis. Patients with pernicious anemia have an excess risk of gastric cancer.[16] Folic acid therapy results in improvement of cervical dysplasia associated with oral contraceptive use.[17] Localized folate deficiency occurs in the oral mucosal cells of cigarette smokers.[18] In addition, dietary deficiencies of vitamin B_{12} and of folic acid have been shown to decrease the bioavailability of SAM *in vivo* (Table 1).[6,19-23] Although almost all of these studies were conducted using animals that were fed diets that were deficient in methionine and/or choline, in addition to lacking vitamin B_{12} or folic acid. It is evident that the superimposition of the vitamin B_{12} or folate deficiency did result in decreased hepatic levels of SAM, increased hepatic levels of SAH, or increased levels of serum homocysteine (Table 1). These findings demonstrate that under certain circumstances, at least, dietary deficiencies of folic acid and of vitamin B_{12} do contribute to a hypomethylating environment *in vivo*.

TABLE 1
The Effects of Vitamin B_{12} and Folic Acid Deficiencies on Hepatic S-adenosylmethionine and Serum Homocysteine

Study	Findings
Vidal & Stokstad, 1974	Vitamin B_{12} deficiency decreased the hepatic SAM levels in rats fed a low methionine diet.[19]
Mikol & Poirier, 1981	Vitamin B_{12} deficiency alone decreases the hepatic levels of SAM in rats.[20]
Shivapurkar & Poirier, 1984	Combined folate and B_{12} deficiencies further lowered the hepatic SAM/SAH ratios in rats fed a methionine- and choline-deficient diet.[6]
Henning *et al.*, 1989	Folate deficiency further lowered the hepatic SAM/SAH ratios in rats fed a low methionine, choline-deficient diet.[21]
Doi *et al.*, 1989	Vitamin B_{12} deficiency decreased the liver contents of SAM, SAM synthase, and methionine synthase in rats.[22]
Lin *et al.*, 1989	Folate deficiency in rats produces a 2 to 4-fold increase in serum homocysteine.[23]

III. Synthesis

Clinical evidence for a causal link between folate/B_{12} deficiency and a hypomethylating environment *in vivo* came from an unexpected quarter: studies on the neuropathy seen in HIV-infected patients (Table 2).[24,25] The neuropathy seen in AIDS patients resembles that seen in experimental animals treated with nitrous oxide.[26] In the pig, such neuropathy has been associated with decreased SAM/SAH ratios.[26] Two groups have examined the levels of SAM and related compounds in the cerebrospinal fluid of HIV-positive patients.[24,25] As shown in Table 2, there were marked decreases in SAM, SAM/SAH ratios, and N^5-CH_3-THFA in the cerebrospinal fluid of HIV patients compared to controls. The drop in N^5-CH_3-THFA is indicative of a folate deficiency leading to SAM insufficiency rather than the reverse.

TABLE 2
Abnormal Levels of S-adenosylmethionine (SAM) and Related Compounds in the Cerebrospinal Fluid of HIV-Positive Patients

Study	Compound	Level[a] in Controls	Level[a] in Patients
R. Surtees *et al.*[24]	Methionine	4.4 ± 0.3	2.9 ± 1.1
	SAM	247 ± 14	118 ± 36[b]
	N^5-CH_3-THFA	90 ± 5	26 ± 7[b]
J.N. Keating *et al.*[25]	SAM	128.0 ± 9.3	60.8 ± 6.9[b]
	SAH	17.6 ± 1.9	31.0 ± 2.4[b]
	SAM/SAH	8.2 ± 1.0	2.1 ± 0.4[b]

[a] Mean ± SE; units are µmole/l for methionine and nmole/l for SAM, SAH, and N^5-CH_3-THFA.
[b] Significantly different from controls ($p<0.01$).

These findings led us to reconsider other situations in which humans may be particularly sensitive to folate deficiency. Folic acid deficiency is fairly common in humans.[27] Indeed, among four species investigated the hepatic levels of tetrahydrofolic acid (THFA) were lowest in humans; further, the hepatic content of dihydrofolate reductase (DHFR) was also much less in humans than in the monkey or the rat (Table 3).[28] One might thus expect humans to be particularly sensitive to toxic agents which stress the folate pool. This is indeed the case with methanol, whose toxic metabolic, formic acid is detoxified by metabolism in the C^1-folate pool. The relative toxicities of methanol to humans, monkeys, rats, and mice is inversely proportional to the capacity of the species to metabolize formic acid via the reduced folate pool.[28] Thus, the limited experimental and clinical evidence available indicates that humans appear to be more sensitive to dietary folate deficiency than are rodents.

TABLE 3
Interspecies Comparisons of Reduced Hepatic Folates and Dihydrofolate Reductase[a]

Compound	Species: Mouse	Rat	Monkey	Human
THFA[b]	42.9 ± 1.2	11.4 ± 0.8	7.4 ± 0.8	6.5 ± 0.3
CHO-THFA	6.4 ± 0.6	4.6 ± 1.3	10.5 ± 0.8	3.3 ± 0.5
N^5-CH_3-THFA	11.6 ± 0.4	9.3 ± 0.6	7.6 ± 1.1	6.0 ± 0.7
Total	60.9 ± 2.1	25.3 ± 0.9	25.5 ± 1.2	15.8 ± 0.8
DHFR	–	19.8 ± 1.3	4.1 ± 0.7	0.7 ± 0.2

[a] From Johlin *et al.*[28]
[b] THFA = Tetrahydrofolic acid in nmole/g ± SE.
[c] DHFR = Dihydrofolate reductase in nmoles product/min/mg protein ± SE.

Conversely, primates seem relatively insensitive to choline deficiency. The hepatotoxicity of choline deficiency is less in baboons than in rats fed the same diet.[29] Low choline intake by humans is associated with biochemical, but not clinical, abnormalities.[11,12] Finally, enteral administration of a low choline, elemental formula to male cirrhotic and non-cirrhotic patients led to low plasma choline concentrations in the former but not in the latter.[30] Thus, the sum of the available evidence makes it reasonable to postulate: 1) that humans and other primates derive a greater portion of their physiological methyl groups through *de novo* biosynthesis than do rodents; and 2) that metabolic disturbances of the folate pool would consequently have significant impact on the bioavailability of SAM in humans.

Toxicological studies with two compounds, methotrexate (MTX) and ethanol, lend credence to these proposals. Chronic and subchronic treatment with MTX produces hepatotoxicity in both rats and humans. Such toxicity is manifested by: fatty liver, hepatic cirrhosis, and fibrosis.[31-33] In addition, like choline deficiency,[34] MTX treatment of rats leads to decreased serum levels of triglycerides.[31] In a limited number of carcinogenicity studies, MTX has exhibited cocarcinogenic activity.[35,36] Further, a number of unexpected cases of tumor formation have been observed in patients treated with MTX, either in combination with other anti-neoplastic agents against primary tumors, or as therapy against non-neoplastic diseases; the development of such tumors has not yet been shown to be of epidemiological significance.[33,36,37] Table 4 illustrates a number of interactions between MTX and methionine metabolism *in vivo*.[38-45] The effects of MTX on

TABLE 4
Interactions Between Methotrexate (MTX) and Methionine Metabolites *In Vivo*

Compound Administered	Affected	Result Noted
MTX	Betaine	Decreased hepatic levels both in normal and in choline-deficient rats.[38]
	Methionine	Decreased plasma levels in patients receiving high dose infusions.[39]
	Homocysteine	Increased serum levels in patients receiving high dose infusions.[39-40]
		Increased serum and hepatic levels in rats.[41]
	SAM	Decreased hepatic levels in rats.[41]
	SAM/SAH	Decreased ratios in the livers of mice after acute high dose.[42]
		Decreased ratios after subchronic treatment of methionine-fed mice.[43]
		Decreased ratios in the livers of rats.[41]
Choline	MTX	Inhibition by choline of the toxicity of MTX to liver but not bone marrow in rats.[44]
		Synergism between choline deficiency and MTX in hepatotoxicity in rats.[45]
MTX+N^5-CH_3 THFA	SAM/SAH	Reversal by N^5-CH_3-THFA of decreased ratios in livers of MTX-treated mice.[43]

betaine, methionine, homocysteine, SAM, and SAM/SAH ratios are fully consistent with what one would expect by the suppression of methionine biosynthesis through a lack of availability of tetrahydrofolic acid caused by the inhibition of DHFR by MTX. The net effect of MTX is to produce a hypomethylating environment in liver. The fact that choline inhibits the hepatotoxicity of MTX indicates that the toxicity of this organ is mediated in part through the bioavailability of methyl groups (Table 4). Finally, the fact that N^5-CH_3-THFA partially protects against the decreased SAM/SAH ratios in the livers of MTX-treated mice further implicates THFA deficiency as being the primary cause of MTX-induced decrease in methyl bioavailability.[43]

Unlike the case with MTX, there is much epidemiological evidence indicating that drinking of alcoholic beverages is causally related to cancer formation in humans.[46] Such studies show that cancers of the oral cavity, pharynx, larynx, and esophagus are associated with alcohol consumption.[46] Of more direct relevance to this presentation is the more well-known association between the consumption of alcoholic beverages and liver cancer in man.[46,47] Deficiencies of folic acid, along with several other vitamins, have long been recognized as a consequence of excess alcohol consumption (Table 5).[15,47] This folate deficiency is the result of several different effects of alcohol on folate metabolism.[47] The link between alcohol ingestion and abnormal methyl group metabolism has been made only relatively recently (Table 5).[48,56] As might be expected from its effects on folate, alcohol ingestion has been associated with decreased methionine biosynthesis via the folate-dependent pathway (Table 5).[56] SAM synthetase has also been shown to be decreased in the livers of alcoholic-cirrhotic patients.[54,55] Such ethanol administration to baboons has been shown to decrease hepatic SAM

TABLE 5
Metabolic Interactions Between Ethanol and Methyl Group Metabolism *In Vivo*

Observations
Folate deficiency is a common feature of alcoholism.[15,47]
Alcohol-induced hepatotoxicity in rats, baboons, and humans is inhibited by exogenous SAM.[48-51]
Dietary ethanol inhibits fetal DNA methylation in mice.[52]
Ethanol administration enhances liver tumor promotion by choline deficiency in diethylnitrosamine-initiated rats.[53]
SAM synthase activity decreases in the livers of cirrhotic patients.[34,55]
Chronic alcohol administration decreases the folate-dependent pathway of methionine biosynthesis, but increases the betaine-dependent pathway in the livers of rats.[56]

content.[49] The drop in hepatic SAM levels, as well as several other parameters of alcohol-induced hepatotoxicity, can be inhibited by treatment with exogenous SAM (Table 5).[48-51] As might be expected from the effects of ethanol on SAM, ethanol treatment has been recently shown to inhibit fetal DNA methylation in mice (Table 5),[52] and to enhance the formation of enzyme-altered foci by choline deficiency in diethylnitrosamine-initiated rats.[53] Thus, although not thoroughly investigated in a systematic manner, the evidence available indicates that chronic alcohol consumption produces many of the lesions associated with physiological methyl group insufficiency. Two other features of alcohol toxicity should be noted. The first is that alcohol is metabolized to a known carcinogen, acetaldehyde which is a reactive electrophile.[46] The second is that choline failed to prevent the toxicity of ethanol in the baboon.[57] The latter finding may indicate that the baboon, like the human, may have low hepatic levels of betaine oxidase and that SAM may be a more effective source of physiological methyl donors in this species.

IV. Conclusions

The present report summarizes the results from several studies providing evidence that: 1) in certain specific circumstances, interference with the *de novo* pathway of methionine biosynthesis can produce a physiological methyl insufficiency *in vivo*; 2) that such insufficiency may be a not infrequent feature in patients with various diseases; and 3) that such methyl insufficiency, like that produced in experimental animals, may increase the risk of cancer development.

References

1. Mikol, Y.B., Hoover, K.L., Creasia, D., and Poirier, L.A., Hepatocarcinogenesis in rats fed methyl-deficient, amino acid-defined diets, *Carcinogenesis*, 4, 1619, 1983.

2. Newberne, P.M., Lipotropic factors and oncogenesis, in *Essential Nutrients in Carcinogenesis*, Poirier, L.A., Pariza, M.W., and Newberne, P.M., Eds., Plenum Press, New York, 1986, 223.

3. Ghoshal, A.K., Sarma, D.S.R., and Farber, A., Ethionine in the analysis of the possible separate roles of methionine and choline deficiencies in carcinogenesis, in *Essential Nutrients in Carcinogenesis*, Poirier, L.A., Pariza, M.W., and Newberne, P.M., Eds., Plenum Press, New York, 1986, 283.

4. Shinozuka, H., Katyal, S.L., and Perera, M.I.R., Choline deficiency and chemical carcinogenesis, in *Essential Nutrients in Carcinogenesis*, Poirier, L.A., Pariza, M.W., and Newberne, P.M., Eds., Plenum Press, New York, 1986, 253.

5. Locker, J., Reddy, T.V., and Lombardi, B., DNA methylation and hepatocarcinogenesis in rats fed a choline-devoid diet, *Carcinogenesis*, 7, 1309, 1986.

6. Shivapurkar, N. and Poirier, L.A., Tissue levels of S-adenosylmethionine and S-adenosylhomocysteine in rats fed methyl-deficient, amino acid-defined diets for one to five weeks, *Carcinogenesis*, 4, 1051, 1983.

7. Hoover, K.L. and Poirier, L.A., Hepatocyte-like cells within the pancreas of rats fed methyl-deficient diets, *J. Nutr.*, 116, 1569, 1986.

8. Bhave, M.R., Wilson, M.J., and Poirier, L.A., c-H-*ras* and c-K-*ras* gene hypomethylation in the livers and hepatomas of rats fed methyl-deficient, amino acid-defined diets, *Carcinogenesis*, 9, 343, 1988.

9. Poirier, L.A., Zapisek, W., and Lyn-Cook, B.D., Physiological methylation in carcinogenesis, in *Mutation and the Environment*, Part D, Wiley-Liss, New York, 1990, 97.

10. Poirier, L.A., Zapisek, W.F., Cronin, G.M., and Lyn-Cook, B.D., Oncogene hypomethylation in the livers of rats fed methyl-deficient, amino acid-defined diets, *Proc. Amer. Assoc. Cancer Res.*, 31, 142, 1990.

11. Baraona, E. and Lieber, C.S., Effects of ethanol on lipid metabolism, *J. Lipid Res.*, 20, 289, 1979.

12. Zeisel, S.H., Choline deficiency, *J. Nutr. Biochem.*, 1, 332, 1990.

13. Eto, I. and Krumdieck C.L., Role of vitamin B_{12} and folate deficiencies in carcinogenesis, in *Advances in Experimental Medicine and Biology*, Vol. 206, Poirier, L.A., Pariza, M.W., and Newberne, P.M., Eds., Plenum Press, New York, 1986, 313.

14. Herbert, V., The role of vitamin B_{12} and folate in carcinogenesis, in *Advances in Experimental Medicine and Biology*, Vol. 206, Poirier, L.A., Pariza, M.W., and Newberne, P.M., Eds., Plenum Press, New York, 1986, 293.

15. Herbert, V., Development of human folate deficiency, in *Folic Acid Metabolism in Health and Disease*, Picciano, M.F., Stokstad, E.L.R., and Gregory, J.F., III, Eds., Wiley-Liss, New York, 1990, 195.

16. Elsborg, L. and Mosbech, J., Gastric cancer as a risk factor in pernicious anaemia, in *Vitamin B12*, Zagalak, B. and Friedrich, W., Eds., Walter de Gruyter, New York, 1979, 1119.

17. Butterworth, C.E., Jr., Hatch, K.D., Gore, H., Mueller, H., and Krumdieck, C.L., Improvement in cervical dysplasia associated with folic acid therapy in users of oral contraceptives, *Am. J. Clin. Nutr.*, 35, 73, 1982.

18. Hine, R.J., Piyathilake, C.J., and Krumdieck, C.L., Evidence of localized folate deficiency in oral mucosal cells of cigarette smokers, *FASEB J.*, 4, A1043, 1990.

19. Vidal, A.J. and Stokstad, E.L., Urinary excretion of 5-methyltetrahydrofolate and liver S-adenosylmethionine levels of rats fed a vitamin B_{12}-deficient diet, *Biochim. Biophys. Acta*, 5, 245, 1974.

20. Mikol, Y. and Poirier, L.A., An inverse correlation between hepatic ornithine decarboxylase and S-adenosylmethionine in rats, *Cancer Lett.*, 13, 195, 1981.

21. Henning, S.M., McKee, R.W., and Swendseid, M.E., Hepatic content of S-adenosylmethionine, S-adenosylhomocysteine, and glutathione in rats receiving treatments modulating methyl donor availability, *J. Nutr.*, 119, 1478, 1989.

22. Doi, T., Kawata, T., Tadano, N., Iijima, T., and Maekawa, A., Effect of vitamin B_{12} deficiency on S-adenosylmethionine metabolism in rats, *J. Nutr. Sci. Vitaminol. (Tokyo)*, 35, 1, 1989.

23. Lin, J-Y., Kang, S-S., Zhou, J., and Wong, P.W.K., Homocysteinemia in rats induced by folic acid deficiency, *Life Sci.*, 44, 319, 1989.

24. Surtees, R., Hyland, K., and Smith, I., Central-nervous-system methyl-group metabolism in children with neurological complications of HIV infection, *Lancet*, 335, 619, 1990.

25. Keating, J.N., Weir, D.G., Trimble, K.C., Mulcahy, F., and Scott, J.M., Methyl transferase inhibition produces brain hypomethylation—a possible cause of AIDS myelopathy, Personal communication, 1990.

26. Weir, D.G., Molloy, A., Keating, J.N., McPartlin, J., Kennedy, S., Blancheflower, J., Rice, D., and Scott, J.M., Hypomethylation produces vitamin B_{12} associated neuropathy in the pig, in *Biomedicine & Physiology of Vitamin B12*, Linnell, J.C. and Bhatt, H.R., Eds., The Children's Medical Charity, London, 1990, 129.

27. Brody, T., Shane, B., and Stokstad, E.L.R., Folic acid, nutritional, biochemical and clinical aspects, in *Handbook of Vitamins*, Machlin, L.F., Ed., Marcel Dekker, New York, 1984, 459.

28. Johlin, F.C., Fortman, C.S., Nghiem, D.D., and Tephly, T.R., Studies on the role of folic acid and folate-dependent enzymes in human methanol poisoning, *Molec. Pharmacol.*, 31, 557, 1987.

29. Hoffbauer, W. and Zaki, F.G., Choline deficiency in baboon and rat compared, *Arch. Pathol.*, 79, 369, 1965.

30. Chawla, R.K., Wolf, D.C., Kutner, M.H., and Bankovsky, H.L., Choline may be an essential nutrient in malnourished patients with cirrhosis, *Gastroenterology*, 1, 203, 1990.

31. Freeman-Narrod, M., Custer, R.P., and Narrod, S.A., Effect of age and choline administration on triglyceride in the liver of methotrexate-treated rats, *Proc. Am. Assoc. Cancer Res.*, 16, 124, 1975.

32. Custer, R.P., Freeman-Narrod, M., and Narrod, S.A., Hepatotoxicity in Wistar rats following chronic methotrexate administration: a model of human reaction, *J. Natl. Cancer Inst.*, 58, 1011, 1977.

33. IACR Monographs on the Carcinogenic Risk of Chemicals to Humans, Vol. 26, *Some Antineoplastic and Immunosuppressive Agents*, 1981, 267.

34. Schieferstein, G.J., *NCTR Final Report for Experiment 6531*, National Center for Toxicological Research, Jefferson, AR, 1991.

35. Shklar, G., Cataldo, E., and Fitzgerald, A.L., The effect of methotrexate on chemical carcinogenesis in hamster buccal pouch, *Cancer Res.*, 26, 2218, 1966.

36. Rogers, A.E., Akhtar, R., and Zeisel, S.H., Procarbazine carcinogenicity in methotrexate-treated or lipotrope-deficient male rats, *Carcinogenesis*, in press, 1990.

37. Harris, C.C., Malignancy during methotrexate and steroid therapy for psoriasis, *Arch. Derm.*, 103, 501, 1971.

38. Barak, A.J. and Kemmy, R.J., Methotrexate effects on hepatic betaine levels in choline-supplemented and choline-deficient rats, *Drug Nutr. Interact.*, 1, 275, 1982.

39. Broxson, E.H., Stork, L.C., Allen, R.H., Stabler, S.P., and Kolhouse, J.F., Changes in plasma methionine and total homocysteine levels in patients receiving methotrexate infusions, *Cancer Res.*, 49, 5879, 1989.

40. Refsum, H., Ueland, P.M., and Kvinnsland, S., Acute and long-term effects of high-dose methotrexate treatment on homocysteine in plasma and urine, *Cancer Res.*, 46, 5385, 1986.

41. Svardal, A.M., Ueland, P.M., Berge, R.K., Aarsland, A., Aarsaether, N., Lønning, P.E., and Refsum, H., Effect of methotrexate on homocysteine and other sulfur compounds in tissues of rats fed a normal or a defined, choline-deficient diet, *Cancer Chemother. Pharmacol.*, 21, 313, 1988.

42. Hilton, M., Effect of high-dose methotrexate (HDMTX) citrovorum factor (CF) rescue on phenylalanine/tyrosine ratios (PHE/TYR) in plasma and on S-adenosylmethionine/S-adenosylhomocysteine ratios (ADOMET/ADOHCY) in livers of mice, *Fed. Proc.*, 46, 2254, 1987.

43. Hilton, M.A., Hoffman, J.L., and Sparks, M.K., Effect of methotrexate with 5-methyltetrahydrofolate rescue and dietary homocystine on survival of leukemic mice and on concentrations of liver adenosylamino acids, *Cancer Res.*, 43, 5210, 1983.

44. Freeman-Narrod, M., Choline antagonism of methotrexate liver toxicity in the rat, *J. Med. Ped. Oncol.*, 3, 9, 1977.

45. Tuma, D.J., Barak, A.J., and Sorrell, M.F., Interaction of methotrexate with lipotropic factors in rat liver, *Biochem. Pharmacol.*, 243, 1327, 1985.

46. IARC Monographs on the Evaluation of Carcinogenic Risks to Humans, Vol. 44, *Alcohol Drinking*, 1988.

47. Rogers, A.E. and Conner, M.W., Alcohol and cancer, in *Essential Nutrients in Carcinogenesis*, Poirier, L.A., Pariza, M.W., and Newberne, P.M., Eds., Plenum Press, New York, 1986, 473.

48. Feo, F., Pascale, R., Garcea, R., Daino, L., Piris, L., Frassetto, S., Ruggiu, M.E., *et al.*, Effect of the variations of S-adenosyl-L-methionine liver content on fat accumulation and ethanol metabolism in ethanol-intoxicated rats, *Toxicol. Appl. Pharmacol.*, 83, 331, 1986.

49. Lieber, C.S., Casini, A., DeCarli, L.M., Kim, C. I., Lowe, N., Sasaki, R., and Leo, M.A., S-adenosyl-L-methionine attenuates alcohol-induced liver injury in the baboon, *Hepatology*, 11, 165, 1990.

50. Vendemiale, G., Altomore, E., Trizio, T., Le Grazie, C., Di Padova, C., Salerno, M.T., Carrieri, V., *et al.*, Effects of oral S-adenosyl-L-methionine on hepatic glutathione in patients with liver disease, *Scand. J. Gastroenterol.*, 24, 407, 1989.

51. Pascale, R., Daino, L., Garcea, R., Frassetto, S., Ruggiu, M.E., Vannini, M.G., Cozzolino, P., and Feo, F., Inhibition by ethanol of rat liver plasma membrane (Na+,K+)ATPase: protective effect of S-adenosyl-L-methionine, L-methionine, and N-acetylcysteine, *Toxicol. Appl. Pharmacol.*, 97, 216, 1989.

52. Garro, A., McBeth, D., Lima, V., and Lieber, C.S., Dietary ethanol inhibits fetal DNA methylation: Implications for fetal alcohol syndrome, *FASEB J.*, 4, A365, 1990.

53. Porta, E.A., Markell, N., and Dorado, R.D., Chronic alcoholism enhances hepatocarcinogenicity of diethylnitrosamine in rats fed a marginally methyl-deficient diet, *Hepatology*, 5, 1120, 1985.

54. Corrales, F., Cabrero, C.M. Pajares, M.A., Ortiz, P., Martin-Duce, A., and Mato, J.M., Inactivation and dissociation of S-adenosylmethionine synthetase by modification of sulhydryl groups and its possible occurrence in cirrhosis, *Hepatology*, 11, 216, 1990.

55. Duce, A.M., Ortiz, P., Cabrero, C., and Mato, J.M., S-adenosyl-L-methionine synthetase and phospholipid methyltransferase are inhibited in human cirrhosis, *Hepatology*, 8, 65, 1988.

56. Barak, A.J., Beckenhauer, H.C., Tuma, D.J., and Badakhsh, S., Effects of prolonged ethanol feeding on methionine metabolism in rat liver, *Biochem. Cell Biol.*, 65, 230, 1987.

57. Lieber, C.S., Leo, M.A., Mak, K.M., DeCarli, L.M. and Sato, S., Choline fails to prevent liver fibrosis in ethanol-fed baboons but causes toxicity, *Hepatology*, 5, 561, 1985.

Chapter 13

Optimal Detection of and Effect of Vitamin D_3 on Extrachromosomal Oncogene Sequences

Daniel D. Von Hoff and Donald R. VanDevanter

Table of Contents

I. Introduction

Gene amplification (GA) is the mechanism by which transformed cells generate multiple copies of discrete regions of their genome, with a resulting increase in titers of gene product(s) coded for within the amplified region.[1,2] GA can produce resistance to antineoplastic drugs in culture, and has been implicated in tumor progression *in vivo*.[1,2] The occurrence of specific oncogene amplifications has also been shown to be of prognostic significance in certain malignancies.[3,4] Amplification of an oncogene sequence can lead to a more aggressive behavior.

Cytogenetic markers of gene amplification include DMs (double minutes; small acentric chromatin bodies) and HSRs (chromosomally-expanded regions).[1,2] DMs are the most frequently observed marker of gene amplification in fresh biopsy specimens, with HSRs more commonly observed in cells passaged in culture.[5]

Recently, new information has become available on the origin of double minutes. Carroll and colleagues[6] and Von Hoff *et al.*[7] have documented that double minutes can be formed by multimerization of submicroscopic circular DNA molecules ranging from 160-750 kbp in size. These submicroscopic circular DNA molecules are called episomes. Episomes carrying amplified oncogenes as well as amplified drug resistance genes have now been described in hamster and human tumor cell lines as well as in primary human tumors.[8-12]

In the present work we will discuss two aspects of episomes. The first is their optional detection. Obviously, to facilitate studies of these circular molecules, methods to optimize their detection are essential. The second aspect of the episome work is strategies to eliminate episomes from tumor cells. If episomes containing amplified oncogenes or amplified drug resistance genes could be eliminated from tumor cells, it could potentially lead to decreased progression of patient tumor (by eliminating amplified oncogenes) or decreased resistance of a patient's tumor to chemotherapy (through elimination of drug resistance genes).

II. Optimal Detection of Episomes

A. Overview

Episomes containing both amplified drug resistance genes and oncogenes have been detected and characterized in tumor cell lines by alkaline lysis[11] followed by agarose gel electrophoresis at high (5.6 V/cm) electric field strengths. This technique specifically detects supercoiled circular episomal DNA, although circular DNA can exist in both supercoiled and relaxed forms (Figure 1). Relaxed and supercoiled circular DNA molecules exhibit different electrophoretic properties, with relaxed circles unable to migrate under certain conditions.[13]

We have compared two different electrophoretic strategies, low voltage (1.7 V/cm) electrophoresis (LoVE) and field-inversion gel electrophoresis (FIGE[14]) to high voltage (5.6 V/cm) electrophoresis (HiVE) with respect to sensitivity of supercoiled episome detection and ability to detect relaxed circular episomes in lysates of the human promyelocytic leukemia cell line HL-60[8] and the PALA-resistant CHO cell line C5R500.[11]

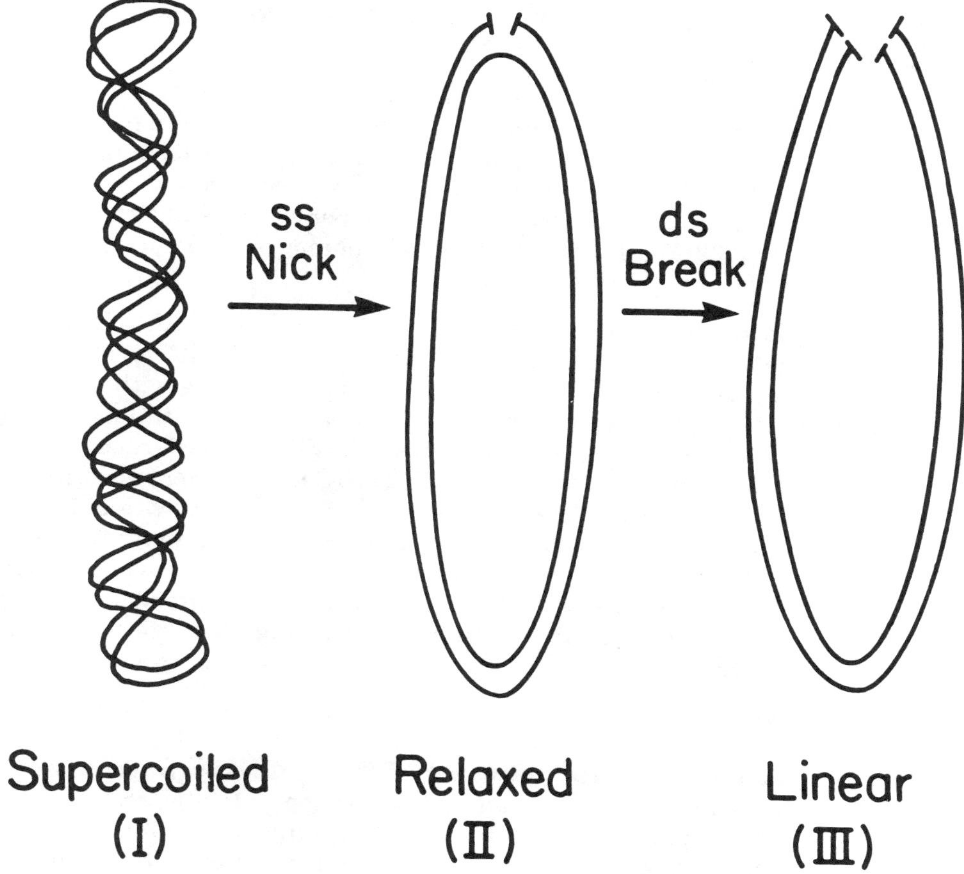

Figure 1. Topological forms of episomal DNA. Episomal DNA molecules can be interconverted between three potential topologic forms: supercoiled (form I), relaxed circular (form II), or linear (form III). These three forms exhibit different electrophoretic characteristics, with large (>50 kbp) relaxed circles incapable of migrating in normal agarose electrophoretic gels.[13] Supercoiled DNA is converted to relaxed circular DNA by the introduction of a single strand nick, and to linear DNA by the introduction of a second nick. The reverse processes require enzyme catalysis and energy.

B. Methods

1. **Cell Culture**. An early passage (p46) of HL60 cells was obtained from Dr. Steve Collins, University of Washington. Cells were initially placed in 96-well titer dishes in RPMI medium enriched with 20% FBS and grown at 37°C in 5% CO_2. After several population doublings, cells were transferred to 6-well dishes, and then to T-25 flasks. Growth medium was then changed to RPMI + 10% FBS, and cells were cut 1:4 every week. The cell line C5R500, a CHO cell line which contains a 250 kbp episomes harboring CAD genes,[11] was obtained from Geoffrey Wahl of the Salk Institute and grown as described previously.[11]

2. **Alkaline Lysis.** HL60 cells (2.0×10^7 cells per tube) and C5R500 cells (4.0×10^6 cells per tube) were lysed under alkaline conditions to isolate circular DNA.[11] DNA pellets were rinsed once with ice-cold 70% ethanol, dried briefly,

and suspended in 20 µl of 50mM sodium acetate, 100mM NaCl, 1mM $ZnSO_4$, pH 4.6 (S_1 nuclease buffer).

3. **S_1 Nuclease Digestion of Alkaline Lysates.** Alkaline lysates from HL60 cells were pooled and spun 10 minutes in a microfuge at 10,000 x g to remove particulates. Cleared lysates were split into 20 µl aliquots in microfuge tubes and treated with 2 µl of S_1 nuclease (Sigma) diluted appropriately in S_1 nuclease buffer for 10 minutes at 37°C. Reactions were stopped by the addition of 3 µl of 0.66 M Tris base, 0.33 M EDTA and an equal volume of 10% sucrose, 0.05% bromophenol blue.

4. **DNA Electrophoresis.** Horizontal 1.0% agarose (BRL UltraPure) electrophoretic gels were run in 45 mM Tris Borate, 1 mM EDTA, pH 8.3 (0.5X TBE) buffer with recirculation. Gels were stained after running with 1.0 µg/ml ethidium bromide and photographed with a red filter while transilluminated by a 300 nm UV source. Low voltage electrophoresis (LoVE) was performed at room temperature for 24 hours at a field strength of 1.7 V/Cm. All other gels were run at 14°C with a field strength of 5.6 V/cm. FIGE was performed with a forward to reverse pulse ratio of 3.0, with pulses ramped linearly from an initial forward pulse time of 3 seconds to a final forward pulse time of 60 seconds over 12 hours. Linear DNA molecular weights were determined with intact chromosomes of *S. cerevisiae* (Beckman) and coliphage lambda DNA digested with HINDIII restriction endonuclease (BRL).

5. **DNA Transfer and Hybridization.** DNA was transferred from agarose gels to nylon-66 membranes (Schleicher and Schuell Nytran) by alkaline capillary transfer. Gels were equilibriated in 0.5 M NaOH, 1.5 M NaCl (transfer buffer) for 30 minutes at room temperature and placed on top of two pieces of wetted 3MM chromatography paper (Whatman) draped into transfer buffer. Nylon-66 membrane was wetted in water and then transfer buffer, placed on top of agarose gels, and covered with two pieces of 3MM paper wetter in transfer buffer. Six inches of paper towels and a 500 g weight were placed on top, and transfers were allowed to proceed overnight. Membranes were hybridized with specific DNA probes labeled with ^{32}P by nick translation kit (Boehringer Mannheim) to a specific activity of greater than 10^8 dpm/µg as previously described.[15] Hybridized membranes were matted with x-ray film (Kodak X-OMAT) between two intensifying screens (DuPont Lightning Plus) and incubated at -70°C to generate autoradiograms.

6. **DNA Probes.** Nylon membranes were probed for c-*myc* sequences using a commercially available (Oncor) probe for the third exon of human c-*myc*. CAD gene sequences were probed with an insert of the CAD-specific plasmid p102F (Geoffrey Wahl).

C. Results

1. **Optimization of Episome Electrophoresis.** Circular DNA molecules can exist in both supercoiled and relaxed topologies which complicates their detection and characterization. Three different electrophoretic strategies were compared for their relative efficiencies in the detection and characterization of episomal DNA from alkaline lysates: HiVE, LoVE, and FIGE. Agarose gel electrophoresis with a high voltage (5.6 V/Cm) gradient (HiVE) has been employed previously to size large supercoiled circular DNA molecules,[8,11] but has

also been reported to arrest migration of relaxed circular molecules.[13] In contrast, electrophoresis with lower voltage (1-2 V/cm) gradients (LoVE) has been reported to allow the migration of relaxed circular DNA molecules which are arrested at higher field strengths.[13] FIGE has been reported to allow the migration of larger relaxed circular DNA molecules,[13] in addition to the resolution of linear molecules between 20 kbp and 1000 kbp.[14]

When identical amounts of HL60 alkaline lysate DNA were electrophoresed under the three separate conditions described above, the most intense c-*myc* signals were obtained under LoVE conditions (Figure 2). In contrast, HiVE afforded the poorest episome detection, requiring extensive autoradiographic exposures to reveal an episome band. FIGE provided slightly less intense c-*myc* episomal signals than LoVE, but with the notable addition of "extra" bands (arrows, Figure 2) within the region in which circular DNA molecules migrate, suggesting that relaxed episomal circles are also migrating in this system.

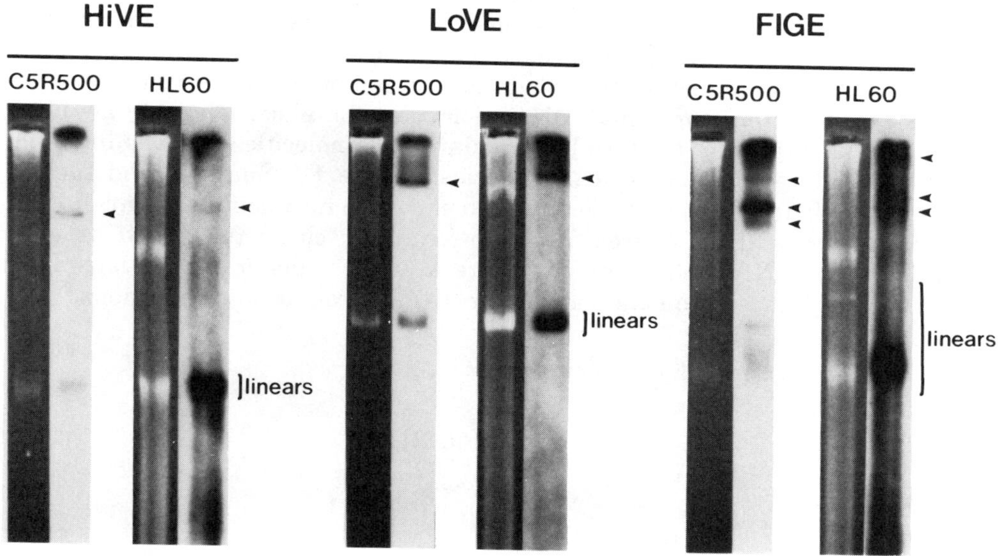

Figure 2. Comparison of HiVE, LoVE, and FIGE electrophoresis of episomal DNA from C5R500 and HL60 cells. Two cell lines containing episomes, C5R500 cells carrying CAD gene episomes[7] and HL60 cells carrying c-*myc* gene episomes[8] were extracted under alkaline conditions (methods) and equal volumes of cell lysates were electrophoresed under HiVE, LoVE, or FIGE conditions. The lysate from 4 x 10^6 cells were loaded on each C5R500 lane, and the lysate from 2 x 10^7 cells was loaded in each HL60 lane. Gels were run as described (methods), ethidium stained and photographed, and DNA from each was transferred to a single nylon membrane. HL60 episomal DNA was detected by membrane hybridization to a radiolabeled c-*myc* specific DNA probe. C5R500 episomal DNA was detected by hybridizing to a CAD specific DNA probe, 102F. Arrows mark circular DNA species. Linear DNA molecules are marked.

C5R500 cell lysates subjected to FIGE also showed the presence of multiple CAD-containing circular DNA molecules (arrows, Figure 2). Interestingly, LoVE appeared to be less efficient than FIGE at detecting the 250 kbp CAD-containing episomes of the cell line C5R500 (Figure 2). This apparent anomaly results because a majority of the circular CAD DNA in these C5R500 lysates existed in the relaxed topological form and could not migrate under LoVE conditions (see below).

Although LoVE provided the most sensitive detection of supercoiled episomes, it also provided the worst size resolution. Note that the 250 kbp CAD episome of C5R500 cells and the slightly larger c-*myc* episome of HL60 cells are better resolved under both HiVE and FIGE conditions than under LoVE conditions (Figure 2). This "compression" of supercoiled circular molecules by LoVE may explain the enhanced autoradiographic signals observed under LoVE conditions. The lack of multiple episomal DNA bands in LoVE gel lanes also suggested that relaxed circular episomes did not migrate under these conditions. Controlled S_1 nuclease digestion of supercoiled HL60 episomes confirmed this conclusion (below).

2. **S_1 Nuclease Generates an Additional HL60 Episomal Band in FIGE Gels.** In order to confirm that additional bands observed in alkaline lysates subjected to FIGE (Figure 2) were relaxed episomes, lysates of HL60 cells were pooled and treated with increasing concentrations of S_1 nuclease to generate relaxed circular c-*myc* episomal DNA molecules for electrophoretic analysis. Single strand nicking of supercoiled circular DNA molecules relieves torsional stress, generating a relaxed circular species (Figure 1). Single-strand specific nucleases (such as S_1) have previously been shown to nick double-stranded DNA in regions with a large degree of single-stranded "character" (such as gene promoters).[16] DNA helix torsional stress (which generates supercoiling) additionally enhances the single-stranded DNA character of such regions.[17]

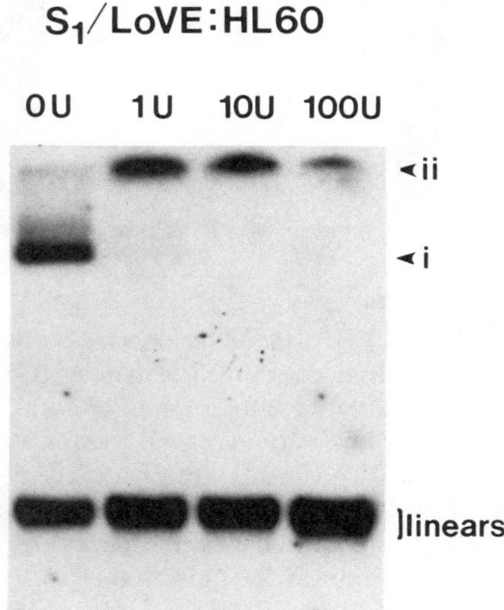

Figure 3. S_1 nuclease digestion of HL60 episomal DNA: LoVE analysis. Alkaline lysates from HL60 cells (2 x 10^7 cells/lane) were treated with 0, 1, 10, or 100 Units of S_1 nuclease for 10 minutes (methods) and electrophoresed under LoVE conditions. DNA was transferred to a nylon membrane and hybridized with a radiolabeled c-*myc*-specific DNA probe. The initial circular DNA species (band "i") was lost following dilute S_1 digestion levels causing the loss of band "ii", with a corresponding increase in linear c-*myc* DNA signal (marked).

LoVE and FIGE analysis of HL60 cell lysates digested with S_1 nuclease showed the conversion of supercoiled c-*myc* episomes (labeled "i" in Figures 3 and 4) to a second DNA species ("ii") which could not migrate under LoVE conditions but could migrate under FIGE conditions. The second DNA structure generated by S_1 nuclease treatment was observed to migrate more slowly under FIGE conditions than the supercoiled HL60 episome (Figure 4). The inability of this second DNA structure ("ii") to migrate under LoVE conditions (Figure 3) and its FIGE migration (which does not match linear DNA molecules within the episome molecular weight range; Figure 4) identify it as a relaxed circular DNA molecule. Increased digestion with S_1 nuclease resulted in degradation of the relaxed episomal species to linear DNA molecules (Figure 3).

The relaxed episomal DNA band generated by S_1 nuclease digestion of supercoiled HL60 episomes matched the migration of one of the additional bands observed in FIGE gels of alkaline lysates (arrows, Figure 2). The third episomal band observed near the origin of FIGE lanes was not reproduced by episome relaxation (compare Figures 2 and 4), leaving its identity undetermined.

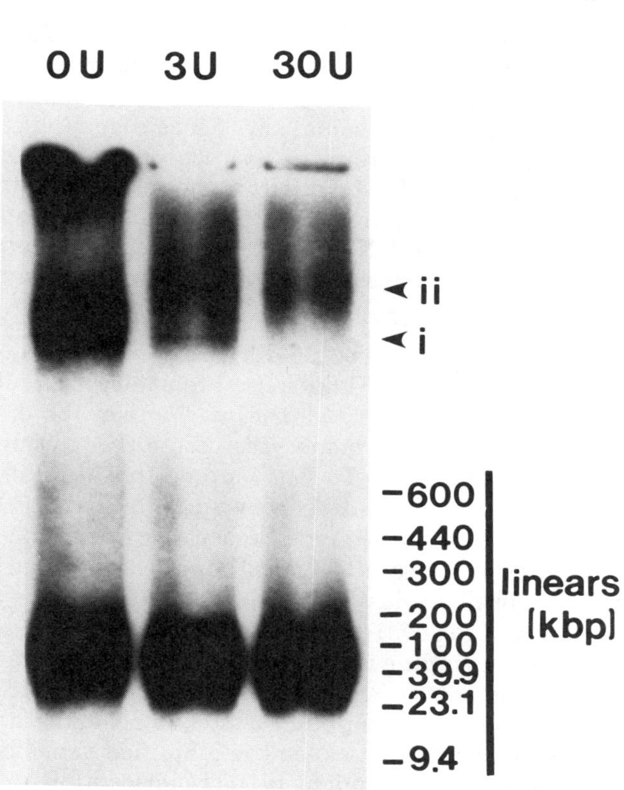

Figure 4. S_1 nuclease digestion of HL60 episomal DNA: FIGE analysis. Alkaline lysates from HL60 cells (2 x 10^7 cells/lane) were treated with 0, 3, or 30 Units of S_1 nuclease for 10 minutes (methods) and electrophoresed under FIGE conditions. DNA was transferred to a nylon membrane and hybridized with a radiolabeled c-*myc*-specific DNA probe. Two circular DNA species could be detected (marked "i" and "ii"), one of which (band "ii") was the S_1 nuclease digestion product of the other. Linear molecular weights are given in kbp.

D. Summary

Optimal detection of supercoiled episomes was achieved by the LoVE technique, while the HiVE technique was least sensitive. Analysis of cell lysates by FIGE[11] demonstrated an intermediate sensitivity in detecting supercoiled episomes, but also revealed "extra" episomal DNA bands, one of which was shown by controlled S_1 nuclease digestion experiments to be relaxed circular episomal DNA. These experiments suggest that a significant portion of episomal DNA in alkaline lysates can exist in the relaxed topologic state, requiring FIGE for detection.

III. Strategy for Elimination of Episomes

A. Overview

As outlined above, if a strategy could be devised to eliminate episomes containing amplified oncogenes or drug resistance genes from a patient's tumor, this might prevent progression (if amplified oncogenes are eliminated) or could reverse drug resistance (if amplified drug resistance genes are eliminated).

Previous work by our group has demonstrated that once episomes are formed (presumably by a deletion event[5]) they multimerize to form double minutes.[6,7] If cells are carried further in passage, the extrachromosomally located double minutes can integrate into a chromosomal site. Once the amplified oncogenes or drug resistance genes are moved from the extrachromosomal (episome or DM) locations (where they are vulnerable to loss from the cell) to an intrachromosomal site, they no longer can be lost from the cell. Therefore, any strategy for elimination of extrachromosomal DNA (in the form of episomes or DMs) from the cell must rely on the amplified genes remaining in that extrachromosomal site(s).

One candidate we had selected as an agent for possible elimination of amplified c-*myc* from HL60 cells was 1,25-dihydroxy vitamin D_3. That agent is known to cause differentiation of HL60 cells (promyelocytic leukemia cells) to form monocytes.[18-21] We reasoned that the mechanism for differentiation of malignant HL60 cells to benign monocytes might be through the loss of extrachromosomally located c-*myc*. To follow up on that thinking, experiments were performed to determine if 1,25-dihydroxy vitamin D_3 (hereafter designated Vit D_3) treatment did not cause an elimination of c-*myc* containing episomes from the cell at concentrations as low as 10^{-8}M. Vit D_3 induces differentiation of nearly 85% of HL60 cells to morphologically and functionally mature monocytes and macrophages.[18] However, as will be noted below, an even more interesting finding arose—namely, the finding that Vit D_3 at 10^{-8}M concentrations caused an inhibition of incorporation of extrachromosomally located amplified c-*myc* into a chromosomal site. Keeping the amplified c-*myc* in an extrachromosomal site could be very helpful as a strategy to keep the amplified genes in an extrachromosomal compartment where they might be more susceptible to elimination by other agents (see below).

B. Methods

1. **Cell Line.** The HL60 cell line (passage 62) from the same source described above was utilized.

2. **Preparation and Irradiation of Cells in Blocks.** Cells were harvested, rinsed with PBS, and suspended in PBS at a density of 2.5 x 10^7 cells/ml. Cell suspensions were mixed with an equal volume of molten (55°C) 1% low melting point agarose (Sea-Plaque, FMC Corporation, Rockland, ME) in PBS and pipetted in 40-µl aliquots (5 x 10^5 cells) into a rubber-based block-forming mold.[23] Blocks were allowed to harden and were placed in 15-ml culture tubes containing 2 ml of 1% Sarkosyl (Sigma Chemical Co.), 100 mM EDTA. Proteinase K (2 mg/ml) was added, the blocks were incubated for 24 h at 55°C, rinsed twice with 10 ml of TE, and stored in TE at 4°C. Blocks were placed in 100 µl of TE in 1.5 ml microfuge tubes, and irradiated by ^{137}Cs source (Gamma Cell 40, Atomic Energy of Canada Ltd., Ottawa, Canada) at a dose of 1.2 Gy/min for 6 min before electrophoresis.

3. **Electrophoresis Technique.** In the present series of experiments, we have utilized a technique which can distinguish between amplified genes located in an extrachromosomal site (on DMs or episomes) versus amplified genes located on an intrachromosomal site (in a homogeneously staining region (HSR) or an abnormal banding region (ABR). The technique used to enable that distinction is the contour-clamped homogeneous electric field or CHEF technique. CHEF electrophoresis was performed using a CHEF-II DR apparatus (Bio-Rad Laboratories, Richmond, CA) in 0.6% agarose gels at 14°C with 60 min pulses for 158 hours at 50 Volts. Molecular weights between 200 and 1000 kbp were determined by electrophoresing the chromosomes of *Sacchromyces cerevisiae* (Beckman Instruments, Inc., Houston, TX). Linearized *Escherichia coli* chromosome was used as a 4800 kbp marker.[22]

4. **Exposure to 1,25-dihydroxy Vitamin D_3.** 1,25-dihydroxy vitamin D_3 was obtained from Hoffman LaRoche, Nutley, NJ. It was dissolved in DMSO for all of the studies. HL60 leukemia cells containing amplified c-*myc* on extrachromosomal sites (exposures and DMs) were exposed to either the vehicle (0.1% DMSO) or to the vehicle plus Vit D_3 at concentrations ranging from 10^{-8} - 10^{-6} M for 10 passages (cells were passaged every 3-4 days). After approximately one month of exposure to the vehicle or vehicle plus Vit D_3 the cells were embedded in agarose blocks, the blocks were prepared as outlined above, and DNA was electrophoresed from the blocks using the CHEF technique outlined above.

C. Results

Figure 5 summarizes the results of this series of experiments. As can be seen in these experiments, passages 73 and 74 HL60 cells with no Vit D_3 added show intense signals in the well of the gel as well as in the zone of compression (designated by a "C") in Figure 5. That amount of c-*myc* signal in these areas indicates the majority of the amplified c-*myc* sequences are positioned in an intrachromosomal site. As can also be seen in the 2 lanes without Vit D_3 added, there are signals in the area of the size of double minutes (1.5 Mbp and approximately 3.0 Mbp). There is less of a signal in these areas in passage 74 than there is in passage 73. What is also very clear in Figure 5 is that when the cells are exposed to 10^{-8} M Vit D_3 there is less of an incorporation of the c-*myc* sequence into the intrachromosomal compartment (i.e., there is less c-*myc* signal in the zone of compression and in the well). In addition, more of the c-*myc* sequence is noted in the area of the double minutes (note signals in 1.5 Mbp and 3.0 Mbp areas). These data indicate Vit D_3 at 10^{-8} M inhibits the incorporation of extrachromosomally located amplified c-*myc* into a chromosomal site.

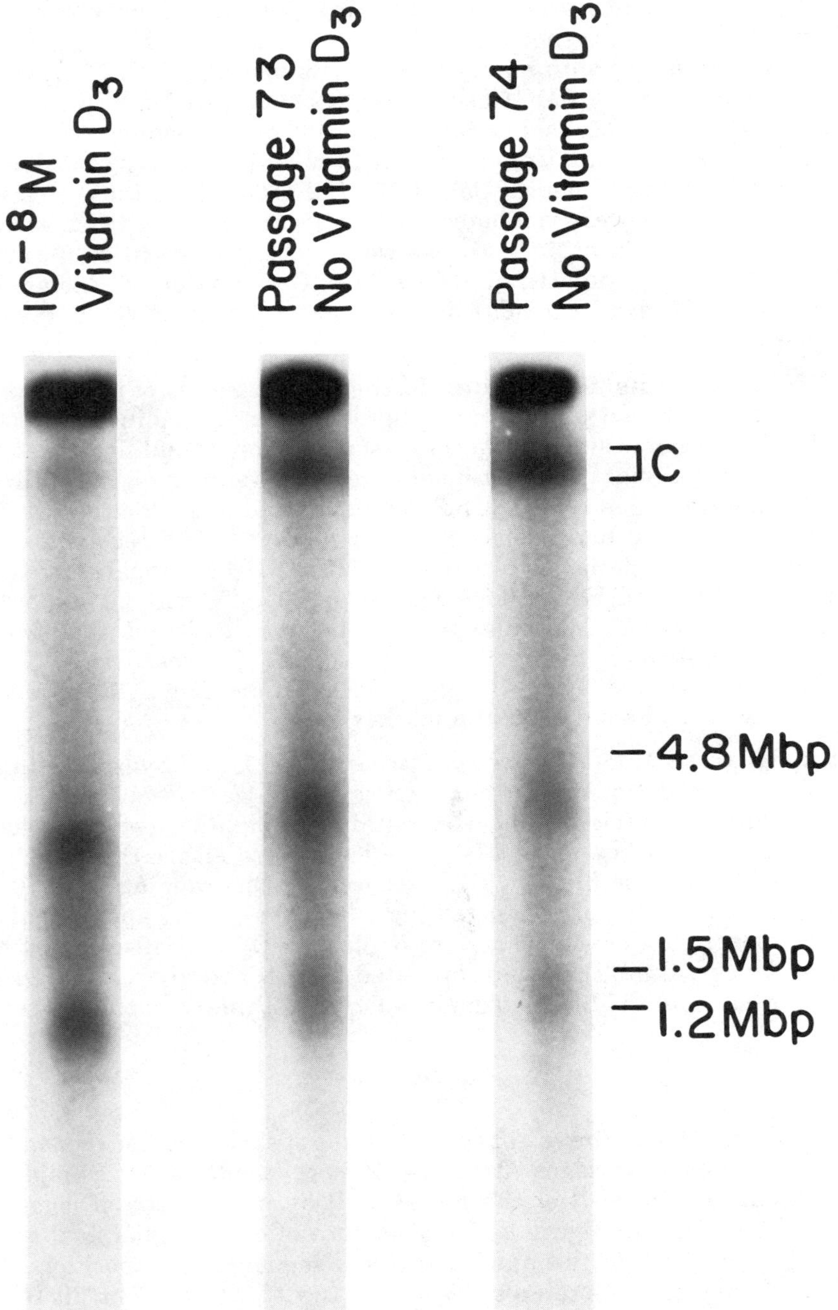

Figure 5. HL60 cells passaged in the presence of either no Vit D_3 or in the presence of Vit D_3 at 10^{-8} M. The cells were embedded in agarose blocks, and gamma irradiated as outlined in the text. The DNA was electrophoresed using the CEHF apparatus under conditions noted in the text. The DNA in the gel was transferred to a nylon membrane. C-*myc* sequences were detected by membrane hybridization to a radiolabeled c-*myc* probe. The "C" designates a zone of compression while the other markers give sizes estimated as noted in the text. The Vit D_3 prevented the extrachromosomally located ($\approx$ 1.5 and 3.0 Mbp) c-*myc* signals from integrating into the chromosomal compartment (designated by the "C" for zone of compression).

IV. Discussion

A. Optimal Detection of HL60 Episomal DNA

We have examined three different electrophoretic strategies for the optimal detection of both supercoiled and relaxed episomal DNA in alkaline lysates of C5R500 and HL60 cells. Normal agarose gel electrophoresis under low electric field strengths (LoVE) provided the most sensitive detection of supercoiled episomal DNA, while higher field strengths significantly reduced episome detection capabilities (Figure 2). Normal agarose electrophoretic gels run under both low and high field strengths showed a single episomal DNA species, while the FIGE technique (which showed intermediate sensitivity) yielded multiple episomal bands (Figure 2).

In contrast to the results obtained with HL60 alkaline lysates above, lysates of the CHO cell line C5R500 provided significantly more episomal DNA signal when electrophoresed under FIGE conditions than when run under LoVE conditions (Figure 2). Careful analysis of C5R500 episomal DNA run under FIGE conditions showed that the brightest episomal CAD band occurred at the position where relaxed episomes were found to migrate (compare the FIGE lane of C5R500 cells in Figure 2 with the locations of bands "i" and "ii" in Figure 4). A much weaker CAD DNA signal was observed at the position where supercoiled episomes migrated (Figure 2). Thus, FIGE provided a greater episome signal than LoVE for C5R500 lysates because a majority of circular CAD DNA in these lysates existed in the relaxed topological form, and could not migrate under LoVE conditions.

Recently, an alternative technique for the detection of circular DNA has been reported which involves the degradation of intact cellular DNA in immobilized in agarose blocks by gamma irradiation.[9,22] Irradiated DNA is then electrophoresed under pulsed-field conditions, and discreet linear DNA bands appearing upon hybridization to specific DNA probes can be attributed to linearization of circular DNA molecules. This technique has been successfully employed to identify and size amplified episomal DNA carrying the multidrug resistance gene *mdr-1* in human KBV-1 cells resistant to velban,[9] and to size DMs carrying amplified dihydrofolate reductase genes in murine 3T6R50 cells resistant to methotrexate.[22] Interestingly, we have found that this technique fails to detect episomal DNA in HL60 cells, presumably because a significant portion of amplified c-*myc* sequences in the HL60 cells studied are carried on much larger (>1000 kpb) DM chromosomes.[7] Under irradiation/pulsed-field conditions in which the 250 kbp CAD episome of C5R500 cells can be clearly detected, only a smear resulting from DM degradation can be detected in HL60 cell lanes (data not shown). For this reason, HL60 DNA irradiation/linearization is not a viable alternative to alkaline lysis for HL60 episome detection.

Analysis of HL60 alkaline lysates electrophoresed under FIGE conditions revealed more than one circular DNA species carrying c-*myc* sequences, while normal electrophoresis showed only a single circular species (Figure 2). It has previously been reported that FIGE is capable of migrating relaxed circular DNA molecules under conditions in which the same molecules are arrested in normal agarose gel electrophoresis,[13] suggesting that additional c-*myc* bands in FIGE gels might be relaxed topological forms of episomal DNA.

Additional evidence that one of the "extra" episomal bands in FIGE gel lanes was a relaxed circular molecule was provided by S_1 nuclease digestions of HL60 episomal DNA, which generated one of the "extra" episomal bands (Figure 4, "ii") observed in FIGE gels of alkaline lysates (Figure 2). Internal proof that S_1 nuclease nicked supercoiled HL60 episomes to relaxed circles was provided by reprobing the nylon membrane of Figure 4 with a mitochondrial-specific DNA probe. Supercoiled 15 kbp mitochondrial DNA (which is also recovered from cells by the alkaline lysis technique[11] was observed to be converted to relaxed circular and linear forms by increasing S_1 nuclease digestion (data not shown). Mitochondrial DNA in alkaline lysates can also be visualized by ethidium bromide staining of electrophoretic gels (note the ethidium staining bands migrating above linear DNA regions in Figure 2).

The identity of the "third" episomal band observed in alkaline lysates run under FIGE conditions (arrows closest to the origin in Figure 2) remains unknown. This species may be: (a) a topological intermediate between fully supercoiled and fully relaxed circular DNA forms, or (b) a supercoiled circle of such high molecular weight that it is incapable of migrating under any electrophoretic conditions but FIGE (perhaps a concatomer of the smaller episome), or (c) a product of irreversible arrest of one of the other circular DNA species during FIGE electrophoresis. Any one of these hypotheses may be correct, and unfortunately, the observation that this species also appears to be lost following S_1 nuclease digestion (Figure 4) does not discriminate between them.

While HL60 is one of only two human tumor cell lines documented to carry episomal oncogene amplification,[8] oncogenes are the most commonly observed genes amplified in human malignancies.[1,2] For this reason, optimization of HL60 episome detection and isolation should prove valuable in the examination of human tumor biopsy specimens for episomal gene amplification. The heterogeneity of c-*myc* amplification structures observed in HL60 cells may accurately reflect the *in vivo* condition, suggesting that simple irradiation/linearization detection techniques might fail to detect small episomal DNA molecules in human tumor biopsy specimens. In contrast, alkaline lysis and agarose gel electrophoresis employing low (1.7 V.cm) electric fields was found to be optimal for detecting small populations of amplified (supercoiled) episomal DNA in heterogeneously amplified cell populations. FIGE appeared to be less sensitive in detecting supercoiled episomal DNA, but had the distinct advantage of also migrating relaxed circular episomal DNA, which can represent a significant portion of episomal DNA in alkaline lysates (as in the case of C5R500 lysates of Figure 2). In addition, a third episomal species (of undetermined structure) was observed in lysates run under FIGE conditions (Figure 2), again suggesting that FIGE may provide a greater possibility of episome characterization than LoVE.

B. Prevention of Integration of Episomes Into a Chromosomal Location

Preliminary work in this area has documented that 1,25-dihydroxy vitamin D_3 at 10^{-8} M concentrations does inhibit incorporation of extrachromosomally located amplified c-*myc* into a chromosomal site. This is a significant finding because if the extrachromosomally located oncogenes can be kept in an extrachromosomal site they can be kept vulnerable to loss from the cells.

Recently, we and others have described pharmacologic strategies to eliminate extrachromosomally located oncogenes and drug resistance genes from human tumor cell lines using hydroxyurea (at easily clinically achievable concentrations).[24–26] Perhaps Vit D_3 could be used to keep the extrachromosomally located genes in that location, vulnerable to the treatment with hydroxyurea for elimination.

There are some cautionary notes on the Vit D_3 work. There are preliminary studies *in vitro* using concentrations of Vit D_3 which while low (10^{-8} M), nonetheless could possibly be associated with hypercalcemia if administered to patients. Therefore, it is imperative that *in vivo* models be developed to test these *in vitro* findings. That model development is ongoing. In addition, testing of combinations of Vit D_3 plus hydroxyurea (to optimize oncogene elimination from cells) is also ongoing.

Acknowledgements

The authors thank Dr. Steve Collins for providing an early freeze of the HL60 cell line, and Dr. Geoffrey M. Wahl for providing the C5R500 cell line and the CAD-specific probe, 102F, as well as for helpful discussions. We also thank Dr. Phillip Serwer for his constructive suggestions.

Supported by the American Institute for Cancer Research grant 88A61 and NIH grant 1U01CA48405-01.

References

1. Stark, G. and Wahl, G.M. Gene amplification, *Annu. Rev. Biochem.*, 53, 447, 1984.

2. Schimke, R.T., Gene amplification drug resistance, and cancer, *Cancer Res.*, 44, 1735, 1984.

3. Slamon, D.J., Clark, G.M., Wong, S.F., Levin, W.J., Ullrich, A., and McGuire, W.L., Human breast cancer: Correlation of relapse and survival with amplification of the HER-2/*neu* oncogene, *Science*, 235, 177, 1987.

4. Brodeur, G.M., Seeger, R.C., Schwab, M., Varmus, H.E., and Bishop, J.M., Amplification of N-*myc* in untreated human neuroblastomas correlates with advanced disease stage, *Science*, 224, 1121, 1984.

5. Wahl, G.M., The importance of circular DNA in mammalian gene amplification, *Cancer Res.*, 49, 1333, 1989.

6. Carroll, S.M., DeRose, M.T., Gaudray, P., Moore, C.M., Needham-VanDevanter, D.R., Von Hoff, D.D., and Wahl, G.M., Double minute chromosomes can be produced from precursors derived from a chromosomal deletion, *Mol. Cell Biol.*, 8, 1525, 1988.

7. Von Hoff, D.D., Forseth, B.J., Clare, N., Hansen, K.L., and VanDevanter, D.R., Double minutes arise from circular extrachromosomal DNA intermediate which

integrate into chromosomal sites in human HL60 leukemia cells, *J. Clin. Invest.*, 85, 1887, 1990.

8. Von Hoff, D.D., Needham-VanDevanter, D.R., Yucel, J., Windle, B.F., and Wahl, G.M, Amplified human MYC oncogenes localized to replicating submicroscopic circular DNA molecules, *Proc. Natl. Acad. Sci. USA.*, 85, 4804, 1988.

9. Ruiz, J.C., Choi, K., Von Hoff, D.D., Roninson, I.B., and Wahl, G.M, Autonomously replicating episomes contain *mdr* 1 genes in a multidrug resistant human cell line, *Mol. Cell Biol.*, 9, 109, 1989.

10. Maurer, B.T., Lai, E., Hamkalo, B.A., Hood, L., and Attardi, G., Novel submicroscopic extrachromosomal element containing amplified genes in human cells, *Nature*, 327, 434, 1987.

11. Carroll, S.M., Gaudray, P., DeRose, M.L., Emery, J.F., Meinkoth, J.L., Nakkin, F., Subler, M., Von Hoff, D.D., and Wahl, G.M, Characterization of an episome produced in hamster cells that amplify a transfected CAD gene at high frequency: functional evidence for a mammalian replication origin, *Mol. Cell. Biol.*, 7, 1740, 1987.

12. VanDevanter, D.R., Piaskowski, V.D., Casper, J.T., Douglass, E.C., and Von Hoff, D.D., Circular extrachromosomal DNA molecules can carry amplified N-*myc* genes in human neuroblastomas *in vivo*, *J. Natl. Cancer Inst.*, 1990, (in press).

13. Levene, S.D. and Zimm, B.H., Separations of open-circular DNA using pulsed-field electrophoresis, *Proc. Natl. Acad. Sci. USA*, 84, 4054, 1987.

14. Carle, G.F., Frank, M., and Olson, M.V., Electrophoretic separations of large DNA molecules by periodic inversion of the electric field, *Science*, 232, 65, 1986.

15. Meinkoth, J. and Wahl, G.M., Hybridization of nucleic acids immobilized on solid supports, *Anal. Biochem.*, 138, 267, 1984.

16. Kroker, W.D. and Kowalski, D.R., Gene-sized pieces produced by digestion of linear duplex DNA with mung bean nuclease, *Biochemistry*, 17, 3236, 1987.

17. Rich, A., Nordheim, A., and Wang, A.H.-J., The chemistry and biology of left-handed Z DNA, *Ann. Rev. Biochem.*, 53, 791, 1984.

18. McCarthy, D.M., San Miguel, J.F., Freake, H.C., Green, P.M., Zola, H., Catorsky, D., and Goldron, J.M., 1,25-Dihydroxy vitamin D_3 inhibits proliferation of human promyelocytic leukemia (HL60) cells and induces monocyte-macrophage differentiation in HL60 and normal human bone marrow cells, *Leukemia Res.*, 7, 51, 1983.

19. Bar-Shavit, Z., Teitelbaum, S.L., Reitsma, P., Hall, A., Peggy, L.F., Trial, J., and Kahn, A.J., Induction of monocytic differentiation and bone resorption by 1,25-dihydroxy vitamin D_3, *Proc. Natl. Acad. Sci. USA*, 80, 5907, 1983.

20. Djulbegovic, B., Christmas, S.E., Evans, G., and Moore, M., Studies of the effect of 1,25 dihydroxycholecalciferol and differentiation of the human promyelocytic leukaemia cell lines HL60, *Biomed. and Pharmacol.*, 40,407, 1986.

21. Daniel, C.P., Parreira, A., Goldman, J.M., and McCarthy, D.M., The effect of 1,25-dihydroxy vitamin D_3 on the relationship between growth and differentiation in HL60 cells, *Leukemia Res.*, 11, 191, 1987.

22. van der Bliek, A.M., Lincke, C.R., and Borst, P., Circular DNA of 3T6R50 double minute chromosomes, *Nucl. Acids Res.*, 16, 4841, 1988.

23. VanDevanter, D.R., Trammell, T.T.M., and Von Hoff, D.D., Simple construction of rubber-based agarose block molds for pulsed-field electrophoresis, *BioTechnique*, 7, 143, 1989.

24. Von Hoff, D.D., Forseth, B., Bradley, T., and Wahl, G., Hydroxyurea can decrease drug resistance gene copy numbers in tumor cell lines, *Proc. Am. Soc. Clin. Oncol.*, 9, 55, 1990.

25. Von Hoff, D.D., Waddelow, T., Forseth, B., Davidson, K., Scott, J., and Wahl, G., Loss of drug resistant gene-containing episomes from tumor cells is accelerated by hydroxyurea, *Cancer Res.*, 1991, (in press).

26. Christen, R.D., Shalinsky, D.R., and Howell, S.B., Hydroxyurea (HU) accelerates the rate of loss of resistance to vinblastine (VBL) in KBV cells, but does not change the sensitivity to cisplatin in cisplatin resistant human ovarian carcinoma cells, *Proc. Am. Soc. Clin. Oncol.*, 9, 55, 1990.

Chapter 14

Anti-Tumor Proliferation Properties of Vitamin E

Kimberly Kline and Bob G. Sanders

Table of Contents

I. Introduction

Various forms of the fat soluble vitamin, vitamin E, have been shown to be effective in inhibiting certain types of chemically-induced and retrovirus-induced tumor growth *in vivo*.[1-6] One possible mechanism that has been proposed for these anti-tumor effects by vitamin E is a direct effect on tumor cell growth. *In vitro* analyses have demonstrated that vitamin E can inhibit the growth of several types of cells, including human neuroblastoma,[7] murine neuroblastoma,[8] murine melanoma,[9] rat neuroblastoma and glioma cells,[10] and avian lymphoid leukemia cells, the subject of this review.[11] Of the various forms of vitamin E tested for antiproliferative effects on tumor cells, the succinated form of natural D-α-tocopherol, referred to by the common names D-α-tocopheryl acid succinate or vitamin E succinate or by its trivial name, RRR-α-tocopheryl acid succinate, has been demonstrated to be the most effective form *in vitro*.

II. Inhibition of Avian Retrovirus-Transformed Lymphoid Tumor Cell Proliferation by Vitamin E Succinate

The effects of vitamin E on the rapidly proliferating cells of the established chicken lymphoid cell line, C4#1 (obtained from Dr. Henry R. Bose, Jr., Department of Zoology, University of Texas at Austin, Austin, TX), transformed by the highly oncogenic replication defective retrovirus, reticuloendotheliosis virus (REV-T) carrying the *v-rel* oncogene, and its replication competent associated helper virus (REV-A) were examined. REV (REV-T/REV-A) transformed cell lines exhibit a lymphoblastoid morphology. Some lines have been characterized as immature B-cells based on the presence of terminal deoxynucleotidyl transferase and weak to moderate expression of B-cell determinants.[12-14] Some lines exhibit weak expression of T-cell markers.[15] C4#1 is the most immature REV-transformed line characterized. Unlike other REV-transformed cell lines that exhibit various states of germline heavy or light immunoglobulin chain gene rearrangments, C4#1 cells do not show any immunoglobulin gene rearrangements.[7]

A. Dose-Dependent Nature of Vitamin E's Effects

Treatment of C4#1 tumor cells for 48 hours with vitamin E succinate ranging in concentration from 0.01 to 10 μg/ml inhibited cellular proliferation without affecting cell viability, with maximal growth inhibition occurring at the 10 μg/ml concentration (Figure 1).

The cytostatic effects of vitamin E succinate on C4#1 tumor cells appear to be reversible in that cells treated for either 24 or 48 hours in the presence of vitamin E succinate exhibited the capacity to recover their ability to proliferate when they were removed from the vitamin E succinate treatment and recultured in the absence of vitamin E succinate. Similar results on the reversibility of vitamin E succinate induced cytostatic effects have been reported by Prasad and coworkers who showed that mouse melanoma, B-16, cells cultured for 4 days with vitamin E succinate exhibited delayed proliferation for 24 hours following

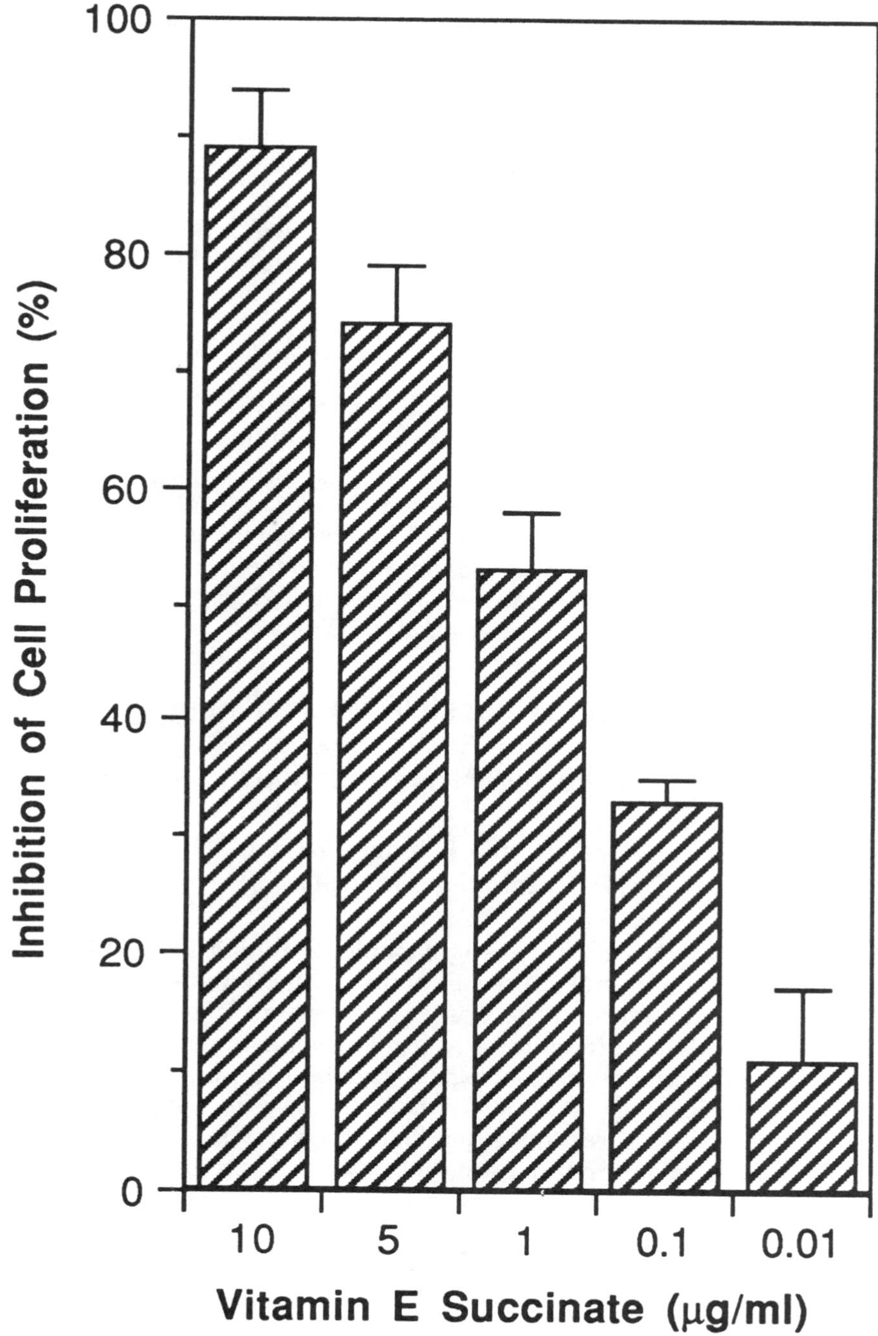

Figure 1. C4#1 tumor cells at 1 x 10^6/ml were cultured with varying concentrations of vitamin E succinate for 48 hrs, tritiated thymidine was added, cells were harvested 18 hrs later, and tritiated thymidine uptake was determined. Data are presented as average percent inhibition of proliferation of cells treated with vitamin E succinate in relation to proliferation of C4#1 tumor cells grown in the presence of equivalent amounts of vehicle ± SD of 3 replicates. Viability of vitamin E succinate and vehicle control-treated cells for all concentrations tested was greater than 90%. (From Kline, K., Cochran, G. S., and Sanders, B. G., *Nutr. Cancer* 14, 27, 1990.

removal of the vitamin E succinate but eventually were capable of growing to confluency.[10]

B. Forms of Vitamin E that Exhibit Anti-Tumor Proliferation Activities *in Vitro*

While various forms of vitamin E have been shown to be potent modulators of chemical and retrovirus-induced tumor growth *in vivo*,[1-6] the succinate ester of vitamin E has been shown to be the most effective form for inhibiting tumor cell growth *in vitro* (Table 1).[7-11,16]

C. Hematopoietic Cell Types that Are Responsive to Vitamin E Inhibition

Investigations of the effects of vitamin E succinate on the proliferative capacity of various transformed avian cell lines of hematopoietic origin as well as quiescent and mitogen-stimulated normal lymphoid cells illustrates that vitamin E's antiproliferative effects are dependent on the cell type and activation-state of the cell under investigation (Table 2).

III. Investigations of Possible Mechanisms Whereby Vitamin E Mediates Its Antiproliferative Activities

A. Does Vitamin E Induce Tumor Cell Differentiation/Maturation?

Because vitamin E succinate was capable of inhibiting C4#1 tumor cell proliferation, it was of interest to see if vitamin E succinate was having an effect on the differentiation state of the C4#1 cells, perhaps inducing the immature lymphoid C4#1 cells to differentiate to a more mature, nonproliferative state. Based on lack of change in morphological parameters, i.e. vitamin E succinate treated cells retain their abnormal lymphoblastoid-like appearance and no change in expression of several avian hematopoietic cell surface membrane markers (Table 3), it does not appear that vitamin E succinate is inducing the differentiation of C4#1 cells to a more mature, nonproliferative stage.

B. Is it an Antioxidant Effect?

Vitamin E's best characterized function is as a lipid-soluble antioxidant in cell membranes, functioning as a free radical scavenger to prevent lipid peroxidation of polyunsaturated fatty acids.[17] Since there are reports that certain cellular activation pathways ultimately initiating cell proliferation involve an obligatory, free-radical-mediated step,[18] it was of interest to ascertain if the anti-tumor proliferative activity of vitamin E might be attributable to its classical antioxidant properties. Several antioxidants, including the lipid-soluble antioxidants, butylated hydroxyanisole (BHA) and butylated hydroxytoluene (BHT) which have been demonstrated to be more effective as free radical scavengers when used in

TABLE 1
Effects of Different Forms of Vitamin E on C4#1 Tumor Cell Proliferation *in Vitro*

Treatment	% Viability[a]	^{3}H-TdR Uptake[b] (cpm)	% Inhibition[c]
Vehicle control	92	69,789 ± 1,465	0
Untreated media control	96	62,811 ± 1,604	
Vitamin E succinate			
10 µg/ml	100	3,285 ± 441	95
5 µg/ml	100	10,246 ± 517	85
D-α-Tocopherol			
100 µg/ml	95	85,823 ± 1,718	0
50 µg/ml	94	94,164 ± 3,718	0
25 µg/ml	95	78,065 ± 3,101	0
12.5 µg/ml	93	75,297 ± 2,223	0
6.25 µg/ml	98	85,276 ± 2,564	0
DL-α-Tocopherol			
100 µg/ml	96	70,458 ± 9,015	0
50 µg/ml	94	95,830 ± 5,869	0
25 µg/ml	95	68,064 ± 2,238	2
12.5 µg/ml	92	91,126 ± 3,600	0
6.25 µg/ml	96	99,096 ± 6,861	0
Vitamin E Acetate			
50 µg/ml	99	95,646 ± 3,795	0
25 µg/ml	98	98,130 ± 3,472	0
10 µg/ml	99	93,870 ± 2,868	0
Trolox			
50 µg/ml	100	70,470 ± 1,485	0
25 µg/ml	94	69,924 ± 4,147	0
10 µg/ml	96	65,337 ± 2,829	0
5 µg/ml	97	70,662 ± 904	0

[a] Cultures of C4#1 tumor cells at 1 x 10^6/ml, not receiving tritiated thymidine, were used to determine cell viability using the trypan blue dye exclusion assay.
[b] C4#1 tumor cells at 1 x 10^6/ml were treated for 24 hours, labeled with tritiated thymidine, harvested 18 hours later, and counted.
[c] % inhibition of proliferation of vitamin E succinate, D-α-tocopherol, DL-α-tocopherol, and vitamin E acetate treated cells were determined in relation to the proliferation of vehicle (ethanol) treated control cells. Trolox treated cells were compared to untreated media control cells.

combination,[19] Trolox, a water soluble analog of RRR-α-tocopherol with a carboxyl group instead of the isoprene side chain which is reported to be an effective antioxidant,[20] and mannitol, a scavenger for hydroxy radicals were tested for antiproliferative activity at nontoxic concentrations (Table 4). These data suggest that the inhibition of tumor cell proliferation by vitamin E succinate is probably unrelated to its antioxidant functions.

TABLE 2
Effects of Vitamin E on the Proliferative Capacity of Various Avian Hematopoietic Tumor Cells and Normal Cells *in Vitro*

Cell Line Designation and Description of Transformed Cell Type or Type of Normal Cell and Activation State		Effects of Vitamin E Succinate on Cellular Proliferative Status
C4#1	REV-transformed immature lymphoid cell	Inhibitory
BB5	REV-transformed immature lymphoid cell	Inhibitory
KBMC	REV-transformed immature B-like cell	Inhibitory
6C2	AEV-transformed erythroblast	Inhibitory
HD11	MC29-transformed macrophage	Inhibitory
Thymic lymphocytes	Unstimulated	Enhancing
Thymic lymphocytes	Mitogen-stimulated	Inhibitory
Splenic lymphocytes	Unstimulated	Enhancing
Splenic lymphocytes	Mitogen-stimulated	Inhibitory
Bursal lymphocytes	Unstimulated	Enhancing
Bursal lymphocytes	Mitogen-stimulated	No effect

C. Does It Involve a Blockage of the Cell Cycle?

Since vitamin E has a cytostatic rather than cytotoxic effect, investigations were carried out to determine if vitamin E succinate was blocking C4#1 cells in the cell cycle. Analyses of DNA content of propidium iodide stained cells using a fluorescence-activated cell sorter showed the vitamin E succinate treated cells to be blocked in the G_0+G_1/early S phase of the cell cycle (Figure 2).

D. Does It Involve Modulation of Oncogene Expression?

Since it was not known whether or not the *v-rel* oncogene was a replication-linked gene, it was of interest to ascertain if C4#1 cells inhibited from proliferating by treatment with vitamin E succinate exhibited any changes in the expression of *v-rel* messenger RNA or in the level of expression of the *v-rel* encoded 59,000 dalton cytoplasmic protein. The levels of *v-rel*-encoded $pp59^{v\text{-}rel}$

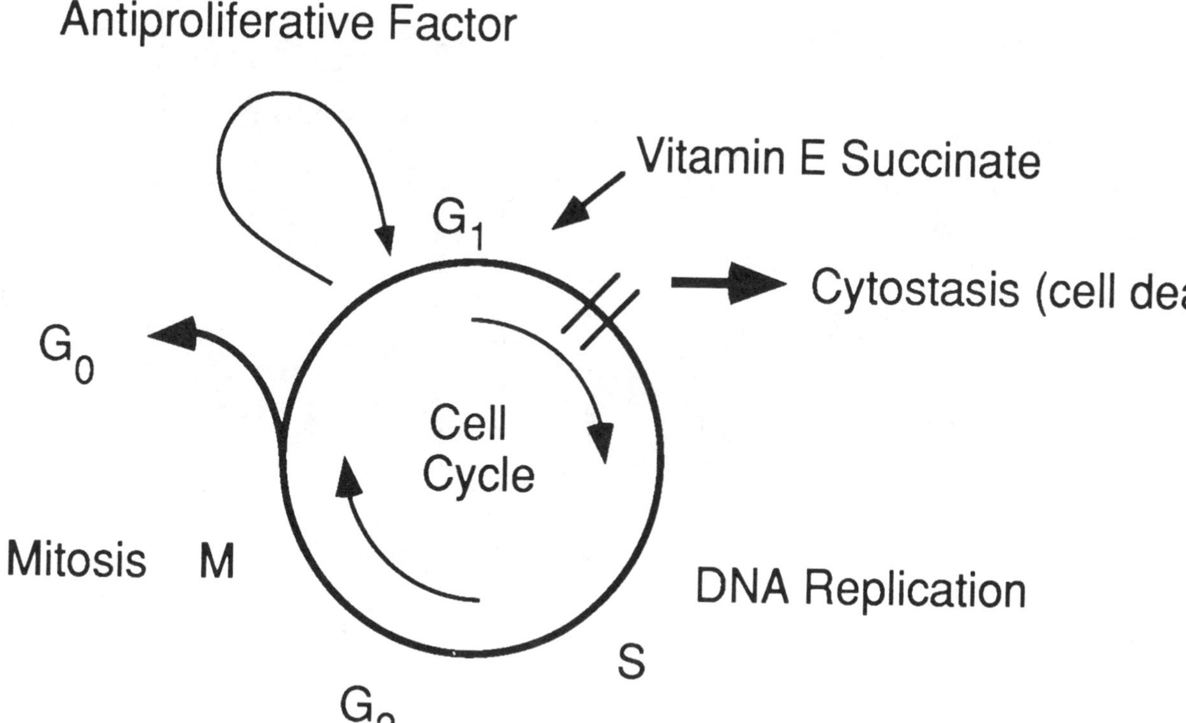

Figure 2. When a cell resting in the G_0 phase is stimulated to undergo proliferation, it proceeds through phases G_1, S (DNA synthesis) and G_2 prior to mitosis (M, cell division). Vitamin E succinate has been shown to block C4#1 cells in the G_0+G_1/early S phase of the cell cycle.

TABLE 3
Cellular Differentiation Status of C4#1 Tumor Cells Treated with Vitamin E Succinate[a]

Differentiation Parameters	Treatments: Vitamin E	Vehicle	Untreated
Hematopoietic-lymphoid markers[b]			
gp50	+	+	+
CFA	+	+	+
MHC class II (Ia)	+	+	+
Surface immunoglobulin	-	-	-
Macrophage specific markers[c]			
CMTD-1	-	-	-
CMTD-2	-	-	-
Con A binding	+	+	+
Rosetting properties[d]			
E rosettes	-	-	-
EA rosettes	+	+	+
Morphology[e]	NC	NC	

[a] C4#1 tumor cells were cultured with 5 and 10 mg/ml of vitamin E succinate, equivalent levels of vehicle or media for 24 and 48 hrs, and analyzed for various phenotypic markers.
[b] +, Positive; -, negative; NC, no change compared with untreated media control cells.
[c] Expression of 4 hematopoietic-lymphoid membrane antigens was determined by radioimmunometric assay using specific polyclonal and monoclonal antibody reagents as described in Materials and Methods.
[d] C4#1 tumor cells were assayed for presence of 2 macrophage-specific antigens and ability to bind peroxidase labeled concanavalin A (Con A).
[e] E rosetting properties of C4#1 tumor cells were determined by analyzing their ability to bind quail red blood cells. EA rosetting properties were determined by analyzing ability of C4#1 tumor cells to bind antibody-sensitized sheep red blood cells.
[f] Morphology was determined by microscopic examination of Wright-Giemsa-stained C4#l cells. (From Kline, K., Cochran, G. S., and Sanders, B. G., *Nutr. Cancer* 14, 27, 1990).

were determined by quantitative Western blot analyses (Figure 3A) and the levels of *v-rel*-specific messenger RNA were determined by dot blot analyses (Figure 3B). No significant differences in levels of pp59$^{v\text{-}rel}$ or *v-rel* messenger RNA were observed among proliferating untreated or vehicle control treated C4#1 tumor cells and C4#1 cells inhibited from proliferating by vitamin E succinate treatment.

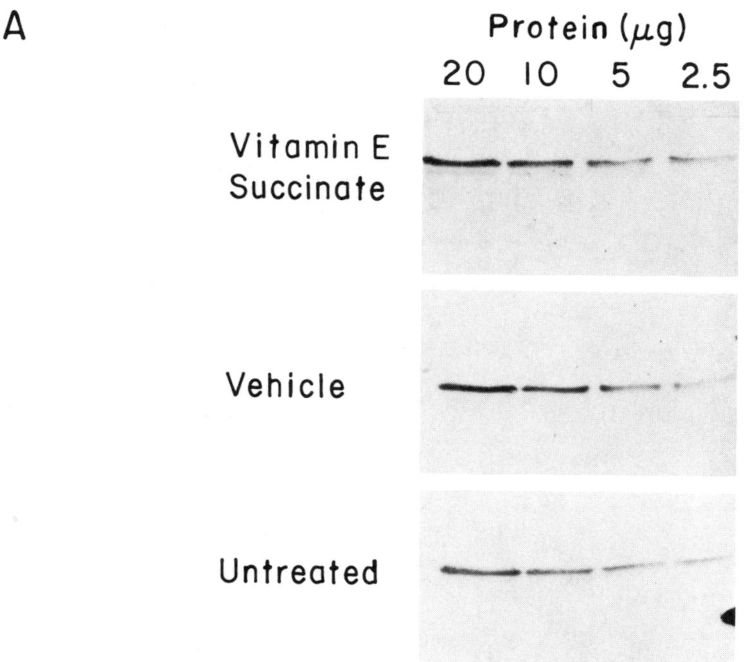

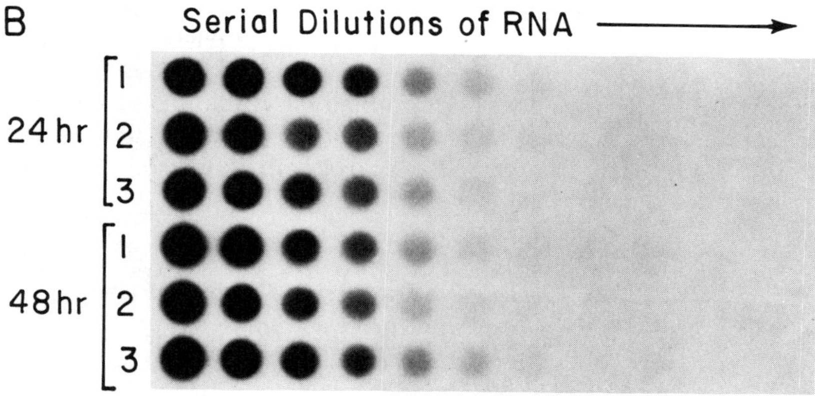

Figure 3. Figure 3A represents the expression of the *v-rel*-encoded protein, $pp^{59v\text{-}rel}$, in C4#1 tumor cells cultured for 20 hours with vitamin E succinate or vehicle control or untreated. Aliquots of whole-cell lysates containing 20, 10, 5, and 2.5 µg total protein were analyzed by one-dimensional sodium dodecyl sulfate-polyacrylamide gel electrophoresis followed by electrophoretic transfer of the separated proteins to nitrocellulose and detection of $pp^{59v\text{-}rel}$ with a monoclonal antibody. The resulting bands were compared following analyses on a modified Helena TLC Quick Scan Densitometer. Figure 3B represents *v-rel* specific RNA expression as analyzed by dot blot hybridization using a radiolabeled probe specific for *v-rel* sequences. C4#1 tumor cells were treated with 10 µg/ml of vitamin E succinate (1), vehicle control (2), or untreated (3) for 24 and 48 hours, RNA was extracted, serially diluted, and collected on filter paper. Washed filters were reacted with a radiolabeled probe specific for *v-rel* sequences, and exposed on Kodak XAR-2 film using an intensifying screen. The autoradiograph presented represents a 17 hour exposure. (From Kline, K., Cochran, G. S., and Sanders, B. G., *Nutr. Cancer* 14, 27, 1990.)

TABLE 4
Antioxidant Effects on C4#1 Tumor Cell Proliferation *in Vitro*

Treatment	% Viability[a]	^{3}H-TdR Uptake[b] (cpm)	% Inhibition[c]
Vehicle control	88	97,936 ± 7,166	0
Untreated media control	100	78,853 ± 6,174	
Vitamin E succinate (10 µg)	92	18,355 ± 1,968	81
BHA (5 µM)	92	95,847 ± 3,339	0
BHT (5 µM)	93	92,717 ± 2,361	0
BHA + BHT (1 µM each)	94	97,667 ± 3,288	0
Mannitol (5 µM)	92	97,975 ± 2,096	0

[a] Parallel cultures, not receiving tritiated thymidine, were used to determine cell viability using the trypan blue dye exclusion assay.
[b] C4#1 tumor cells at 1 x 10^{6}/ml were treated for 24 hours, labeled with tritiated thymidine, harvested 18 hours later, and amount of tritiated thymidine uptake determined.
[c] % inhibition of proliferation was determined for vitamin E succinate, BHA, and BHT treated cells in relation to proliferation of vehicle (ethanol) treated cells. % inhibition of mannitol treated cells was determined in relation to proliferation of untreated media control cells.

E. Does It Involve Increased Activity of an Antiproliferative Factor?

One mechanism for uncontrolled cell growth involves the lack of production of soluble, autocrine-acting, antiproliferative factors or the inability of tumor cells to receive and process such antiproliferative signals. In an effort to determine if vitamin E succinate's growth inhibitory effect might involve upregulating the expression of an antiproliferative factor, conditioned media from treated C4#1 cells were analyzed (Figure 4).

Results suggest that there is an antiproliferative factor in the conditioned media of C4#1 tumor cells treated with vitamin E succinate and that this antiproliferative factor is not vitamin E succinate. Further studies showing that boiling the conditioned media for 10 minutes did not inactivate the antiproliferative factor and that acid treatments activate the factor indicate that the vitamin E induced antiproliferative factor shares certain physical characteristics with transforming growth factor β (TGF-β). TGF-β is a potent autocrine growth inhibitor of hematopoietic cells, including lymphocytes.[21-25]

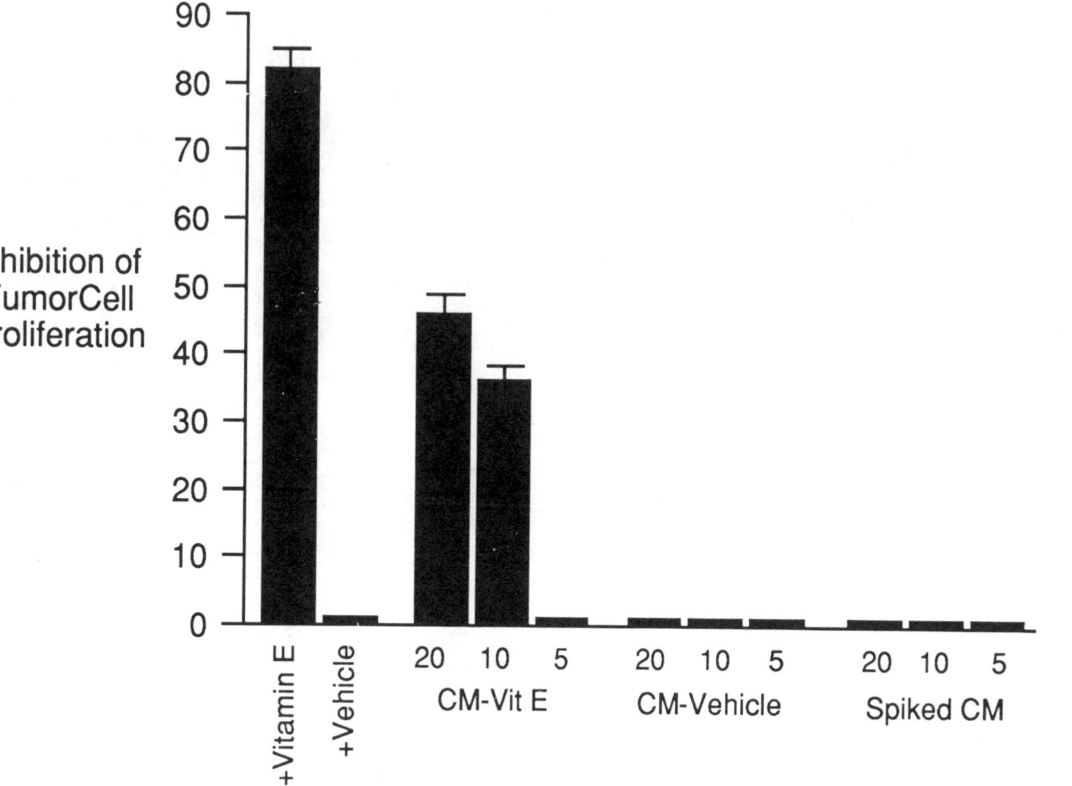

Figure 4. Conditioned media (CM) from C4#1 cells 24 hours after treatment with vitamin E succinate or vehicle were concentrated down using Millipore centrifuge concentrators with a 10,000 dalton molecular weight cut-off. Concentrated conditioned media were then tested at different concentrations on untreated C4#1 cells. Unlike conditioned media from vehicle treated cells (CM-Vehicle) or conditioned media from vehicle treated cells to which vitamin E succinate was intentionally added prior to concentration (spiked CM), conditioned media from vitamin E succinate treated cells inhibited the proliferation of untreated C4#1 cells in a dose-dependent manner.

IV. Evidence for a Cytosolic Vitamin E Binding Protein in C4#1 Tumor Cells

It was of interest to ascertain if vitamin E might be mediating its antiproliferative activities via a mechanism similar to two other fat soluble vitamins, namely, retinoic acid (vitamin A metabolite) and 1,25-dihydroxyvitamin D (active metabolite of vitamin D), which involve cytosolic receptors that, after binding to their respective vitamins, are translocated into the nucleus where DNA binding domains on the receptor mediate a variety of gene regulatory events.[26-29] An affinity chromatography approach was used in an effort to determine if C4#1 cells contained a cytosolic vitamin E binding protein. As illustrated in Figure 5, this method successfully isolated 32,000 dalton molecules from rat liver cytosol that exhibit the same molecular weight as the reported vitamin E binding protein as well as molecules of approximately 65-70,000 daltons from C4#1 cytosol and chicken liver cytosol.[30-33]

V. Model for Vitamin E Mediated Inhibition of Tumor Cell Proliferation

Figure 6 illustrates a hypothetical model for how vitamin E succinate inhibits tumor cell proliferation. This model addresses the underlying mechanisms by which vitamin E acts as a potent inhibitor of hematopoietic-tumor cell proliferation.

VI. Summary and Conclusions

Nutritional modulation of antitumor mechanisms leading to the destruction of tumor cells with no effect on normal cells and minimal toxic side effects to the patient is the ultimate goal of nutrition-immunology-cancer research. The studies reviewed here show that vitamin E succinate is a potent, and potentially important, antitumor agent in that it prevents the growth of a wide range of tumor cells of hematopoietic origin. Vitamin E succinate also has the unique property of enhancing the proliferation of resting splenic and thymic lymphocytes but inhibiting the proliferation of mitogen stimulated T lymphocytes. Understanding how vitamin E succinate enhances the proliferation of normal resting lymphocytes, inhibits tumor cell growth, and inhibits the proliferation of mitogen stimulated T lymphocytes may be fundamental to our understanding of the role vitamin E plays as a modulator of retrovirus-induced immune dysfunctions and malignant cell growth. The growth-inhibitory properties of vitamin E appear to be mediated by mechanisms other than its classical functional role as an antioxidant. It appears that vitamin E succinate does not induce tumor cells to differentiate into a non-proliferative state, rather, the tumor cells appear to be blocked in the cell cycle prior to DNA synthesis. The tumor cells, perhaps due to their arrested state in a specific cell cycle stage, produce and secrete an antiproliferative factor that is capable of inhibiting proliferation of other tumor cell types. The activity of the antiproliferative factor is enhanced by boiling and by acid/neutralization treatments, properties similar to the well established antiproliferative factor, TGF-β. A model for explaining how vitamin E succinate

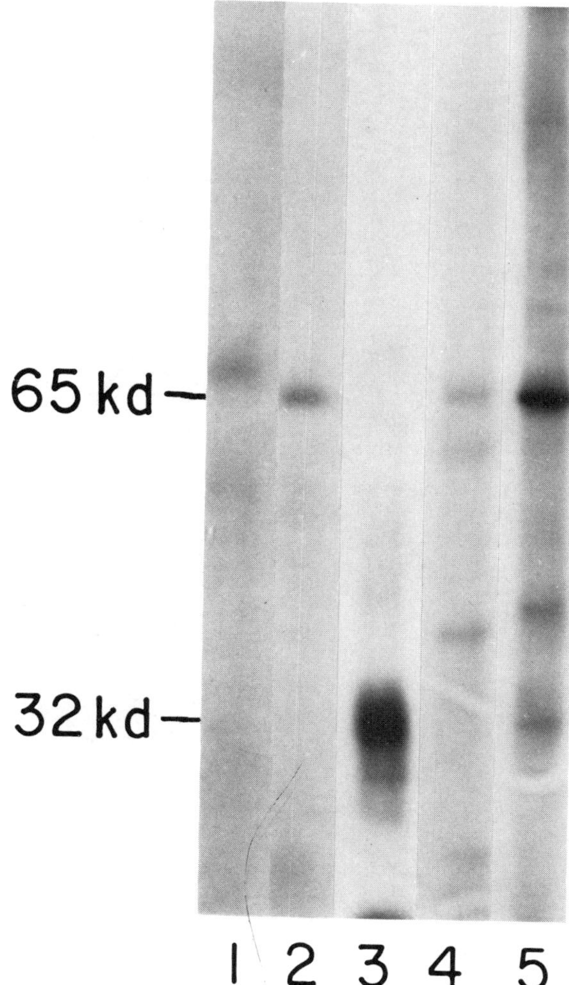

Figure 5. Autoradiographs of one-dimensional sodium dodecyl sulfate-polyacrylamide gel electrophoretic analyses of radioiodinated cytosolic proteins isolated by affinity chromatography using EAH-Sepharose conjugated to vitamin E succinate. Reduced or nonreduced samples analyzed in lanes 1-5 were: C4#1 cytosolic proteins purified two times by affinity chromatography-reduced; C4#1 cytosolic proteins purified two times by affinity chromatography-nonreduced; rat liver cytosolic proteins purified one time by affinity chromatography-nonreduced; C4#1 cytosolic protein purified one time by affinity chromatography and one time by HPLC-DEAE chromatography-nonreduced; and chicken liver cytosolic proteins purified one time by affinity chromatography and one time by HPLC-DEAE chromatography-nonreduced.

might mediate its antiproliferative effects postulates that vitamin E binds to a cytosolic vitamin E binding protein which is then transported to the nucleus where gene activation of an antiproliferative factor occurs. Alternatively, there is the possibility, that vitamin E may be functioning by mediating the conversion of an inactive precursor of the antiproliferative factor to its biologically active state. Although not proven, support for the model comes from studies showing the presence of a vitamin E binding protein of approximately 65,000 kilodaltons in tumor cells responsiveness to vitamin E's antiproliferative effects.

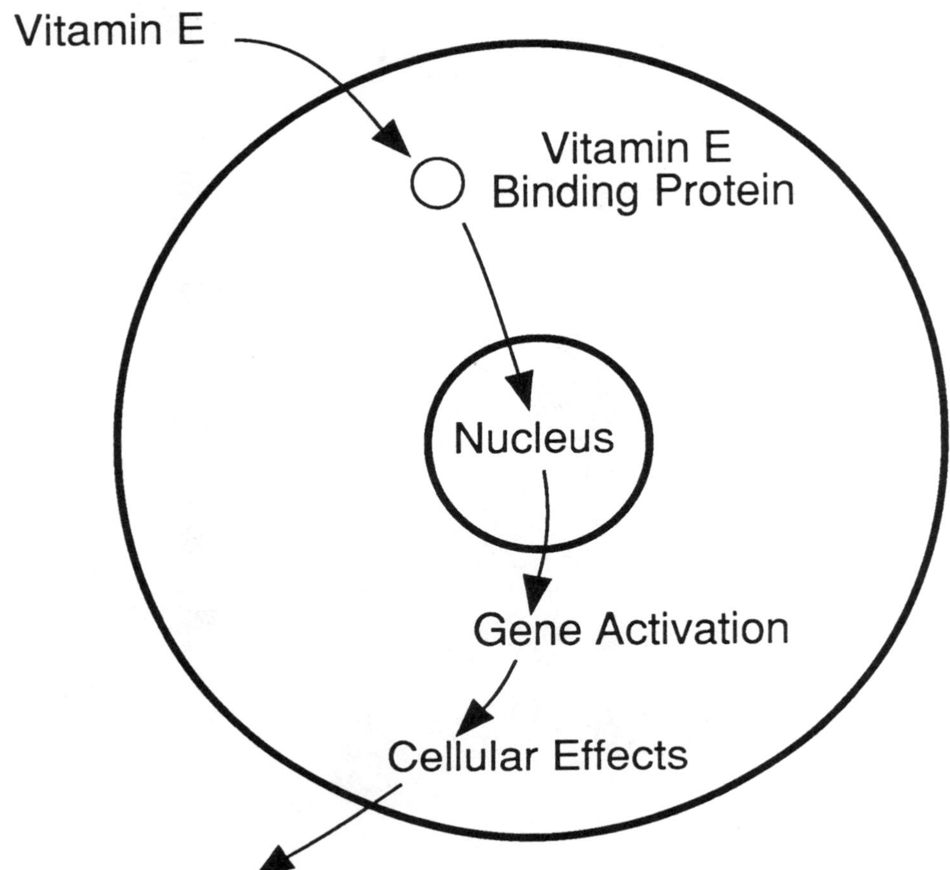

Figure 6. A hypothetical model for vitamin E mediated antiproliferative effects. Vitamin E passes through the cell surface membrane and interacts with its cytosolic receptor which is then translocated into the nucleus where it binds to DNA, an event that causes either gene activation or gene repression. One biological consequence is either increased levels of a soluble antiproliferative factor or increased activity of a soluble antiproliferative factor which blocks cells in the cell cycle.

Acknowledgements

The research was supported by the American Institute for Cancer Research (Washington, D.C.) Grant No. 87A69 (K. Kline and B. Sanders) and by U.S. Public Health Service Grant No. CA-45422 (K. Kline) awarded by the Department of Health and Human Services, National Institutes of Health (Bethesda, MD).

References

1. Kline, K. and Sanders, B.G., Modulation of immune suppresion and enchanced tumorigenesis in retrovirus tumor challenged chickens treated with vitamin E, *In Vivo*, 3, 161, 1989.

2. Slaga, T.J. and Bracken, W.M., The effects of antioxidants on skin tumor initiation and ary hydrocarbon hydroxylase, *Cancer Res.*, 37, 1631, 1977.

3. Cook, M.G. and McNamara, P., Effect of dietary vitamin E on dimethylhydrazine-induced colonic tumor in mice, *Cancer Res.*, 40, 1329, 1980.

4. Haber, S.L. and Wessler, R.W., Effect of vitamin E on carcinogenicity of methylcholanthrene, *Proc. Soc. Exp. Biol. Med.*, 111, 774, 1962.

5. Newmark, H.L. and Mergens, W.J., Alpha-tocopherol (vitamin E) and its relationship to tumor induction and development, in *Inhibition of Tumor Induction and Development,* Zedeck, M.S. and Lipkins, M., Eds., Plenum, New York, 1981, 127.

6. Newberne, P.M. and Suphakarn, V., Nutrition and cancer: a review, with emphasis on the role of vitamins C and E and selenium, *Nutr. Cancer*, 5, 107, 1983.

7. Helson, L., Verma, M., and Helson, C., Vitamin E and human neuroblastoma, in *Modulation and Mediation of Cancer by Vitamins*, Meyskens, F.L. and Prasad, K.N., Eds., Karger, Basel, 1983, 258.

8. Slack, R. and Proulx, P., Studies on the effects of vitamin E on neuroblastoma NIE 115, *Nutr. Cancer*, 12, 75, 1989.

9. Prasad, K.N. and Edwards-Prasad, J., Effects of tocopherol (vitamin E) acid succinate on morphological alterations and growth inhibition in melanoma cells in culture, *Cancer Res.*, 42, 550, 1982.

10. Prasad, K.N., Edwards-Prasad, J., Ramanujam, S., and Sakamoto, A., Vitamin E increases the growth inhibitory and differentiating effects of tumor therapeutic agents on neuroblastoma and glioma cells in culture, *Proc. Soc. Exp. Biol. Med.*, 164, 158, 1980.

11. Kline, K., Cochran, G.S., and Sanders, B.G., Growth-inhibitory effects of vitamin E succinate on retrovirus-transformed tumor cells in vitro, *Nutr. Cancer*, 14, 27, 1990.

12. Sanders, B.G., Allison, J.P., and Kline, K., Monoclonal antibody to chicken fetal antigens on normal erythroid cells and hematopoietic-lymphoid tumor cell lines, *Cancer Res.*, 42, 4532, 1982.

13. Barth, C.F. and Humphries, E.H., A nonimmunosuppressive helper virus T, *J. Exp. Med.*, 167, 89, 1988.

14. Kline, K., Allison, J.P., and Sanders, B.G., Chemical and immunological characterization of developmentally expressed chicken erythroid surface membrane antigens, *Develop. Biol.*, 91, 389, 1982.

15. Beug, H., Muller, H., Drieser, S., Doederlein, G., and Graf, T., Hematopoietic cells transformed in vitro by REV-T avian reticuloendotheliosis virus express characteristics of very immature lymphoid cells, *Virology*, 115, 295, 1981.

16. Prasad, K.N., Rama, B.N., and Detsch, R.M., Modification of tumor cell response in vitro by vitamin E, in *Vitamins and Cancer, Human Cancer Prevention by Vitamins and Micronutrients*, Meyskens, F.L. and Prasad, K.N., Eds., Humana, Clifton, New York, 1986, 93.

17. Tappel, A.L., Vitamin E and free radical peroxidation of lipids, *Ann. N.Y. Acad. Sci.*, 203, 12, 1972.

18. Chaudhri, G., Hunt, N.H., Clark, I.A., and Ceredig, R., Antioxidants inhibit proliferation and cell surface expression of receptors for interleukin-2 and transferrin in T lymphocytes stimulated with phorbol myristate acetate and ionomycin, *Cell. Immunol.*, 115, 204, 1988.

19. Hoffeld, J.T., Agents which block membrane lipid peroxidation enhance mouse spleen cell immune activities in vitro: relationship to the enhancing activity of 2-mercaptoethanol, *Eur. J. Immunol.*, 11, 371, 1981.

20. Thiriot, C., Durand, P., Jasseron, M.P., Kergonou, J.F., and Ducousso, R., Radiosensitive antioxidant membrane-bound factors in rat liver microsomes: I. The roles of glutathione and vitamin E, *Biochem. Int.*, 14, 1, 1987.

21. Sporn, M.B., Roberts, A.B., Wakefield, L.M., and De Crombrugghe, B., Some recent advances in the chemistry and biology of transforming growth factor-β, *J. Cell Biol.*, 105, 1039, 1987.

22. Massague, J., The TGF-β family of growth and differentiation factors, *Cell*, 49, 437, 1987.

23. Roberts, A.B., Flanders, K.C., Kondaiah, P., Thompson, N.L., Van Obberghen-Schilling, E., Wakefield, L., Rossi, P., De Crombrugghe, B., Heine, U., and Sporn, M.B., Transforming growth factor-β: biochemistry and roles in embryogenesis, tissue repair and remodeling, and carcinogenesis, *Recent Prog. Horm. Res.*, 44, 157, 1988.

24. Ellingsworth, L., Nakayama, D., Dasch, J., Segarini, P., Carrillo, P., and Waegell, W., Transforming growth factor beta 1 (TGF-β:1') receptor expression on resting and mitogen-activated T cells, *J. Cell. Biochem.*, 39, 489, 1989.

25. Stoeck, M., Miescher, S., MacDonald, H.R., and Fliedner, V.V., Transforming growth factors beta slow down cell-cycle progression in a murine interleukin-2 dependent T-cell line, *J. Cell. Physiol.*, 141, 65, 1989.

26. Haussler, M.R., Vitamin D receptors: Nature and function, *Ann. Rev. Nutr.*, 6, 527, 1986.

27. Rigby, W.F.C., The immunobiology of vitamin D, *Immunol. Today,* 9, 54, 1988.

28. Minghetti, P.P. and Norman, A.W., 1,25 $(0H)_2$-vitamin D_3 receptors: gene regulation and genetic circuitry, *FASEB J.*, 2, 3042, 1988.

29. DeLuca, H.F., The vitamin D story: a collaborative effort of basic science and clinical medicine, *FASEB J.*, 2, 224, 1988.

30. Kaplowitz, N., Yoshida, H., Kuhlenkamp, J., Slitsky, B., Ren, I., and Stolz, A., Tocopherol-binding proteins of hepatic cytosol, *Ann. N.Y. Acad. Sci.*, 570, 85, 1989.

31. Catignani, G.L., An α-tocopherol binding protein in rat liver cytoplasm, *Biochem. Biophys. Res. Commun.,* 67, 66, 1975.

32. Murphy, D.J. and Mavis, R.D., Membrane transfer of α-tocopherol -influence of soluble α-tocopherol -binding factors from the liver, lung, heart, and brain of the rat, *J. Biol. Chem.*, 256, 10464, 1981.

33. Behrens, W.A. and Madere, R., Occurrence of a rat liver α-tocopherol binding protein in vivo, *Nutr. Rep. Int.*, 25, 107, 1982.

Chapter 15

Vitamin E Effects on Avian Retrovirus-Induced Immune Dysfunctions

Kimberly Kline

Table of Contents

I. Introduction

Retrovirus-induced tumorigenesis is a complicated multistep process that transforms normal cells into tumor cells that exhibit uncontrolled proliferation and that have the unique ability to escape immune destruction. One factor involved in retrovirus infections which enhances the ability of retrovirus transformed tumor cells to escape destruction by the host's immune response system is that retrovirus infection induces a severe immune suppressed state in the infected host. Retrovirus infections of avians,[1] felines,[2] mice,[3,4] and humans[5,6] have been shown to induce immune dysfunctions which precede the onset of the neoplasms and continue throughout the tumorigenic process.

Retrovirus-induced immune dysfunctions are complex, involving disruption of a wide variety of immune mediated events. Mechanisms whereby retroviruses mediate immune disruption include: direct elimination of host immune cells, enhancement of host immune suppressor cell activity, and disruption of the production of soluble immune regulatory substances.[1,7,8]

A goal in the prevention and treatment of cancers is to enhance tumor immunity, with the expectation that enhanced immunity may lead to successful containment or destruction of tumor cells. Nutritional status, especially deficiency or supplementation of specific dietary components, has been shown to have a major impact on immune response system functionality.[9-11] One nutrient of interest in regard to immune enhancing effects is vitamin E.[12,13] Studies in several laboratories have shown that various forms of vitamin E treatment, *in vivo* and *in vitro*, can enhance both cellular and humoral immunity.[12,14-24] Vitamin E is thought to function as a potent immune modulator by increasing the production of immune enhancing cytokines[25,26] and by down regulating the immunosuppressive arachidonic acid cascade metabolite, prostaglandin E_2 (PGE_2).[27-30]

Studies to be reported on here have focused on the effects of vitamin E administered either *in vivo* or *in vitro* to modulate avian retrovirus induced immune dysfunctions in a chicken animal model. Studies conducted *in vivo* demonstrated potent ameliorating effects by synthetic vitamin E (all-rac-α-tocopherol) on retrovirus-induced immune dysfunctions.[31] Follow-up *in vitro* studies designed to ask if the vitamin E effects involved direct effects on immune cells as well as to address cellular and molecular mechanisms for the vitamin E effects were then conducted.[32]

II. Forms of Vitamin E Used

Vitamin E is a generic term for fat-soluble compounds that exhibit the biological activity of natural vitamin E, RRR-α-tocopherol.[33,34] There are two groups of naturally occurring, d-stereoisomers of vitamin E, the tocopherols and the tocotrienols that differ due to the saturated or unsaturated state of the side chain, respectively. Members in each of these groups are designated α, β, γ or δ depending on the number and position of methyl groups attached to the chroman nucleus. In addition to these naturally occurring forms of vitamin E there are commercial preparations of vitamin E and synthetic analogs such as all-rac-α-tocopherol (a mixture of eight stereoisomers), and the vitamin E esters (RRR-α-tocopheryl acetate, RRR-α-tocopheryl succinate, all-rac-α-tocopheryl acetate and all-rac-α-tocopheryl succinate). The various forms of vitamin E differ in stability (especially oxidative inactivation), solubility and biological activity expressed as International Units.[34]

Investigations of the effects of vitamin E on retrovirus-induced immune dysfunctions and tumorigenesis in chickens have involved intraperitoneal injections of vitamin E as all-rac-α-tocopherol dissolved in 95% ethanol then suspended in 10% polyethylene glycol 6000 at 1:9 volume/volume and *in vitro* addition of vitamin E as RRR-α-tocopheryl succinate in a final concentration of 0.5% ethanol. Vehicle and untreated controls were included in all experiments. The chemical formula, terminology and characteristics, including biological activity, of RRR-α-tocopherol as well as the two forms of vitamin E used in these studies are depicted in Figure 1.

III. Avian Retrovirus Immune Dysfunction Model Systems

The avian immune dysfunction model systems investigated involve acute oncogenic avian retroviruses that induce a rapid, severe, generalized immune suppression and cause lethal cancers in a matter of weeks.[8,35,36] Two avian retrovirus-induced immune disorder states were investigated: reticuloendotheliosis virus induced lymphoid leukosis with immunosuppression and avian erythroblastosis virus induced erythroleukemia with immunosuppression. These two avian retroviruses induce similar immune dysfunctions.[8,36,37] The cascade of immunodeficiencies induced by the avian erythroblastosis virus is summarized in Figure 2.

The *in vivo* studies involved challenge with tumor cells transformed by the replication defective avian retrovirus, reticuloendotheliosis virus, REV-T (reticuloendotheliosis virus-transforming) along with its naturally occurring replication competent helper virus, REV-A (reticuloendotheliosis associated virus). Challenge with REV-T/REV-A transformed tumor cells causes a profound immunosuppression as well as a fatal visceral reticuloendotheliosis in young chickens with a latent period of 7-20 days.[1,7,37] Several REV-transformed cell lines that exhibit an abnormal lymphoblastoid morphology and that express both B and T cell specific cell surface markers have been established.[39-41] The REV cell line, designated BB5, which is a virus producing cell line that exhibits partially rearranged immunoglobulin genes, and both B and T cell specific markers was used to induce immune dysfunctions and tumorigenesis in the *in vivo* vitamin E studies.

The highly oncogenic-replication defective avian retrovirus, avian erythroblastosis virus, AEV-R along with its naturally occurring subgroup B replication competent helper virus (avian erythroblastosis-associated-virus, AEAV) was used to induce a severe immune suppressed state for the *in vitro* analyses.[36,42]

IV. Assays Used to Examine Immune Dysfunctions

Immune status of normal uninfected or tumor challenged chickens with or without vitamin E supplementation was assayed by determining the ability of spleen cells to proliferate when cultured with the T cell mitogens, concanavalin

RRR-α-tocopherol

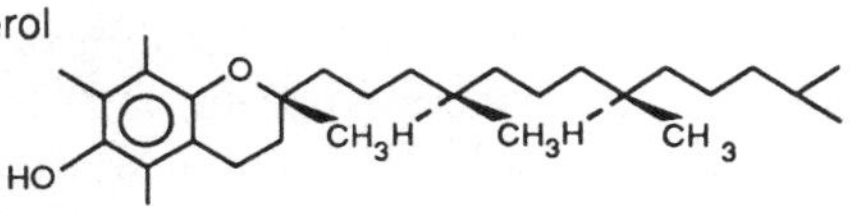

Common names: d-α-tocopherol, Natural Vitamin E
Trivial name: RRR-α-tocopherol
Chemical name: 2,5,7,8-tetramethyl-2-(4',8',12'-trimethyltridecyl)-6-chromanol
Molecular weight: 430.69
Biological activity: 1.49 IU/mg
Empirical formula: $C_{29}H_{50}O_2$

RRR-α-tocopheryl succinate

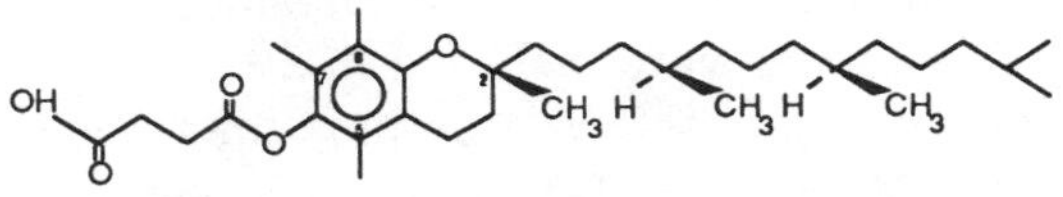

Common names: d-α-tocopheryl acid succinate, Vitamin E Succinate
Trivial name: RRR-α-tocopheryl succinate
Chemical name: 2,5,7,8-tetramethyl-2-(4',8',12'-trimethyltridecyl)-6-chromanol succinate
Molecular weight 530.8
Biological activity: 1.21 IU/mg
Empirical formula: $C_{33}H_{54}O_5$

all-rac-α-tocopherol

d-α-tocopherol (2R 4'R 8'R)

l-α-tocopherol (2S 4'R 8'R)

2R 4'R 8'S-α-tocopherol

2S 4'R 8'S-α-tocopherol

2R 4'S 8'R-α-tocopherol

2S 4'S 8'R-α-tocopherol

2R 4'S 8'R-α-tocopherol

2S 4'S 8'S-α-tocopherol

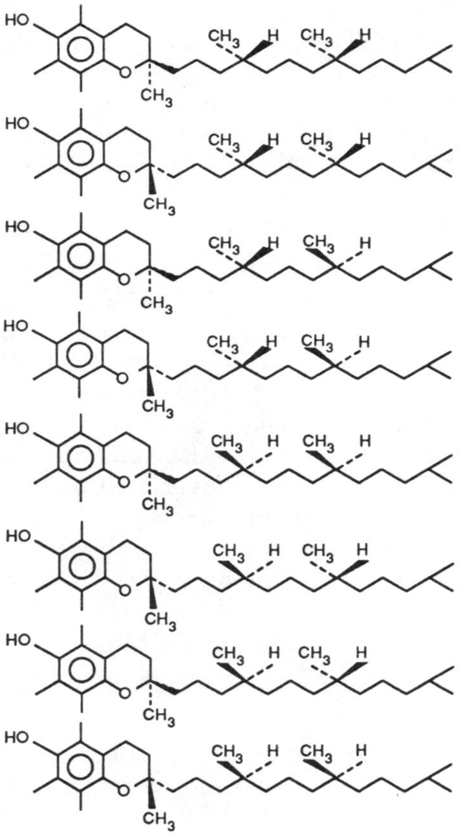

Common name: dl-α-tocopherol
Trivial name: all-rac-α-tocopherol
Structure: A mixture of eight stereoisomers
Molecular weight: 430.69
Biological activity: 1.10 IU/mg
Empirical formula: $C_{29}H_{50}O_2$

Figure 1. Chemical formulas and general characteristics of RRR-α-tocopherol (D-α-tocopherol or natural vitamin E), RRR-α-tocopheryl succinate (the succinate ester of RRR-α-tocopherol), and all-rac-α-tocopherol (synthetic vitamin E that is composed of eight isomeric forms). The biological activity is expressed in International Units (IU). An International Unit is equivalent to 1 mg all-rac-α-tocopheryl acetate. This figure is a modification of information obtained from reference 33.

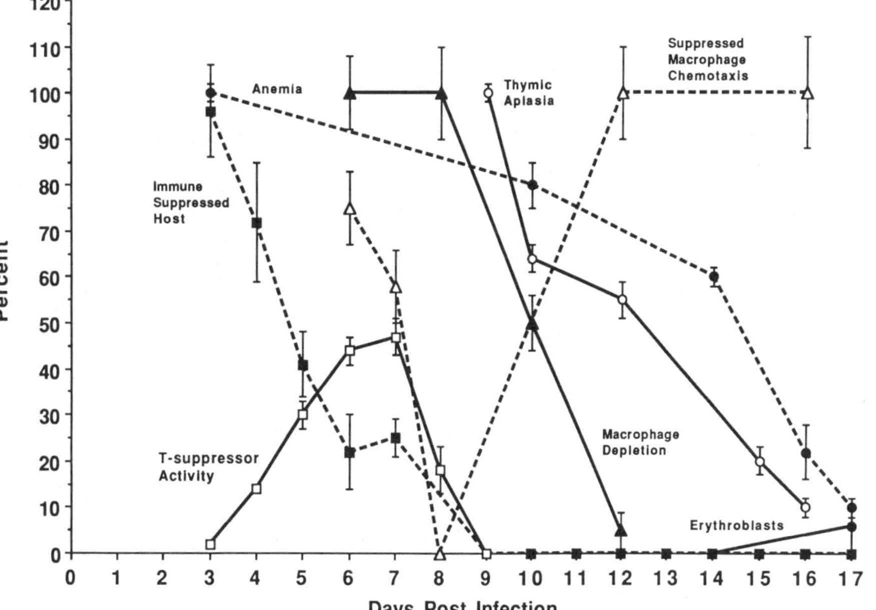

Figure 2. The C-type retrovirus, avian erythroblastosis virus (AEV), causes a fatal erythroblastic anemia within 2-3 weeks after infection. As early as 4 days following infection and continuing until death, spleen cells from AEV-infected chickens give depressed responses to concanavalin A, phytohemagglutinin and pokeweed mitogen (Immune Suppressed Host).[1,36] Abnormal suppressor T cell activity is detectable 4 days following viral inoculation, reaches peak levels of suppression on days 6-7 and disappears by day 9 (T-suppressor Activity).[36] Macrophage chemotactic dysfunction appears to be biphasic with an initial defect disappearing about the same time as the decline in abnormal T suppressor cell activity, followed by a rapid reappearance of macrophages unable to migrate to potent chemoattractants which remain for the duration of the tumorigenic process (Suppressed Macrophage Chemotaxis).[38] Macrophages elicited into the peritoneal cavity begin to decrease in numbers after the first week, with complete nonresponsiveness occurring by day 12 (Macrophage Depletion).[38] Thymic atrophy begins approximately 8 days following AEV infection and involves structural disruption and reduction in number of thymocytes (Thymic Aplasia).[36] AEV-infected chickens gradually become anemic, with hematocrit values falling to less than 50% of normal by 2 weeks post-infection (Anemia). Tumor cells are detectable in the peripheral blood beginning approximately 2 weeks post-infection, 2-3 days prior to death (Erythroblasts).

A (Con A) or phytohemagglutinin (PHA-P) in a well established serum-free mitogen assay system for chicken lymphocytes.[43,44] The assay for T suppressor cell activity involved co-culturing spleen cells from REV-tumor cell challenged or AEV-infected chickens with spleen cells from normal uninfected, untreated chickens in a standard mitogen co-culture assay system.[43,44] Inhibition of mitogen-stimulated cellular proliferation of the normal spleen cells by the test cells is indicative of the presence of abnormal suppressor cells or suppressor factors. Previous investigations had established that suppressor T cell activity was involved in the two systems under investigation.[8,36] Standard chemotactic assays were used to determine the ability of vitamin E to modulate retrovirus induced macrophage migration dysfunctions.[45] Sephadex illicited peritoneal exudate cells (PEC) composed of greater than 90% macrophages were used in the chemotactic analyses.

V. Effects of *in Vivo* Vitamin E Supplementation on Immune Parameters of Uninfected and Retrovirus-Infected Chickens

A. Splenic T Cell Responses to Mitogen Stimulation

The ability of spleen cells obtained from vitamin E treated, uninfected chickens to proliferate when stimulated by the T cell mitogens, Con A or PHA, was enhanced 28 and 42%, respectively (Figure 3-Uninfected). The Con A and PHA mediated proliferative responses of splenic lymphocytes from vitamin E treated-tumor challenged chickens were not as suppressed as the responses of vehicle treated-tumor challenged chickens: 54% versus 75% and 74% versus 96%, respectively (Figure 3-T cell Proliferation).[31]

B. Abnormal T Suppressor Cell Activity

Co-culture analyses for detection of suppressor cell activity showed that vitamin E treated-tumor challenged chickens, in comparison to vehicle treated-tumor challenged chickens, exhibited greatly reduced suppressor cell activity (Table 1 and Figure 3-T_s Cell Activity). More specifically, the ability of splenic lymphocytes obtained from vitamin E treated-tumor challenged chickens to suppress Con A and PHA mediated blastogenic responses of splenic lymphocytes from normal chickens in co-culture was greatly reduced in comparison to co-cultures of splenic lymphocytes obtained from vehicle treated-tumor challenged chickens: 0% versus 50% and 13% versus 57%, respectively.

C. Cancer Progression

Amelioration of retrovirus induced immune suppression was not accompanied by amelioration of the tumorigenic process.[31] Chickens treated with either vitamin E or vehicle, starting at 3 days after hatching and continuing throughout the experiment, were challenged with BB5 tumor cells at 10, 19, or 33 days post-hatch and monitored daily for body weight and survival. In all three tumor challenge groups, the vitamin E treated chickens died in a shorter length of time

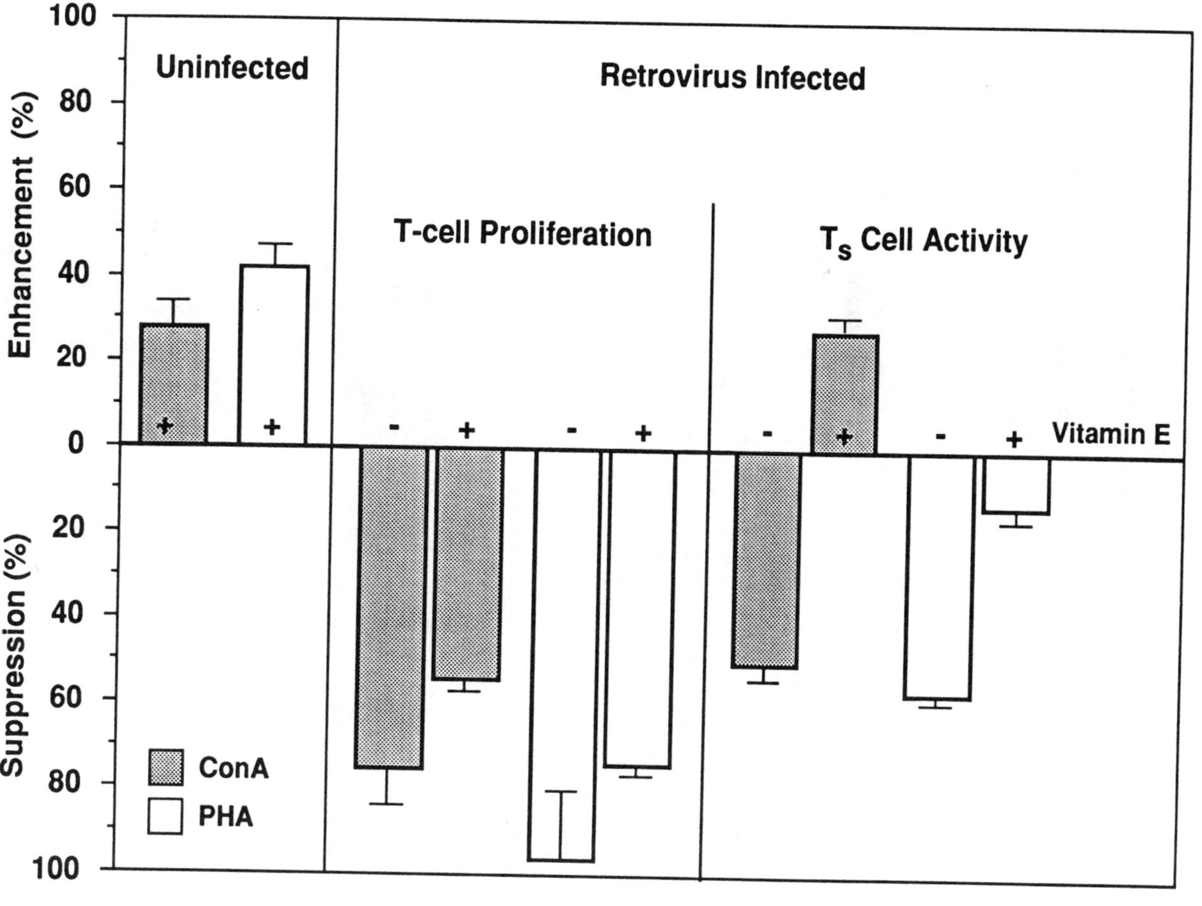

Figure 3. Summary of effects of *in vivo* supplementation with vitamin E (all-rac-α-tocopherol) on T cell responses to mitogen-stimulation and degree of T suppressor cell activity. Vitamin E supplementation is indicated by a "+" and vehicle treatments are indicated by a "–".

TABLE 1
Elimination of Tumor-Induced Suppressor Cell Activity by Vitamin E Treatment[a]

Co-Culture Analyses of Splenic Mitogen-Induced Spleen Cell Proliferative Responses[a]

Treatment[b]	Tumor challenge[c]	+Con A (cpm)	Percent suppression	+PHA (cpm)	Percent suppression
Vitamin E	+	50,160 ± 1,334[c]	0	30,772 ± 1,020	13
Vehicle	+	18,248 ± 664	50	15,056 ± 334	57
Vehicle	-	36,444 ± 875		35,240 ± 509	

[a] Suppressor cell activity in co-culture was examined 6 days following tumor challenge. Co-culture analyses were performed at a 1:1 ratio. Percent suppression was determined by dividing the tritiated thymidine uptake of vitamin E and vehicle treated-tumor challenged chickens by the tritiated thymidine uptake of vehicle treated-unchallenged chickens.
[b] Chickens (10/treatment group) were treated with intraperitoneal injections of vitamin E as all-rac-α-tocopherol at 0.1 mg/gm body weight or the equivalent of vehicle at 2 day intervals, starting 3 days post-hatch and continuing throughout the experiment.
[c] Chickens were challenged with $1x10^4$ BB5 tumor cells at 22 days post-hatch and sacrificed for analyses 6 days following tumor cell challenge.
[d] Mean tritiated thymidine uptake in cpm of triplicate cultures of spleen cells (minus background counts). Each data point represents the average derived from analyses of 10 individual chickens for each treatment group. Tritiated thymidine uptake was analyzed 66 hours after culture initiation and 18 hours after addition of isotope.
Modified from Kline, K. and Sanders, B.G., *In Vivo*, 3, 161, 1989.

and exhibited other signs of more advanced disease such as greater decrease in body weight, greater spleen weight and greater number of tumor foci in the spleen as well as greater incidence of liver foci than did the age-matched, vehicle control treated chickens (Table 2).

TABLE 2
Enhanced Tumor Progression in Vitamin E Treated-Tumor Challenged Chickens

Age of Chicken at Tumor Challenge (in days)	Tumor Progression[a] (Compared to vehicle treated-tumor challenged controls)
10	Enhanced
19	Enhanced
33	Enhanced

[a] Tumor progression was measured by several parameters including: spleen size and weight, number of tumor foci in spleen, number of tumor foci in liver, degree of thymus atrophy, presence of tumor cell infiltration into the thymus, whole body weight, and time of death.

VI. Effects of *in Vitro* Vitamin E Treatment on Retrovirus-Induced Immune Dysfunctions

Considering the complexity of the *in vivo* situation, it was unknown whether vitamin E was having a direct effect on cells of the immune response system, thus *in vitro* analyses were conducted to determine whether or not vitamin E was directly affecting immune cells and if so to address possible mechanisms whereby vitamin E was mediating its immunomodulating effects.

Cells from AEV-infected chickens or normal cells inhibited directly by addition of purified virus in culture were used for the *in vitro* studies. Previous studies in the lab had characterized the kinetics of AEV-induced immune suppression.[36] Suppressed mitogen-induced responsiveness by spleen cells from AEV-infected chickens is evident 4 days following AEV-inoculation with more pronounced suppression being evident on the 5th and succeeding days. Inability of spleen cells from AEV-infected chickens to respond to Con A and PHA remains until the death of the chickens at approximately 14 days following AEV inoculation (Figure 4, left panel). The ability of spleen cells from AEV-infected chickens to suppress mitogen induced proliferation of spleen cells from normal chickens is evident 4 days following AEV-inoculation; however, the suppression is transient with the highest degree of suppression occurring 6-7 days following AEV inoculation.[36]

Based on this profile of AEV-induced immune suppression, spleen cells from 6-day-post AEV-infected chickens were chosen for the *in vitro* vitamin E succinate treatment studies. The T cell mitogen-induced proliferative responses are greatly suppressed (60-80%), and suppressor T cell activity is at its maximum (40-50%) at this time point in the tumorigenic process (Figure 4, left panel).

A. Suppressed Splenic T Cell Responses to Mitogen Stimulation

Spleen cells from 6-day-post AEV-infected chickens cultured without any treatments exhibited 63% and 62% suppression of ability to proliferate in response to either Con A or PHA, respectively. In contrast, replica cultured cells treated with vitamin E succinate exhibited total amelioration of retrovirus-induced suppression for both mitogens, *i.e.* 100% enhancement of suppressed host (Figure 4, right panel).

B. Abnormal T Suppressor Cell Activity

Treatment of co-cultures of spleen cells from AEV-infected chickens and normal chickens with vitamin E succinate at culture initiation, caused a reduction in the degree of suppression observed in comparison to vehicle treated co-cultures.[32] A 94% and 59% reduction in suppression was observed for vitamin E succinate-treated co-cultures stimulated with Con A and PHA, respectively (Figure 4, right panel).

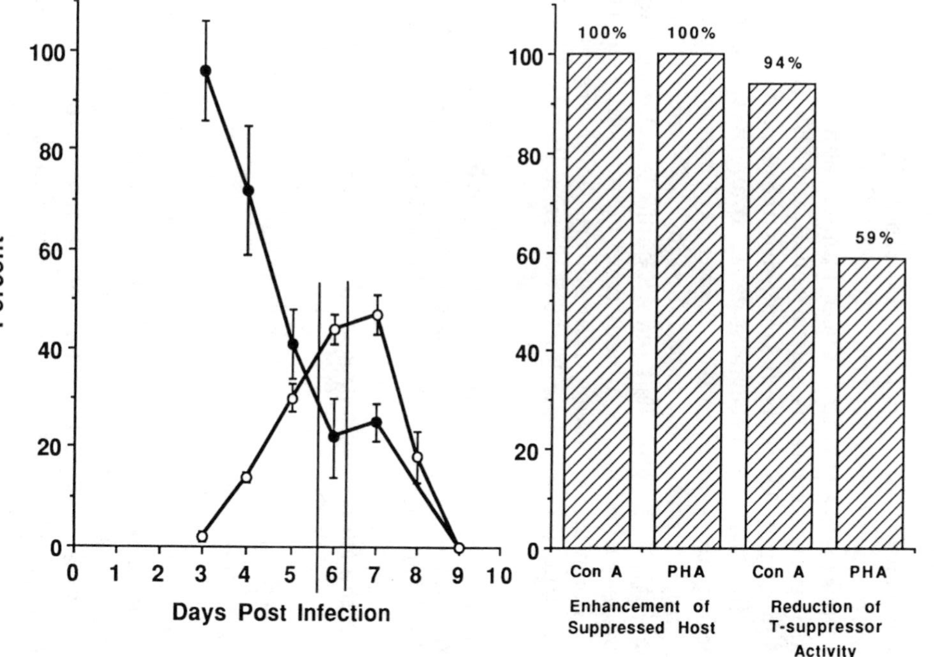

Figure 4. Summary of *in vitro* treatments with vitamin E succinate on AEV-induced immune dysfunctions.[32] The left panel depicts percent decrease of mitogen-induced T cell responses (closed circles) and increased percentage of abnormal T suppressor cell activity (open circles) observed in AEV-infected chickens compared to age-matched uninfected controls. Day 6 post-infection was chosen as the best time point for analyzing vitamin E succinate's effects on both depressed T cell responsiveness to mitogens and abnormal T suppressor cell activity. The right panel summarizes the ability of vitamin E succinate to ameliorate the functional abnormalities of spleen cells from AEV-infected chickens when added directly in culture at the beginning of the respective assays. Vitamin E succinate totally ameliorated both reduced Con A and reduced PHA responsiveness (*i.e.* induced a 100% enhancement in responsiveness compared to vehicle treated cultures). Furthermore, vitamin E succinate was able to reduce abnormal T suppressor cell activity detected in co-culture assays using Con A and PHA stimulation by 94% and 59%, respectively.

C. Decreased Macrophage Chemotaxis

Since macrophages play an important role in immunoregulation, it was of interest to determine if vitamin E succinate could ameliorate the decrease in PEC chemotaxis observed in AEV infection.[38] Studies with PEC from normal chickens showed that vitamin E succinate enhances PEC migration toward lipopolysaccharide (LPS)-activated chicken serum which served as a source of the chemoattractant C5a when compared to untreated and vehicle treated cells.[46] PEC from normal chickens, cultured with vitamin E succinate at 0.1 and 1.0 µg/ml, exhibited 54% and 52% enhancement of chemotaxis, respectively (Figure 5). When the effects of vitamin E succinate on PEC from AEV-infected chickens were analyzed, 0.1 and 1.0 µg/ml concentrations were shown to ameliorate (78% and 40%, respectively) AEV-induced suppression of PEC chemotaxis. Exposure of PEC from normal chickens to either purified AEV or UV-inactivated AEV, *in vitro*, inhibits chemotaxis in a dose-dependent manner.[38] Vitamin E succinate treatments alleviated UV-inactivated AEV-induced inhibition of PEC chemotaxis compared to untreated controls, 62% and 40%, respectively (Figure 5).

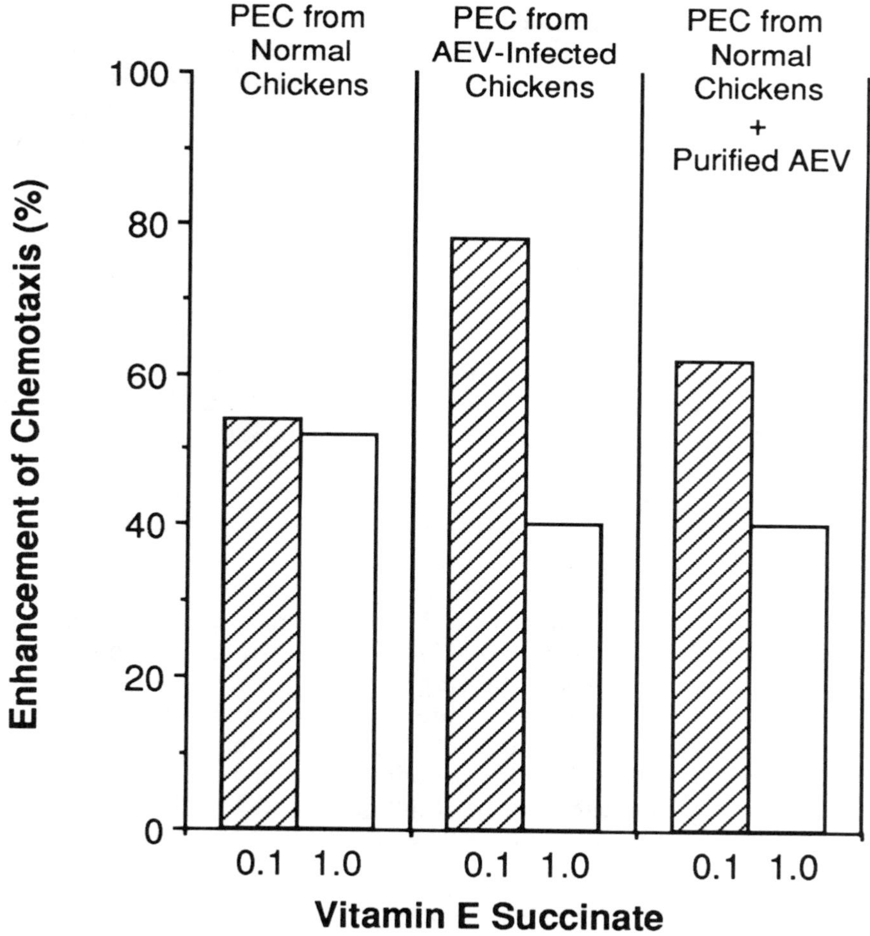

Figure 5. Effects of vitamin E succinate on macrophage chemotaxis.

VII. Model of Vitamin E's Possible Immunomodulatory Activities in Amelioration of Retrovirus-Induced Immune Dysfunctions

A hypothetical model for the immunomodulatory actions by vitamin E is presented in Figure 6. In this model, helper virus immunosuppressive products are proposed to disrupt normal macrophage and/or T-lymphocyte functions resulting in elevated levels of immunosuppressive PGE_2 and reduced levels of immunoenhancing IL-2 cytokines. Elevated levels of PGE_2 are proposed to induce the formation of T suppressor cells.[47] Vitamin E is postulated to ameliorate the immune dysfunctions by interacting with macrophages and/or T lymphocytes, resulting in the down-regulation of PGE_2 and up-regulation of IL-2.[13,27-30]

A. Immunomodulatory Effects on Cytokine Production

Support for the above model is derived from studies showing that the suppressed Con A and PHA mitogen-induced proliferation of spleen cells from 6 days post-AEV-infected chickens can be partially ameliorated by the addition of exogenous interleukin-2 (IL-2).[36] Further support for this model is derived from studies showing that production of IL-2 in the presence of vitamin E succinate enhances the response of cells in the IL-2 bioassay 41% above the response produced by IL-2 produced in the traditional manner, *i.e.* without vitamin E succinate present (Figure 7).[48]

B. Effects on Arachidonic Acid Cascade Metabolite Production

The possibility that vitamin E may play a role in modulating the arachidonic acid cascade has been proposed.[50] The association of vitamin E with arachidonic acid in cell membranes and the possibility that its antioxidant properties might influence free radical mediated reactions in the activation and inactivation of enzymes which catalyze key reactions in the arachidonic acid cascade raise the possibility that vitamin E may influence the spectrum of biologically active compounds produced.[50] Arachidonic acid metabolites such as prostaglandins, thromboxanes and prostacyclins produced by the cyclooxygenase pathway and leukotrienes and lipoxins produced by the lipoxygenase pathway, exhibit both stimulatory and inhibitory activities in regard to various immune functions.[51] Support for the involvement of prostaglandin E_2 (PGE_2), a potent immune response inhibitor, in AEV-induced immune dysfunctions is derived from studies showing that PEC from uninfected chickens can be induced to produce elevated levels of PGE_2 when cultured in the presence of purified AEV (PGE_2 levels 71% above PGE_2 levels from background levels produced by PEC not exposed to virus).[52] Pretreatment of PEC with various concentrations of vitamin E succinate prior to the addition of purified AEV reduces the level of PGE_2 secreted in a dose dependent manner (Figure 8).

A summary of the effects of avian retrovirus infections on lymphocyte and macrophage functions, including cytokine production, and the effects of vitamin E on these retrovirus-induced immune dysfunctions is given in Table 3.

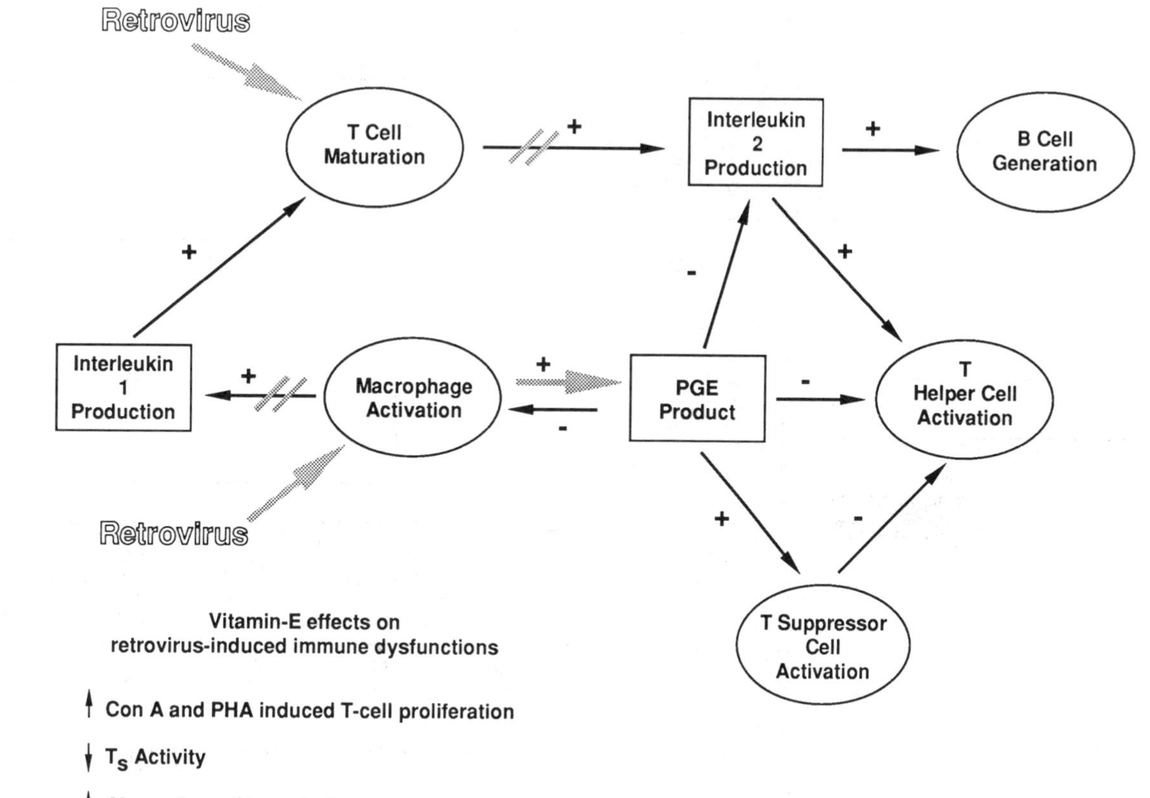

Figure 6. Hypothetical model for the immunomodulatory actions of vitamin E in amelioration of retrovirus induced immune dysfunctions.

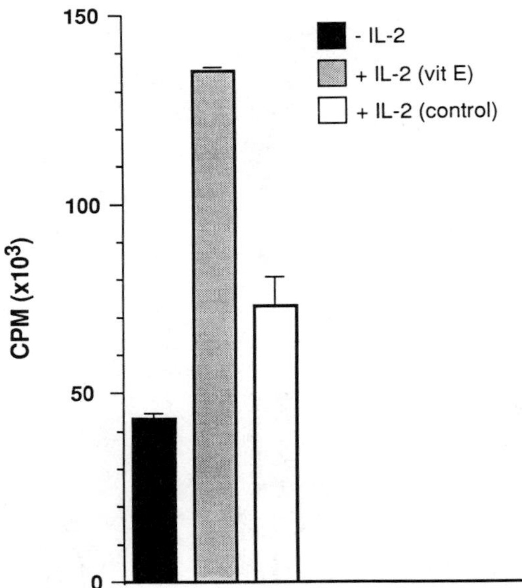

Figure 7. Vitamin E succinate enhances the production of IL-2. The production and the biological assay of chicken IL-2 was performed using previously described procedures.[38] It is unlikely that the enhancement of T-cell blast proliferation was mediated by the presence of vitamin E succinate since the conditioned media is concentrated/dialyzed using Millipore centrifuge concentrators with a 10,000 dalton molecular weight cut-off.

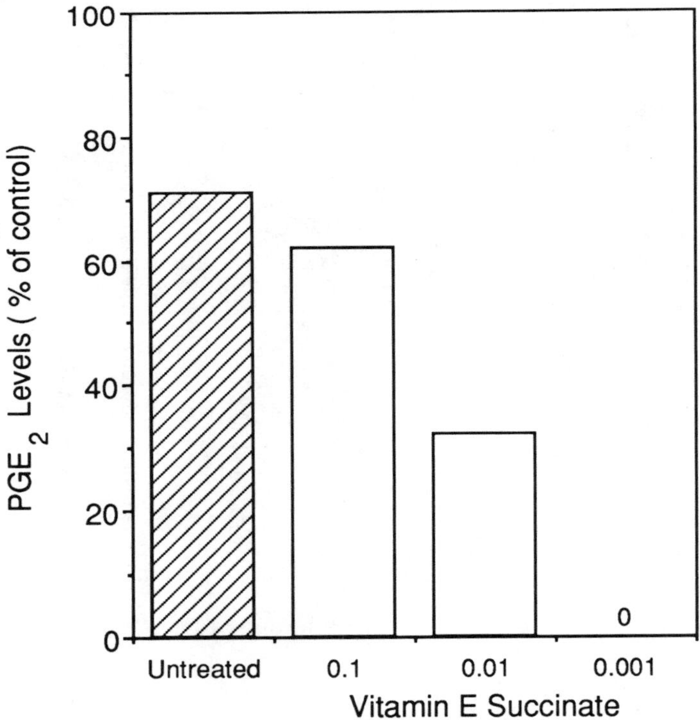

Figure 8. Summary of data that illustrates that exposure of PEC obtained from normal chickens to AEV results in the release of the immunosuppressive compound PGE_2 and that treatment with vitamin E succinate inhibits this virally mediated PGE_2 release in a dose-dependent manner.

TABLE 3
Vitamin E Modulation of Retrovirus Induced Immune Dysfunctions

Immune Functions	Retrovirus Infection	Vitamin E Treatment
Lymphocytes		
T cell mitogen-induced proliferation	D	I
T suppressor cell activity	I	D
IL-2 production	D	I
Macrophages		
Chemotaxis	D	I
Phagocytosis	D, N	No change
PGE_2 production	I	D

D = Decreased, I = Increased, N= Normal
From Kline, K., Rao, A., Romach, E. H., Kidao, S., Morgan, T. J., and Sanders, B. G. *Ann. N. Y. Acad. Sci.* 587, 294, 1990.

VIII. Summary and Conclusions

Vitamin E (all rac-α-tocopherol) supplementation, *in vivo*, has been shown to enhance mitogen-mediated splenic T lymphocyte proliferation of normal chickens, reduce retrovirus-induced suppression of host T lymphocyte responsiveness to mitogen stimulation, and reduce retrovirus-induced T suppressor cell activity, but, unfortunately, to enhance tumorigenesis. Treatment of spleen cells from retrovirus infected chickens with vitamin E succinate, *in vitro*, has been shown to reduce retrovirus-suppressed splenic T cell mitogen mediated responses, reduce T suppressor cell activity, and to enhance chemotaxis of retrovirus-suppressed macrophages. A model has been proposed that retroviruses directly disrupt normal macrophage and T-lymphocyte functions resulting in elevated levels of immunosuppressive PGE_2 and reduced levels of immunoenhancing IL-2 cytokines. Vitamin E is postulated to ameliorate the immune dysfunctions by interacting directly with macrophages and/or T lymphocytes, resulting in the down-regulation of PGE_2 and up-regulation of IL-2. Support for the model is derived from studies showing that vitamin E succinate down-regulates the production of PGE_2 and up-regulates the production of IL-2 in *in vitro* model systems.

Acknowledgements

The research was supported by the American Institute for Cancer Research (Washington, D.C.) Grant No. 87A69 (K. Kline and B. Sanders) and by U.S. Public Health Service Grant No. CA-45422 (K. Kline) awarded by the Department of Health and Human Services, National Institutes of Health (Bethesda, MD).

References

1. Rup, B.J., Holzer, J.D., and Bose, H.R., Jr., Helper viruses associated with avian acute viruses inhibit the cellular immune response, *Virology,* 116, 61, 1982.

2. Cockerell, G.L., Hoover, E.A., Krakowka, S., Olsen, R.G., and Yohn, D.S., Lymphocyte mitogen reactivity and enumeration of circulating B and T cells during feline leukemia virus infection in the cat, *J. Natl. Cancer Inst.*, 57, 1095, 1976.

3. Fowler, A.K., Reed, C.O., Weislow, O.S., and Hellman, A., Inhibition of lymphocyte transformation by disrupted murine oncornavirus, *Cancer Res.*, 37, 4531, 1977.

4. Wood, G.W., Suppression of moloney sarcoma virus immunity following sensitization with attentuated virus, *Cancer Res.*, 35, 4552, 1976.

5. Dent, P.B., Immunodepression by oncogenic viruses, *Progr. Med. Virol.*, 14, 1, 1972.

6. Mims, C.A., Interactions of viruses with the immune system, *Clin. Exp. Immunol.*, 66, 1, 1986.

7. Bose, H.R., Jr., Reticuloendotheliosis virus and disturbance in immune regulation, *Microbiol. Sci.*, 1, 107, 1984.

8. Storms, R.W. and Bose, H.R., Jr., Avian retroviruses, in *Virus-Induced Immunosuppression*, Friedman, H., Berdinelli, M., and Spector S., Eds., Plenum Press, New York, 1989, 375.

9. Gross, R.L. and Newberne, P.M., Role of nutrition in immunologic function, *Physiol. Rev.*, 60, 188, 1980.

10. Chandra, R.K., *Nutrition and Immunology*, Alan R. Liss, Inc., New York, 1988, 1.

11. Bendich, A. and Chandra, R.K., *Micronutrients and Immune Functions,* Vol. 587, New York Academy of Sciences, New York, 1990, 3.

12. Tengerdy, R.P., The role of vitamin E in immune response and disease resistance, *Ann. N.Y. Acad. Sci.*, 587, 24, 1990.

13. Bendich, A., Antioxidant vitamins and immune responses, in *Nutrition and Immunology,* Chandra, R.K., Ed., Alan R. Liss, Inc., New York, 1988, 125.

14. Prasad, K.N., Rama, B.N., and Detsch, R.M., Modification of tumor cell response in vitro by vitamin E, in *Vitamins and Cancer,* Meyskens, F.L., Jr. and Prasad, K.N., Eds., Humana Press, Clifton, New Jersey, 1986, 93.

15. Watson, R.R., Retinoids and vitamin E: Modulators of immune functions and cancer resistance, in *Vitamins and Cancer,* Meyskens, F.L., Jr. and Prasad, K.N., Eds., Humana Press, Clifton, New Jersey, 1986, 439.

16. Black, M.M., Zachrau, R.E., Dion, A.S., and Katz, M., Stimulation of prognostically favorable cell-mediated immunity of breast cancer patients by high dose vitamin A and vitamin E, in *Vitamins, Nutrition and Cancer*, Prasad, K.N., Ed., Karger, Basel, 1986, 134.

17. Corwin, L.M. and Shloss, J., Influence of vitamin E on the mitogenic response of murine lymphoid cells, *J. Nutr.*, 110, 916, 1980.

18. Kurek, M.P. and Corwin, L.M., Vitamin E protection against tumor formation by transplanted murine sarcoma, *Nutr. Cancer*, 4, 128, 1982.

19. Sheffy, B.E. and Schultz, R.D., Influence of vitamin E and selenium on immune response mechanisms, *Fed. Proc.*, 38, 2139, 1979.

20. Tanaka, J., Fujiwara, H., and Toriso, M., Vitamin E and immune response enhancement of helper T-cell activity by dietary supplementation of vitamin E in mice, *Immunol.*, 38, 727, 1979.

21. Tengerdy, P. and Brown, J.C., Effect of vitamin E and A on humoral immunity and phagocytosis in *E. coli* infected chickens, *Poult. Sci.*, 56, 957,1977.

22. Tengerdy, R.P., Effect of vitamin E on immune response, in *Vitamin E*, Machlin, L., Ed., Marcel Dekker, Inc., New York, 1980, 429.

23. Tengerdy, R.P., Effect of vitamin E on immune responses, *Basic Clin. Nutr.*, 1, 429, 1980.

24. Yasunaga, T., Kato, H., Ohgaki, K., Inamota, T., and Hgikasa, T., Effect of vitamin E as immunopotentiation agent for mice at optimal dosage and its toxicity at high dosage, *J. Nutr.*, 112, 1075, 1982.

25. Kline, K., Cochran, G.S., Huggins, E.R., Morgan, T.J., Rao, A., and Sanders, B.G., Vitamin E modulation of retrovirus-induced immune dysfunctions and tumor cell proliferation, *Ann. N.Y. Acad. Sci.*, 570, 470, 1989.

26. Kline, K., Rao, A., Romach, E.H., Kidao, S., Morgan, T.J., and Sanders, B.G., Vitamin E effects on retrovirus induced immune dysfunctions, *Ann. N. Y. Acad. Sci.*, 587, 294, 1990.

27. Meydani, S.N., Meydani, M., Verdon, C.P., Shapiro, A.C., Blumberg, J.B., and Hayes, K.C., Vitamin E supplementation suppresses prostaglandin E2 synthesis and enhances the immune response of aged mice, *Mech. Aging Dev.*, 34, 191, 1986.

28. Meydani, S.N., Meydani, M., Barklund, P.M., Lie, S., Miller, R.A., Cannon, J.G., Rocklin, R., and Blumberg, J.B., Effect of vitamin E supplementation on immune responsiveness of the aged, *Ann. N.Y. Acad. Sci.*, 570, 283, 1989.

29. Machlin, L., Vitamin E and prostaglandins, in *Tocopherol, Oxygen and Biomembranes,* deDuve, C. and Hayaishi, O., Eds., Elsevier/North Holland Biomedical Press, New York, 1978, 179.

30. Tengerdy, R.P., Heinzerling, R.H., and Mathias, M.M., Effect of vitamin E on disease resistance and immune response, in *Tocopherol, Oxygen and Biomembranes,* deDuve, C. and Hayaishi, O., Eds., Elsevier/North Holland Biomedical Press, New York, 1978, 191.

31. Kline, K. and Sanders, B.G., Modulation of immune suppression and enhanced tumorigenesis in retrovirus tumor challenged chickens treated with vitamin E, *In Vivo*, 3, 161, 1989.

32. Kline, K. and Sanders, B.G., RRR-α-tocopheryl succinate enhances T cell mitogen-induced proliferation and reduces suppressor activity in spleen cells derived from AEV-infected chickens, *Nutr. Cancer*, in press.

33. Horwitt, M.K., The forms of vitamin E, in *Vitamin E Abstracts*, Vitamin E Research & Information Service, LaGrange, Illinois, vii, 1987.

34. Machlin, L.J., Vitamin E, in *Handbook of Vitamins*, Machlin, L.J., Ed., Marcel Dekker, Inc., New York, 1984, 99.

35. Sevioan, M.R., Larose, N., and Chamberlain, D.M., Avian lymphomatoses VI: a virus of unusual potency and pathogenicity, *Avian Dis.*, 8, 336, 1964.

36. Rao, A., Kline, K., and Sanders, B.G., Immune abnormalities in avian erythroblastosis virus-infected chickens, *Cancer Res.*, 50, 4764, 1990.

37. Rup, B.J., Spence, J.L., Hoelzer, J.D., Lewis, R.B., Carpenter, C.R., Rubin, A.S., and Bose, H.R., Jr., Immunosuppression induced by avian reticuloendotheliosis virus: mechanism of induction of the suppressor cell, *J. Immunol.*, 123, 1362, 1979.

38. Rao, A., Mechanisms of immune suppression by avian erythroblastosis virus, *Ph.D. Dissertation Thesis*, University of Texas, Austin, 1989.

39. Beug, H., Muller, H., Drieser, S., Doederlein, G., and Graf, T., Hematopoietic cells transformed in vitro by REV-T avian reticuloendotheliosis virus express characteristics of very immature lymphoid cells, *Virol.*, 115, 295, 1981.

40. Lewis, R.B., McClure, J., Rup, B., Niesel, D.W., Garry, R.F., Hoelzer, J.D., Nazerian, K., and Bose, H.R., Jr., Avian reticuloendotheliosis virus: identification of the hematopoietic target cell for transformation, *Cell,* 25, 421, 1981.

41. Shibuya, T., Chen, I., Howatson, A., and Mak, T.W., Morphological, immunological, and biochemical analyses of chicken spleen cells transformed in vitro by reticuloendotheliosis virus strain T, *Cancer Res.*, 42, 2722, 1982.

42. Beard, J.W., Avian virus growths and their etiological agents, in *Advances in Cancer Research,* Haddow, A. and Weinhouse, S., Eds., Academic Press, New York, 1963, 1.

43. Kline, K. and Sanders, B.G., Developmental profile of chicken splenic lymphocyte responsiveness to Con A and PHA and studies on chicken splenic and bone marrow cells capable of inhibiting mitogen-stimulated blastogenic responses of adult splenic lymphocytes, *J. Immunol.,* 125, 1792, 1980.

44. Kline, K. and Sanders, B.G., Suppression of Con A mitogen-induced proliferation of normal spleen cells by macrophages from chickens with hereditary muscular dystrophy, *J. Immunol.*, 132, 2813, 1984.

45. Lohr, K.M. and Snyderman, R., In vitro methods for the study of macrophage chemotaxis, in *Manual of Macrophage Methodology*, Herscowitz, H.B., Holden, H.T., Bellanti, J.A., and Ghaffar, A., Eds., Marcel Dekker Inc., New York, 1981, 301.

46. Romach, E.H., Rao, A., Sanders, B.G., and Kline, K., submitted manuscript, 1990.

47. Chouaib, M., Chatenoud, L., Klatzmann, D., and Fradelizi, D., The mechanisms of inhibition of human IL 2 production II. PGE_2 induction of suppressor T lymphocytes, *J. Immunol.*, 132, 1851, 1984.

48. Kidao, S., Sanders, B.G., and Kline, K., unpublished data, 1990.

49. Kromer, G., Schauenstein, K., and Wick, G., Avain lymphokines: an improved method for chicken IL-2 production and assay. A Con A erythrocyte complex induces higher T cell proliferation and IL-2 production than does free mitogen, *J. Immunol. Methods,* 73, 273, 1984.

50. Reddanna, P., Whelan, J., Burgess, J.R., Eskew, M.L., Hildenbrandt, G., Zarkower, A., Scholz, R.W., and Reddy, C.C., The role of vitamin E and selenium in arachidonic acid oxidation by way of the 5-lipoxygenase pathway, *Ann. N. Y. Acad. Sci.*, 570, 136, 1989.

51. Ninnemann, J.L., Prostaglandins and immunity, *Immunol. Today*, 5, 170, 1984.

52. Romach, E.H., Sanders, B.G., and Kline, K., unpublished data.

Chapter 16

Relationships Between Potassium and Cancer

Maryce M. Jacobs and Roman J. Pienta

Table of Contents

I. Introduction

Much has been written on the physiological and biochemical importance of potassium, but few reports have attempted to elucidate the influence potassium has on the cancer process. Epidemiologic studies, human cancer case reports, experimental animal studies, and cell culture studies have suggested that the level of potassium might influence carcinogenesis. In general, high potassium is associated with decreased risk of cancer and with the inhibition of tumor growth. Many studies have extended their observations to include the relative concentrations of potassium and other electrolytes (cations) or to include potassium to sodium ratios. Generally, a high potassium to sodium ratio is associated with decreased cancer incidence. Conversely, a higher sodium to potassium ratio with a higher absolute sodium concentration is associated with a higher risk of cancer.

The levels of potassium reported may be from diet, intracellular or extracellular fluids, serum or plasma. It is important to make these distinctions. For example, high dietary or serum potassium is associated with decreased tumor growth, while high potassium mucous secretions from the lower intestinal tract have been associated with increased tumor growth.

This chapter reviews reports in humans, animals, and cell cultures that illustrate the relationships between potassium and other electrolytes and the carcinogenic process. Some indications of the mechanisms of potassium action are suggested where sufficient data are available. While many articles have been written about potassium, few, if any, have compiled the research observations that indicate the important role that potassium might have to lower cancer risk and to potentially be incorporated into cancer treatment protocols.

II. Human Studies: Epidemiology and Case Reports

A. Epidemiology

Correa *et al.*[1] performed a nutritional survey of 120 food items in the diet of the inhabitants of four villages in the rural area of Narino, Colombia exhibiting different levels of risk (*i.e.*, low risk of 40/100,000 and high risk of 150/100,000) for gastric cancer and its precursor lesions. The survey showed a higher consumption of fava beans in the villages with high risk for stomach cancer and a higher consumption of fresh fruits and vegetables where the rates for gastric cancer were lower. A low intake of animal proteins and high intake of cereals did not discriminate between the different risk levels. Although sodium consumption was generally high in all villages, there was a tendency for higher cancer risk where families consumed more than 50% of the adequate amount of salt (NaCl). The Na:K ratio was much higher in the high-risk villages. The data showed a deficit of potassium in the highest risk villages, reflecting the inverse correlation between potassium and sodium intake and the high risk asssociated with excess intake of salt and lower intake of potassium. The authors concluded that several factors were involved in the incidence of gastric cancer. They suggested that the excess intake of salt acted as an irritant to the gastric mucosa, producing acute injury necrosis followed by regeneration of the mucosa, and that the presence of a mutagen in the gastric lumen following the nitrosation of fava beans in the intestine (Piacek-Llanes and Tannenbaum[2]) played a role in the cancer process. The role of potassium per se was not discussed.

A study was undertaken in Evans County, Georgia by Grim *et al.*,[3] to test the hypothesis that hypertension was more prevalent among blacks because of their greater intake of sodium than that of whites. Surprisingly, it was found that, to the contrary, white males consumed more sodium than did black males. The dietary intake of potassium was 2.3 times higher for white males and 1.6 times higher for white females. The cancer mortality per 100,000 per year for all cancers was 243 for black men and 156 for white men in Evans County compared to rates of 152 and 154, respectively, in the state. The cancer mortality rates for black women were comparable for Evans County and the state and were higher than the rates for white women.

Macquart-Moulin[4] conducted a case-control study of colorectal cancer in the Marseilles region of southern France. The study included 399 cases and a corresponding number of age- and sex-matched controls. Food intake over the previous year was determined by a dietary history questionnaire. The study showed a lower consumption of vegetables and oil among cancer cases but no differences in the consumption of meat, bread, eggs or butter. Although the intake of several nutrients, particularly potassium, iron, magnesium, vitamins B_2, B_6, C, and vegetable fiber was lower among cancer cases, only potassium retained significance for both cancers of the colon or rectum when these nutrients were analyzed jointly and adjusted for the other. Potassium intake was strongly and inversely associated with the risk of colorectal cancer.

An epidemiological study by Jansson[5] of the geographic distribution of cancers of the colon and rectum showed an especially high mortality rate for colorectal cancer in the northeastern part of the United States. However, it was found that within this area, Seneca County, New York had an unexpectedly low rate for not only colon and rectal cancers but for most other cancers. The low rates of cancer were thought to be related to the unique geographic and geochemical nature of the area in which large deposits of salt underlie the Finger Lakes region resulting in higher concentrations of sodium chloride and potassium chloride ions in the water and soil of the region.

Jansson's[6] study indicated that cancer risks were reduced when intracellular potassium levels were elevated, while cancer risks were increased when intracellular sodium levels were increased. In a further study, Jansson[7] compiled data from a number of independent studies that included geopathological, dietary, gerontological, and geophysical information, data on electrolyte concentrations in healthy and tumor cells, and data on the potassium status of patients with various diseases. Analysis of these data revealed a common finding in the relationship of intracellular concentrations of potassium and sodium to cancer risk. The level of intracellular potassium was negatively correlated to cancer rates. Decreased cancer risks were associated with increased intracellular potassium concentrations and decreased sodium concentrations. Conversely, increased cancer risks were associated with increased intracellular sodium concentrations and decreased intracellular potassium concentrations. The ratio of the concentrations of potassium to sodium ions appeared to be more important than the individual ion concentrations.

It has been postulated by Pantellini[8] that potassium cations play a role in the salification of the hydrogen bonds in all living structures. Accordingly, the lack of salification in DNA and RNA bases leads to opening of the valences and distortion of the genetic information resulting in the formation of cancer. Theoretically, where the environmental potassium is high, lower rates of cancer might be expected.

B. Case Reports

1. **Electrolyte Concentrations in Tissues and Cells.** There is increasing evidence that a relationship exists between cancer and the levels of various elements in the human body.[9] Using atomic absorption spectrophotometry, Ranade and Panday[10] determined the concentrations of potassium, calcium, magnesium, and sodium in normal and neoplastic tissues. Surgically resected specimens of normal, uninvolved, or involved tissues were obtained from various sites including oral cavity, respiratory and gastrointestinal tracts, breast, reproductive organs, bone marrow, and diverse types of neoplasms. The concentration of potassium was found to be higher than in noncancerous counterparts in all cancerous tissues except bone marrow, where leukemic bone marrow contained lower levels of potassium. The mean values for calcium were found to be significantly enhanced only in cancerous bone marrow. The mean concentrations of magnesium were similar for oral regions, bone marrow, esophagus and sarcoma, and slightly higher in cancerous tissues of the breast, rectum-colon, stomach and respiratory organs, but lower than values found in normal samples. The mean values for sodium in cancerous and non-cancerous tissues were not significantly different for oral regions, esophagus, respiratory organs, and respiratory organs. Higher concentrations of sodium were seen in cancerous tissues of breast, bone marrow, rectum-colon, stomach, and sarcoma, when compared to uninvolved areas.

Zs.-Nagy *et al.*[11] used energy dispersive x-ray microanalysis to measure intranuclear potassium, sodium, and chloride concentrations of cells from tumor tissue samples taken from patients suffering from invasive urogenital cancers. The cancers were categorized into either keratinizing, transitional cell, or hypernephroid carcinoma. Intact urothelium from patients having no malignant processes, or proximal and distal tubular cell nuclei from rat kidney cells served as controls for comparison. The analyses showed that in all three types of cancer cells, the average nuclear sodium content increased more than three-fold while potassium content decreased 32, 16, and 13%, respectively. The chloride content increased, but to a lesser extent than did the sodium. The intracellular Na:K ion ratios were more than five-fold higher in the cancer cells than in the non-cancerous control cells.

Smith *et al.*[12] performed elemental x-ray microanalysis on hepatocytes of normal, young adult A/J mice and on the tumor cells and hepatocytes from tumor-bearing mice that had been injected with H6 hepatoma cells. Nuclear and cytoplasmic concentrations of potassium, magnesium, phosphorus, sodium, sulfur, and chlorine were determined. Normal hepatocytes and hepatocytes from hepatoma-bearing mice differed very little in their elemental concentrations. Hepatocytes from the hepatoma-bearing mice showed a decrease in magnesium from normal hepatocytes. However, sodium and chlorine concentrations were more than double those of normal hepatocytes.

Romeu *et al.*[13] studied the variation in the content of potassium, copper, zinc, iron, calcium, magnesium, and sodium in the tissues of inbred C57BL/6 mice following the injection and growth of Lewis lung carcinoma cells. Tissues from various organs and tumor masses were examined. Tissue potassium, calcium, magnesium, and sodium remained relatively unchanged, while copper, zinc, and iron showed a progressive decrease in their tissue concentrations as tumor growth progressed. Liver zinc increased as metastasis increased. Sodium was the only metal to be actively concentrated by the tumor mass.

Potassium is primarily an intracellular cation, and total body potassium (TBK) is a measure of total body cellular mass.[14] TBK can be measured *in vivo* noninvasively by a whole-body counter since natural potassium contains measurable amounts of the radioisotope ^{40}K. Using this technique, Chandra *et al.*[15] were able to measure TBK and the predicted normal total potassium (Kp) for a number of patients with chronic lymphocytic leukemia (CLL). They found that both the absolute TBK and the relative excess of total body potassium (TBK/Kp) were related to the stage of the disease. Both TBK and TBK/Kp increased with increasing clinical stages of the disease. Following successful therapy, the clinically monitored reduction in leukemic cell mass was accompanied by reductions in TBK and TBK/Kp. The study showed that the level of TBK/Kp is a useful indicator of total body leukemia burden and that by quantifying the intracellular content of the leukemic cell it may be possible to determine the actual number of malignant cells in the patient.

Weight loss in cancer patients is well known. It has been shown that this weight loss is accompanied by a decrease in TBK and total body nitrogen (TBN) (Moore *et al.*,[16] Cohn *et al.*[17]). Cohn *et al.*[18] showed that the loss of TBK and TBN are due predominantly to the loss of skeletal muscle.

In a study of 23 patients with cachexia resulting from either malignant or benign inflammatory disease, Watson and Sammon[19] showed that these patients were anemic, overhydrated, and deficient in potassium. Both TBK and intracellular potassium were lower (17% and 25%, respectively) than predicted values based on height, weight, age, and sex.

The ratio of TBN/TBK may serve as the best indicator of recent or ongoing catabolism or anabolism of the neoplastic process.[20] Patients who lost weight showed a decrease in TBN and TBK but an increase in the TBN/TBK ratio, *i.e.*, a relative decrease in potassium. On the other hand, patients who maintained or gained weight showed an increase in TBN and TBK but exhibited a decrease in the TBN/TBK ratio, *i.e.* a relative increase in potassium.

It is well known that hypercalcemia and hypokalemia often coexist.[21,22] In a study of 28 cases of hypercalcemia associated with malignant disease, 11 cases were shown to have low plasma potassium concentrations below 3.4 mEq/L.[23]

2. **Potassium Depletion**. Mucus-secreting tumors of the large intestine resulting in a depletion of body potassium have been reported. McKittrick and Wheelock[24] described a case in which an 82-year-old woman was found to have a villous pappiloma of the rectum which secreted up to 2.2 liters of clear, slightly mucoid fluid containing up to 11 grams of sodium chloride. Serum chloride fell to 70 mEq/L and serum potassium fell to 1.32 mEq/L; blood nonprotein nitrogen was 135 mg/100 ml. Following repletion of fluid and electrolytes, and resection of the rectal tumor, serum electrolytes, including potassium, returned to normal.

Cooling and Marrack[25] described a case in which a woman complained of passing water through the rectum for five years. Sigmoidoscopy and barium enema failed to reveal any evidence of a tumor. The symptoms persisted and eight years later she entered the hospital after complaining of vomiting, abdominal discomfort and failure to pass fecal matter for 4 days. She continued to pass rectal fluid at 4 to 6 pints per day. Her serum potassium level was 2.2 mEq/L and was not improved by oral administration of 144 grams of potassium citrate. Electrolyte determination of the rectal fluid showed a tenfold increase in potassium over sodium. Sigmoidoscopy revealed a granulomatous polypoid mass and a hemicolectomy was performed to remove a villous tumor of the sigmoid colon. All electrolytes returned to normal after removal of the tumor.

Shnitka *et al.*[26] presented two cases and reviewed an additional 16 cases of villous tumors. These were characterized by clinical symptoms including dehydration, hyponatremia, hypokalemia, prerenal azotemia, and metabolic acidosis resulting from the copious secretion of watery mucus from the villous tumor. The authors regarded the excessive loss of mucus, rich in both potassium and sodium as the reason for the serum electrolyte depletion.

Crane[27] reported high concentrations of sodium and potassium in mucus from the large intestine of patients with adult coeliac disease and a villous papilloma located at the rectosigmoid junction. His observation of high concentrations of potassium and a potassium:sodium ratio as high as 46:1 demonstrated the ease with which potassium may be depleted from the body by the excretion of large quantities of mucus. He pointed out the need for replacement of potassium in diseases such as villous tumors, obstruction of the large bowel, ulcerative colitis, and steatorrhea, where large amounts of mucus is excreted. Parks[28] suggested that the gross disturbances in serum electrolytes was due not to the change in electrolyte composition of the mucus secreted by the villous tumor, but principally to the massive increase in the quantity of fluid eliminated.

Davies and Daly[29] examined the relationship between potassium depletion and the size at which villous adenomas of the large bowel undergo malignant transformation. Their study suggested that in potassium-depleted patients, premalignant lesions are prone to undergo malignant transformation at an earlier biologic time than in patients without depleted potassium. They concluded that although the causal relationship of low potassium concentration and malignancy is uncertain, it supports the notion that potassium depletion plays a role in the loss of growth control leading to malignant transformation.

Roy and Ellis[30] described two cases of circulatory collapse due to dehydration and hypokalemia caused by villous tumors of the colon, one in a 70-year-old man, the other in a 56-year-old woman. Electrolyte analysis showed extremely high potassium content in the rectal fluid. The ratio of potassium in the rectal fluid to that in the serum was 8.8 (28 mEq/L versus 3.2 mEq/L) in the man and 5.2 (17.6 mEq/L versus 3.4 mEq/L) in the woman. Following resection of their tumors both patients recovered and their electrolyte levels returned to normal.

A retrospective analysis by Paice *et al.*[31] of biochemical data from 58,167 patients at the Glasgow Royal Infirmary showed that 21% developed hypokalemia (less than 3.5 mMol/L) during hospitalization. Serum potassium levels were less than 3.0 mMol/L in 5.2% of these patients. Patients with leukemia and lymphoid tumors and those with gastrointestinal malignancies were among those most frequently experiencing hypokalemia. Hypokalemia was more common in women, and there was a positive correlation between hyperkalemia and hospital mortality. Hypokalemia was associated with drug and intravenous fluid administration in 56% of the patients. Drug-related hypokalemia was most commonly seen with diuretics and following the use of steroids, insulin, and hematinics. There was no significant association of hypokalemia with cardiovascular disease.

3. **Potassium and Other Electrolyte Disturbances in Human Leukemias**. In a retrospective study of 506 serum potassium and serum calcium values of 51 patients who had died from acute leukemia, Hocker and Reizenstein[32] found that 35% (6/17) of the patients had constant hypocalcemia and almost 24% (4/17) had intermittent hypocalcemia. No patient had constant hypokalemia but 58% (23/40) had intermittent hypokalemia. These hypokalemia samples were significantly associated with high fever and systemic antibiotics, with intestinal antibiotics, blood transfusions, and possibly with corticosteroids. The authors concluded that potassium for newly formed leukemia cells might be derived from the plasma and may be a contributing reason for the hypokalemia, as has been suggested for other neoplastic cells.[33]

Flahavan *et al.*[34] reported consistently higher potassium levels in lymphocytes from patients with chronic lymphatic leukemia (CLL) than in those from normal subjects. The ratio of K:Na in CLL lymphocytes was 3.94 when compared with normal leukocytes. The raised potassium content of CLL lymphocytes was attributed to the possible increased activity of Na/K ATPase or from increased potassium binding on the surface of CLL cells.

Parker *et al.*[35] reported on a case of acute monocytic leukemia (AML) in which the patient's serum potassium was extremely low (1.0 mMol/L). Despite the low plasma potassium the patient was excreting 57 mMol/L of potassium in the urine. TBK, as measured by whole body counting of ^{40}K, was 2.5 mol. The expected value was 2.0 ± 0.16 mol. The high TBK was explained by the additional potassium present in the leukemic cell mass.

Ringelhann[36] reported a case of pseudohyperkalemia in a patient with acute myeloid leukemia. During measurement of blood electrolytes at the terminal stage of the disease, the potassium level was very high (10.2 mEq/L). Although the patient exhibited no symptoms of hyperkalemia, a repeated test showed a similar high value. An investigation of the source of the increased potassium level showed that serum potassium rose 30 minutes after venipuncture, and increased further at 2 hours. It was found that the plasma protein rose when the patient's white cells were incubated after centrifugation. It was unclear whether the high potassium content of the leukemic cells and its release into the plasma was a result of the antileukemia treatment the patient had received. Red cells similarly treated did not release potassium.

4. **Potassium and Cystic Breast Disease**. Secreto *et al.*[37] and Bradlow *et al.*[38] identified two major biochemical subpopulations of cystic breast disease: Type I in which the breast cyst fluid (BSF) has high potassium ion, low sodium ion, and high dehydroepiandrosterone (DHA-S) concentrations, and Type II, in which BSF has low potassium ion, high sodium ion, and low DHA-S. Preliminary data suggest that patients with gross cystic breast disease are at greater risk for developing cancer if they have Type I cysts.

III. Potassium Inhibition of Transplantable Tumors in Experimental Animals

A preliminary report by Chawdhurry *et al.*[39] presented data showing a therapeutic effect of treatment with various combinations of monovalent potassium-, divalent calcium-, and trivalent ferric-ions with lactose on the survival of Swiss mice injected with a transplantable fibrosarcoma. It was found that treatment with large doses of lactose in combination with small doses of the cations produced a cancericidal effect. Treatment produced selective necrosis of the tumors, after which complete healing took place, and mice survived for more than a year. Treatment was by various routes. Intraperitoneal, oral, or intramuscular treatment resulted in 50-67%, 75%, and 80-100% survivors, respectively. Since the authors did not identify the salts or the concentrations used in the treatment protocol, it is difficult to draw any definitive conclusions regarding the therapeutic effect they reported.

In a study to determine if dietary magnesium depletion affected the growth of established transplantable rat mammary adenocarcinoma, Mills *et al.*[40] showed that depletion had no effect on plasma concentrations of potassium, zinc, or sodium. Rats with tumors had increased potassium and decreased sodium levels, independent of dietary effects. In tumors from magnesium-depleted rats, growth was inhibited 46%, magnesium concentration decreased 40%, and tumor necrosis was 50% greater.

The effect of cesium chloride and potassium chloride on the lifespan of female Sprague-Dawley rats inoculated with Novikoff's hepatoma (NH) was studied by Messiha and Stocco.[41] Rats treated with CsCl for 12 days prior to or immediately after inoculation with 1.0 ml of viable NH cells showed an increase in mortality compared to corresponding controls. Conversely, increasing the dose of NH cells to 2.0 ml resulted in a delay of toxicity as evidenced by a decrease in mortality. Treatment in the drinking water consisted of either distilled water, 0.2% CsCl, 0.02% KCl alone or combined with 0.2% CsCl. Treatment with CsCl alone resulted in a delay and decrease of the mortality curve. Treatment with KCl alone resulted in a decreased mortality score. Cumulative mortality scores at the end of the experiment, 32 days post-inoculation, were 50% for the KCl-treated group, 67% for the CsCl-treated group, and 83% for the water controls. Paradoxically, combined treatment with KCl and CsCl resulted in 100% mortality within 20 days of inoculation with NH cells suggesting a critical intercellular balance between Cs and K ions on the inhibitory effects observed.

Weanling rats were placed on synthetic control diet or a diet deficient in either potassium or magnesium or both elements for 1-3 weeks, after which they were inoculated with approximately one million Yoshida ascites tumor cells or Walker 256 carcinoma cells.[42] Restricted dietary intakes were given to prevent nutritional differences between the groups. Reduction in tumor size occurred with magnesium deficiency alone (up to 40%), potassium deficiency alone (30-60%), and combined deficiency (45-85%). There was a positive correlation between tumor size and the combined concentrations of magnesium and potassium in plasma or muscle. There was a significant loss (20%) of potassium from tumors, only from combined dietary deficiency, and a correlation between concentrations of magnesium and potassium in both Yoshida and Walker 256 tumors but not in muscle tissue. The authors concluded that the removal of potassium from tumor tissues by dietary depletion of both magnesium and potassium may affect the replication and survival of tumor cells by inhibiting metabolic activity and causing loss of intracellular potassium.

IV. Potassium Inhibition of Chemically-Induced Tumors in Experimental Animals

In a preliminary report, Jacobs[43] showed that supplementation of the drinking water with potassium chloride inhibited the incidence of gastrointestinal tumors induced by 1,2-dimethylhydrazine (DMH) in Sprague-Dawley rats. Male rats were injected weekly with 20 mg DMH/kg body weight for 20 weeks. Potassium was provided in the drinking water from one week before initiation of DMH treatment and was continued until the animals were sacrificed 14 weeks after the last treatment. Rats in the KCl-supplemented group ingested approximately 288 mg potassium per day, compared to approximately 180 mg per day in the unsupplemented group. The incidence of DMH-induced small intestinal tumors was significantly ($p<0.05$) reduced from 40% (8/20) in the unsupplemented group to 5% (1/20) in the KCl-supplemented group. The incidences of tumors of the colon and of the Zymbal gland were also reduced but to a lesser extent not statistically significant. Liver glutathione transferase activity was increased in KCl-supplemented animals suggesting that inhibition of DMH-induced carcinogenesis by potassium may be attributed in part to the enhancement of a detoxification pathway.

Fukushima *et al.*[44] reported on the significance of L-ascorbic acid (AA) and urinary electrolytes for the promotion of rat urinary carcinogenesis initiated by oral administration of N-butyl-N-(4-hydroxybutyl)nitrosamine (BBN). Administration of 5% sodium L-ascorbate (SA), the sodium ion form of AA, significantly promoted urinary bladder carcinogenesis, whereas administration of 5% AA did not. Urine from SA-treated rats had an elevated pH, an increase of sodium ion concentration, and increases in AA and its metabolite dehydroascorbic acid. Treatment with 5% AA and 3% K_2CO_3 promoted BBN bladder carcinogenesis, whereas treatment with 5% AA and 5% $CaCO_3$ or 5% $MgCO_3$ did not, indicating the importance of urinary sodium or potassium ion concentration and pH in the modulation of bladder carcinogenesis by AA.

V. Potassium Effects on Cells in Culture

High potassium concentrations were shown to alter the morphology and the ability of transformed 6m2 cells (a clone of rat kidney cells infected with a temperature-sensitive mutant of Moloney sarcoma virus) to grow (Lai and Becker[45]). Approximately 60% of the transformed cells reverted to a normal morphology in the presence of 94.8 mM potassium (normal culture medium contains 5.36 mM potassium) in isotonic medium at 39°C, the permissive temperature for transformation, whereas 100% reverted to normal at 72 mM in hypertonic medium. Hypertonic high-potassium medium was prepared by the addition of potassium, as KCl, to normal medium without removal of an equivalent amount of sodium. These conditions also resulted in a reduction of the capacity of the reverted cells to grow in soft agar. It was postulated that NaK-ATPase might play a role in reversal of the transformation process.

To test the hypothesis that the intracellular concentration of sodium is higher in transformed cells than in their normal counterparts, and higher in rapidly dividing cell populations than in slowly dividing cells, Cameron *et al.*[46] examined the intracellular contents of a number of representative cells. Energy dispersive x-ray microanalysis was used to determine concentrations of potassium, sodium, magnesium, phosphorus, sulfur, and chlorine. The 22 cell populations included tumor cells (two hepatomas and two mammary adenocarcinomas), nontumorous counterparts (hepatomas from two species and lactating mammary cells from two species), rapidly dividing cells (enterocytes from the crypts of the small and large intestines, neonatal cells, thymocytes), and slowly dividing cells (pancreatic acinar cells, smoothe muscle cells, and hepatocytes). Statistical analysis of the data showed that the concentration of sodium and chlorine ions was significantly higher in tumor cells than in any of the other normal cell populations. There were no significant differences in the concentrations of potassium, magnesium, phosphorus, or sulfur in tumor or normal cells. Rapidly dividing cell types showed significant increases in the concentrations of potassium, sodium, magnesium, phosphorus, and chlorine. The magnitude of differences in sodium and chlorine concentrations between the rapidly and slowly dividing cell types was not as great as between the tumor cell types and their nontumorous counterpart cell types. Comparisons between tumor cell types and rapidly dividing cell types revealed that sodium and chlorine were in higher concentration in the tumor cell types while potassium, magnesium, and phosphorus were in higher concentration in the rapidly dividing cell types. The authors concluded that high intracellular sodium and chlorine concentrations are associated with mitogenesis and that higher sodium and chlorine concentrations are associated with carcinogenesis. Furthermore, an elevated intracellular concentration of potassium and of magnesium is associated with the maintenance of a high rate of mitotic activity in nontumor cells but not necessarily in tumor cells.

VI. Mechanisms of Action of Potassium

It has been postulated that altered surface properties of tumor cells may cause a loss of growth control mechanisms. The accumulation of potassium ions in malignant cells may be such a mechanism which is partly responsible for the uncontrolled growth of these cells.

Zs.-Nagy *et al.*[47] determined the intracellular concentrations of sodium and potassium in human thyroid tumors of varying malignancy. Energy dispersive x-ray analysis was used to examine specimens of benign adenomas, and differentiated and anaplastic carcinomas of the thyroid. Na:K ion ratios were then calculated and compared to those found in normal thyroid epithelial cells. The data showed a progressive increase in the Na:K ion ratio with increasing malignancy from benign adenoma to differentiated, then anaplastic carcinoma of the thyroid. The results further support the theory of Cone[48] in which the sustained depolarization of the cell membrane results in an increase in the rate of cell division.

Glick and Githens[49] demonstrated that removal of sialic acid from the cell membrane of L1210 leukemia cells by incubation with neuraminidase inhibited potasium ion transport across the membrane. Sodium ion transport and glucose uptake were not significantly inhibited by the same treatment suggesting that transport in general was not affected by sialic acid, and that potassium transport in particular was not regulated by the action of membrane-bound sialic acid on glucose utilization.

Greenhouse and Coe[50] reported that Ehrlich ascites cells depleted of potassium ion and then exposed to potassium for 2 minutes prior to the addition of glucose exhibit a higher initial rate of glycolysis, a lower glucose-6-P accumulation, and a higher fructose-1-6-P_2 accumulation than depleted cells incubated in a potassium-free medium. Both the potassium ion transport and the effect of potassium ion on glycolysis are blocked by ouabain. In the presence of potassium ion the velocities of the glycolytic enzymes, fructose-6-phosphate kinase, lactic acid dehydrogenase, and hexokinase are accelerated immediately after the addition of glucose. The initial stimulation of glycolysis by potassium ion was shown not to be due to an increased rate of ATP hydrolysis associated with potassium ion transport.

Intracellular potassium ion concentration plays an important role in regulation of the rate of glycolysis in Ehrlich ascites tumor cells. Moroff and Gordon[51] showed that in these cells depletion of cellular potassium resulted in an initial decline of ATP with a concomitant increase in ADP and AMP content. Further incubation of the cells resulted in a fall in ATP content to negligible levels and degradation of AMP as manifested by a fall in total adenine nucleotides. The ATP reduction in potassium-depleted cells was prevented by incubation of the cells in a potassium-containing medium. Addition of potassium after preincubation of the potassium-depleted cells did not restore adenine nucleotide levels. However, addition of glutamine to the potassium-depleted cells restored the ATP content. The study suggested that potassium ion depletion does not directly interfere with oxidative phosphorylation and that in a potassium-deficient state the availability of endogenous substrates for mitochondrial oxidation is the limiting factor.

Nissen *et al.*[52] measured the rate of oxygen consumption in freshly prepared mouse neuroblastoma C-1300 cells and in corresponding cells that were cultivated with and without 20% calf serum, which is known to suppress differentiation. Fresh cells and cells grown in serum-depleted serum showed relatively intense respiration, wheras proliferating cultivated cells had a low rate of oxygen intake. Increased potassium concentration in the medium had no effect on cultivated, differentiated cells but completely abolished the uptake of oxygen by fresh neuroblastoma cells. It was noted that the inhibitory effect of excess potassium disappeared completely during differentiation and that cultivated differentiated neuroblastoma cells were virtually unaffected by the excess potassium.

Spaggiare *et al.*[53] investigated the components of unidirectional potassium ion influx and efflux in mouse 3T3 cells and SV40-transformed 3T3 cells in either sparse exponential or dense stationary growth phases. Total unidirectional potassium ion influx and efflux was observed to be twice that of the transformed cells at all densities investigated, showing that transformation specifically decreases unidirectional potassium ion flux. Both cell lines possessed a component of potassium ion flux that was sensitive to ouabain as well as components of potassium ion influx and efflux sensitive to furosemide, suggesting a one-to-one potassium ion exchange mechanism. Potassium ion influx mediated by the ouabain-sensitive component was significantly reduced when 3T3 cells in the exponential and density-inhibited phase were compared, but not in the transformed cells at equivalent cell densities, suggesting that this component of potassium ion influx was correlated with growth. The furosemide component accounted for about 20% of the total unidirectional potassium ion influx and efflux in sparse culture of both 3T3 and transformed cell lines. At high densities, where inhibition of growth occurs in 3T3 cells but not in the transformed cells, the furosemide sensitive component doubled in both cell lines, indicating that the apparent potassium ion exchange mechanism is dependent upon cell density rather than cell growth.

Ernst and Adam[54] reported that intracellular potassium concentration in 3T3 cells showed a sharp decrease at cellular densities leading to inhibition of cell proliferation. The decrease in potassium concentration was not observed in SV40 transformed-3T3 cells at similar cell densities. The authors speculated that the processes of stimulation of quiescent 3T3 cells or of cell density-dependent inhibition of their proliferation are mediated by changes in potassium transport characteristics which lead to increased or decreased intracellular concentrations, respectively.

Johnson and Weber[55] reported no significant differences in potassium ion influx or ouabain binding between growing normal chick embryo cells and Rous sarcoma virus-transformed chick embryo cells. Potassium ion influx was growth related but not transformation specific since ouabain binding and ouabain-sensitive potassium ion influx was almost 2-fold lower in density inhibited cells. The potassium content of transformed cells was 1.4-fold higher than in growing normal and density-inhibited cells. Similarly, sodium levels were 2- to 4-fold higher in transformed cells than in normal or density-inhibited cells. The rate of potassium ion efflux was 1.3 to 1.5 times higher in growing normal cells than in density-inhibited or transformed cells. However, based on the absolute number of potassium ions, efflux was similar in normal and transformed chicken embryo cells because of the larger potassium pool in transformed cells.

Neoplastic diseases may directly or indirectly affect renal structure and function resulting in derangements in fluid and electrolyte metabolism. Hyperkalemia may be seen in patients with malignant disorders when there is adrenal insufficiency secondary to metastasis of tumors or deposition of amyloid associated with other neoplasms, and when there is renal failure due to obstruction of ureters, infiltration of the kidney, or sludging of the tubules with urea during chemotherapy.[56] Excessive losses of potassium in the urine may occur in patients with tumor cells that produce adrenocorticotrophic hormone (carcinoma of lung, esophagus, prostate, parotid, thymus, thyroid, breast, ovary, pancreas, bronchial adenoma, pheochromcytoma, ganglioma, paraganglioma, carcinoid, melanosarcoma), renin (Wilms' tumor, hemangiopericytoma, carcinoma of the lung), and aldosterone (adrenal adenoma, adrenal carcinoma). Excess urinary losses of potassium have been reported in patients with Hodgkins disease,[57] multiple myeloma,[58-61] and myelocytic leukemia.[62]

VII. Potassium in Nutritional or Dietary Cancer Therapy

Parsons *et al.*[63] reported the regression of tumor growth in some patients with terminal cancer following depletion of magnesium and potassium by a combination of dietary adjustment and hemodialysis. In these patients daily diets were adjusted to provide less than 5 mg of magnesium compared with 70-100 mg absorbed from a normal diet. Three dialysis sessions per week reduced plasma concentrations of potassium and magnesium to the desired concentrations of 3 mM potassium per liter and 0.8 mg of magnesium per ml. Striking clinical improvement was frequently observed immediately following dialysis suggesting the removal of toxic factors although none were identified in the spent dialysis fluid.

Hocken[64] attempted to repeat the therapeutic effect of magnesium and potassium depletion observed by Parsons.[63] In his study, eight patients who had already received conventional anticancer chemotherapy were treated with a combination of oral sodium cellulose phosphate and sodium phase resonium cationic binding resins to reduce serum potassium and magnesium levels. A free diet was allowed. Depletion was considered achieved when the level of serum potassium could be maintained at or below 3.0 mM/L and the magnesium at or below 0.6 mM/L. Depletion was achieved and maintained for five and one-half to seven weeks in four patients and for two weeks in four other patients. In none of the eight patients did depletion of magnesium and potassium influence the course of primary tumor or any secondary lesions. The results were contrary to those reported by Parsons[63] and were ascribed to the treatment of previously treated cancers. Patients treated by Parsons[63] had not previously received conventional anticancer therapy.

Hyperalimentation provided enterally or parenterally can replete most malnourished cancer patients.[65] Rudman *et al.*[66] were able to treat the weight loss of 11 underweight adults whose body weight was less than 85% of ideal by intravenous hyperalimentation. The infusions provided the following amounts of nutrient per kilogram of body weight: 15 g glucose, 0.40 g N, 0.018 g P, 2.4 mEq K, 3.0 mEq Na, 2.3 mEq Cl, 0.5 mEq Mg, 0.45 mEq Ca, and 50 ml water. Patients gained weight at an average weight of 9.0 g/kg. The data showed that the retention of individual elements was not independent of each other. Withdrawal of either N, P, Na, or K impaired or abolished retention of the other elements. Removal of N halted retention of P, K, Na, and Cl; withdrawal of K stopped retention of N and P; withdrawal of N or P interrupted retention of all other elements. Weight gain occurs in one or more body compartments, namely, protoplasm, extracellular fluid, adipose tissue, and bone. Repletion of protoplasm and extracellular fluid in undernourished adults is retarded or abolished if N, P, Na, or K is lacking. Repletion of bone occurs in the absence of N or K, but not in the absence of Na or P. Weight gains during hyperalimentation lacking N, P, K, or Na consisted predominantly of adipose tissue.

A number of nutritional or "metabolic" therapies claiming cures for cancer and various other diseases by detoxifying the body or enhancing the immune system have been reported.[67,68] Gerson[69,70] developed a nutritional program combined with vigorous purging that he claimed was a successful therapy for advanced cancers. The therapy program, still available in Mexico, consists of a diet high in potassium, low in sodium, with no fats or oils, with minimal amounts of animal protein, with juices of raw vegetables and fruits, and with raw liver. A recent review[71] of the literature concluded there is no evidence that the Gerson method results in objective benefit in the treatment of cancer in humans, and discourages cancer patients from seeking treatment with this procedure.

VIII. Summary

Epidemiological studies have identified geographic areas having both high and low risk for colorectal cancers and other cancers. Subsequent studies have shown a correlation between potassium intake and cancer risk. Increased potassium intake is asssociated with decreased cancer risks, whereas, increased sodium intake is associated with increased cancer risk. Levels of intracellular potassium are inversely correlated to cancer rates. However, the ratio of potassium to sodium appears to be more important than the levels of individual electrolytes. There is a strong relationship between cancer and the levels of intracellular potassium. Generally, intracellular potassium concentrations are higher in noncancerous tissues than in cancerous tissues. Leukemic bone marrow appears to be an exception. Conversely, intracellular sodium is higher in tumor cells than in normal cells. Consequently, intracellular sodium to potassium ratios are generally higher in cancer cells due to this increase in intracellular sodium.

Both hyperkalemia and hypokalemia occur in people with cancer although hypokalemia occurs more frequently. Hyperkalemia can occur following chemotherapy for rapidly growing tumors, when tumor lysis occurs and large amounts of intracellular electrolytes are released into the bloodstream. Total body potassium has been shown to increase with increasing clinical stages of malignancy or during the progression from benign to malignant tumors. Since potassium is primarily intracellular, total body potassium is a good measure of the tumor burden in a patient with malignant disease. Hypokalemia develops as a result of either a decreased intake of or increased loss of potassium. Hypokalemia occurs in patients with both acute and chronic leukemias. Weight loss and catabolism also result in losses of potassium and sodium via the urine. Hypokalemia often accompanies mucus-secreting villous tumors of the large intestine. Excess loss of large amounts of rectal fluid by patients with these colorectal tumors is responsible for the depletion of body potassium. Resection of the tumors results in a return of serum electrolytes to normal. In potassium-depleted patients, villous tumors of the large bowel are prone to become malignant at an earlier stage than in patients whose potassium is not depleted. This suggests that potassium depletion plays a role in the loss of growth control leading to malignant transformation of the tumor.

A correlation of increased proliferation with intracellular Na:K ratio has been described for various cell types including normal animal cells, transformed cells, normal rapidly or slowly dividing cells, and cancer cells of invasively growing human tumors. Cancer cells have an increased cellular sodium concentration and an increased Na:K ratio.

Patients with gross cystic breast disease are considered to be at greater risk for developing breast cancer if the cyst fluid is high in potassium, low in sodium, and high in dehydroepiandrosterone.

Transplantable or chemically-induced tumors in rodents have been shown to be inhibited by potassium administered parenterally, in the diet, or in the drinking water. High concentrations of potassium in the culture medium was shown to cause virus transformed rat cells to revert to normal morphology and growth characteristics.

Altered surface properties of tumor cells may cause a loss of growth control mechanisms. The accumulation of potassium ions in malignant cells may reflect such a mechanism. It has been postulated that sustained depolarization of the cell membrane due to an increase in the sodium:potassium ratio is involved in the regulation and control of cell division during both normal and cancerous growth of tissues.

Intravenous hyperalimentation with increased potassium has been used to treat hypokalemia and to increase muscle mass in patients wasted by malignant disease. A number of nutritional or dietary cancer therapy regimens have been attempted. However, efforts to cure malignancies by the use of diets rich in potassium have questionable merit and require further study.

References

1. Correa, P., Cuello, C., Fajardo, L.F., Haenszel, W., Bolanos, O., and de Ramirez, B., Diet and gastric cancer: Nutrition survey in a high-risk area, *J. Natl. Cancer Inst.* 70, 673, 1983.

2. Piacek-Llanes, B.G. and Tannenbaum, S.R., Formation of an activated n-nitroso compound in nitrite treated fava beans (*Vicia faba*), *Carcinogenesis* 3, 1379, 1982.

3. Grim, C.E., Luft, F.C., Miller, J.Z., Meneely, G.R., Battarbee, H.D., Hames, C.G., and Dahl, L.K., Racial differences in blood pressure in Evans County, Georgia: Relationship to sodium and potassium intake and plasma renin activity, *J. Chron. Dis.*, 33, 87, 1980.

4. Macquart-Moulin, G., Riboli, E., Cornee, J., Charnay, B., Berthezene, P., and Day, N., Case-control study on colorectal cancer and diet in Marseilles, *Int. J. Cancer*, 38, 183, 1986.

5. Jansson, B., Seneca County, New York: An area with low cancer mortality rates, *Cancer*, 48, 2542, 1981.

6. Jansson, B., Geographic mapping of colorectal cancer rates: A retrospect of studies, 1974-1984, *Cancer Detect. and Prevent.*, 8, 341, 1985.

7. Jansson, B., Geographic cancer risk and intracellular potassium/sodium ratios, *Cancer Detect. and Prevent.*, 9, 171, 1986.

8. Pantellini, V.G., Hydrogen (H) bonds and their salification by potassium (K) in the structuring of living matter, *Med. Biol. Environ.*, 4, 467, 1978.

9. Pories, W.J., vanRij, A.M., Mansour, E.G., and Flynn, A., Trace element profiles in cancer patients, *Biol. Trace Elements Res.*, 1, 229, 1979.

10. Ranade, S.S. and Panday, V.K., Major metals in human cancer: Calcium, magnesium, sodium and potassium, *Sci. Total Environ.*, 41, 79, 1985.

11. Zs.-Nagy, I., Lustyik, G., Zs.-Nagy, V., Zarandi, B., and Bertoni-Freddari, C., Intracellular Na^+:K^+ratios in human cancer cells as revealed by energy dispersive x-ray microanalysis, *J. Cell. Biol.*, 90, 769, 1981.

12. Smith, N.R., Sparks, R.L., Pool, T.B., and Cameron, I.L., Differences in the intracellular concentration of elements in normal and cancerous liver cells as determined by x-ray microanalysis, *Cancer Res.* 38, 1952, 1978.

13. Romeu, A., Arola, L., and Alemany, M., Essential metals in tissues and tumor of inbred C57BL/6 mice during the infective cycle of Lewis lung carcinoma, *Cancer Biochem. Biophys.*, 9, 53, 1986.

14. Forbes, G.B. and Hursh, J.B., Age and sex trends in lean body mass calculated from ^{40}K measurements: With a note on theoretical basis for the procedure., *Ann. N.Y. Acad. Sci.*, 110, 255, 1963.

15. Chandra, P., Sawitsky, A., Chanana, A.D., Cohn, S.H., Rai, K.R., and Cronkite, E.P., Correlation of total body potassium and leukemic cell mass in patients with chronic lymphocytic leukemia, *Blood*, 53, 594, 1979.

16. Moore, F.D., Olesen, K.H., McMurrey, J.D., Parker, H.V., Ball, M.R., and Boyden, C.M., Eds., Chronic wasting disease and anabolic recovery, in *The Body Cell Mass and its Supporting Environment: Body Composition in Health and Disease*, W.B. Saunders Co., Philadelphia, London, 1963, 173.

17. Cohn, S.H., Vartsky, D., Yasumura, S., Sawitsky, A., Zanzi, I., Vaswani, A., and Ellis, K.J., Compartmental body composition based on total-body nitrogen, potassium, and calcium, *Am. J. Physiol.*, 239 (Endocrinol. Metab.2), E524, 1980.

18. Cohn, S.H., Gartenhaus, W., Sawitsky, A., Rai, K., Zanzi, I., Ellis, K.J., Yasumura, S., Cortes, E., and Vartsky, D., Compartmental body composition of cancer patients by measurement of total body nitrogen, potassium, and water, *Metabolism*, 30, 222, 1981.

19. Watson, W.S. and Sammon, A.M., Body composition in cachexia resulting from malignant and nonmalignant diseases, *Cancer*, 46, 2041, 1980.

20. Cohn, H., Gartenhaus, W., Vartsky, D., Sawitsky, A., Zanzi, I., Vaswani, A., Yasumura, S., Rai, K., Cortes, E., and Ellis, K.J., Body composition and dietary intake in neoplastic disease, *Am. J. Clin. Nutr.*, 34, 1997, 1981.

21. Sanderson, P.H., Renal potassium wasting in hypercalcaemia, *Br. Med. J.*, 1, 679, 1967.

22. Azzopardi, J.G. and Whittaker, R.S., Bronchial carcinoma and hypercalcaemia, *J. Clin. Pathol.*, 22, 718, 1969.

23. Zilva, J.F. and Nicholson, J.P., Plasma phosphate and potassium levels in the hypercalcemia of malignant disease, *J. Clin. Endocrinol. Metab.*, 36, 1019, 1973.

24. McKittrick, L.S. and Wheelock, F.C., Jr., *Carcinoma of the Colon*, Charles C. Thomas, Springfield, Ill., 1954, 61.

25. Cooling, C. and Marrack, D., Potassium-secreting tumour of the colon, *Proc. Royal Soc. Med.*, 50, 272, 1957.

26. Shnitka, T.K., Friedman, M.H.W., Kid, E.G., and McKenzie, W.C., Villous tumors of the rectum and colon characterized by severe fluid and electrolyte loss, *Surg. Gynecol. Obstet.*, 112, 609, 1961.

27. Crane, C.W., Observations on the sodium and potassium content of mucus from the large intestine, *Gut*, 6, 439, 1965.

28. Parks, A.G., Changes in general condition during evolution of villous tumors of the rectosigmoid, *Proc. Royal Soc. Med.*, 5, 441, 1968.

29. Davies, R.J. and Daly, J.M., Potassium depletion and malignant transformation of villous adenomas of the colon and rectum, *Cancer*, 53, 1260, 1984.

30. Roy, A.D. and Ellis, H., Potassium-secreting tumours of the large intestine, *Lancet*, 1, 759, 1959.

31. Paice, B.J., Paterson, K.R., Onyanga-Omara, F., Donnelly, T., Gray, J.M.B., and Lawson, D.H., Record linkage study of hypokalemia in hospital patients, *Postgrad. Med J.*, 62, 187, 1986.

32. Hocker, P. and Reizenstein, P., Calcium and potassium disturbances in acute leukemia, *Blut*, 29, 398, 1974.

33. Lawson, D.H., Murray, R.M., Parker, J.L.W., and Hay, G., Hypokalemia in megaloblastic anaemias, *Lancet*, 2, 588, 1970.

34. Flahavan, E., Smyth, H., and Thornes, R.D., Increased potassium in lymphocytes from patients with chronic lymphatic leukaemia, *Br. J. Cancer*, 28, 354, 1973.

35. Parker, A.C., Lambie, A.T., Housley, E. and Simpson, J., Plasma-potassium levels in leukemia, *Lancet*, 1, 392, 1975.

36. Ringelhann, B., Laszlo, E., and Vajda, L., Pseudohyperkalemia in acute myeloid leukemia, *Lancet*, 1, 928, 1974.

37. Secreto, G., Recchione, C., Ballerini, P., Callegari, L., Fariselli, G., Attili, A., and Moglia, D., Cations and active androgens in breast cyst fluid, *Ann. N.Y. Acad. Sci.*, 586, 88, 1990.

38. Bradlow, H.L., Fleisher, M., Breed, C.N., and Chasalow, F.I., Biochemical classification of patients with gross cystic breast disease, *Ann. N.Y. Acad. Sci.*, 586, 12, 1990.

39. Chowdhury, J.R. and Chowdhury, H., Cancericidal effect of certain salt combination in transplanted mouse fibrosarcoma, *J. Indian Med. Assoc.*, 62, 333, 1974.

40. Mills, B.J., Broghamer, W.L., Higgins, P.J., and Lindeman, R.D., Inhibition of tumor growth by magnesium depletion of rats, *J. Nutr.*, 114, 739, 1984.

41. Messiha, F.S. and Stocco, D.M., Effect of cesium and potassium salts on survival of rats bearing Novikoff hepatoma, *Pharmacol. Biochem. Behavior*, 21 (Suppl. 1), 31, 1984.

42. Young, G.A. and Parsons, F.M., The effects of dietary deficiencies of magnesium and potassium on the growth and chemistry of transplanted tumours and host tissues of the rat, *Europ. J. Cancer*, 13, 103, 1977.

43. Jacobs, M.M., Potassium inhibition of DMH-induced small intestinal tumors in rats, *Nutr. Cancer*, 14, 95, 1990.

44. Fukushima, S., Shirai, T., Hirose, M., and Ito, N., Significance of L-ascorbic acid and urinary electrolytes in promotion of rat bladder carcinogenesis, in *Diet, Nutrition and Cancer*, Y. Hayashi *et al.*, Eds., Japan Sci. Soc. Press, Tokyo/VNU Sci. Press, Utrecht, 1986, 159.

45. Lai, C-N. and Becker, F.F., Potassium-induced reverse transformation of cells infected with a temperature-sensitive transformation mutant virus, *J. Cell. Physiol.*, 125, 259, 1985.

46. Cameron, I.L., Smith, N.K.R., Pool, T.B., and Sparks, R.L., Intracellular concentration of sodium and other elements as related to mitogenesis and oncogenesis, *in vivo*, *Cancer Res.*, 40, 1493, 1980.

47. Zs.-Nagy, I., Lustyik, G., Lukacs, G., Zs.-Nagy, V., and Balazs, G., Correlation of malignancy with the intracellular Na^+:K^+ ratio in human thyroid tumors, *Cancer Res.*, 43, 5395, 1983.

48. Cone, C.D., Jr., Unified theory on the basic mechanism of normal mitotic control and oncogenesis, *J. Theor. Biol.*, 30, 151, 1971.

49. Glick, J.L. and Githens, S., III, Role of sialic acid in potassium transport in L1210 leukaemia cells, *Nature*, 208, 88, 1965.

50. Greenhouse, W.V. and Coe, E.L., The effect of potassium depletion on the initial kinetics of glycolysis in ascites tumor cells, *Biochim. Biophys. Acta*, 329, 183, 1973.

51. Moroff, G. and Gordon, E.E., Effect of K^+ deficiency on oxidative metabolism in Ehrlich ascites tumor cells, *Biochim. Biophys. Acta*, 325, 406, 1973.

52. Nissen, C., Ciesielski-Treska, J., Hertz, L., and Mandel, P., Regulation of oxygen consumption in neuroblastoma cells: Effects of differentiation and of Potassium., *J. Neurochem.*, 20, 1029, 1973.

53. Spaggiare, S., Wallach, M.J., and Tupper, J.T., Potassium transport in normal and transformed mouse 3T3 cells, *J. Cell. Physiol.*, 89, 403, 1976.

54. Ernst, M. and Adam, G., Dependence of intracellular alkali-ion concentrations of 3T3 and SV40-3T3 cells on growth density, *Cytobiologie*, 18, 450, 1979.

55. Johnson, M.A. and Weber, M.J., Potassium fluxes and ouabain binding in growing, density-inhibited and Rous sarcoma virus-transformed chicken embryo cells, *J. Cell. Physiol.*, 101, 89, 1979.

56. Glassock, R.J., Friedler, R.M., and Massry, S.G., Kidney and electrolyte disturbances in neoplastic diseases, *Contr. Nephrol.*, 7, 2, 1977.

57. Geary, C.C., Platts, M.M., and Stewart, A.K., Hypokalemia of unknown etiology complicating Hodgkin's disease, *Br. Med J.*, 2, 507, 1966.

58. Sirota, J.H. and Hamerman, D.J., Renal function studies in an adult with Fanconi syndrome, *Am. J. Med.*, 16, 138, 1954.

59. Dragsted, P.J. and Hjoith, N., The association of Fanconi syndrome and malignant disease, *Dan. Med. Bull.*, 3, 177, 1956.

60. Engle, R.L. and Wallis, L.A., Multiple myeloma and the adult Fanconi syndrome, *Am. J. Med.*, 22, 5, 1957.

61. Ben-Ishary, D., Dreyfuss, F., and Ullman, T.D., Fanconi syndrome with hypouricemia in an adult, *Am. J. Med.*, 31, 793, 1961.

62. Muggia, F.M., Heineman, H.O., Farhaug, M., and Osserman, E.F., Lysozymuria and renal tubule dysfunction in monocytic and myelomonocytic leukemia, *Am. J. Med.*, 47, 351, 1969.

63. Parsons, F.M., Anderson, C.K., Clark, P.B., Edwards, G.F., Ahmad, S., Hetherington, C., and Young, G.A., Regression of malignant tumours in magnesium and potassium depletion induced by diet and haemodialysis, *Lancet*, 1, 243, 1974.

64. Hocken, A.G., Magnesium and potassium depletion in patients with cancer, *New Zealand Med. J.*, 25 April, 275, 1984.

65. Blackburn, G.L., Maini, B.S., Bistrian, B.R., and McDermott, W.V., Jr., The effect of cancer on nitrogen, electrolyte, and mineral metabolism, *Cancer Res.*, 37, 2348, 1977.

66. Rudman, D., Millikan, W.J., Richardson, T.J., Bixler, T.J, II, Stackhouse, W.J., and McGarrity, W.C., Elemental balances during intravenous hyperalimentation of underweight adult subjects, *J. Clin. Invest.*, 55, 94, 1975.

67. Miller, N.J. and Howard-Ruben, J., Unproven Methods of cancer management, Part 1: Background and historical perspectives, *Oncol. Nursing Forum*, 10, 46, 1983.

68. Michelmore, P., Beware of health hucksters, *Reader's Digest*, January, 1989, 114.

69. Gerson, M., *A Cancer Therapy: Results of Fifty Cases*, 3rd Ed., Ashland, Oregon, World Wide Publishing Corp., 1977.

70. Gerson, M., The cure of advanced cancer by diet therapy: A summary of 30 years of clinical experimentation, *Physiol. Chem. Phys.*, 10, 449, 1978.

71. American Cancer Society, Unproven methods of cancer management: Gerson method, *CA*, 40, 252, 1990.

List of Poster Abstracts

Effects of Selenium in Cultured L1210 and MCF7 Cells: Evidence that Selenium Induces Apoptotic, Programmed Cell Death

H.J. Thompson, N.W. Gibson, K. Adlakha, P.J. Schedin, A.C. Wilson and M.A. Witt
AMC Cancer Research Center,
1600 Pierce Street, Denver, CO 80214

It is known that mammary tumor occurrence in both the rat and mouse following carcinogen administration (DMBA, 7,12-dimethylbenz(a)anthracene and MNU, 1-methyl-l-nitrosourea) is reduced by dietary selenium. We have studied, *in vitro*, the mechanism of action of selenium using two tumor cell lines, one from a mouse leukemia (L121O) and the other from human breast (MCF7). Combined morphological and molecular data provide evidence that selenium induces programmed cell death in these tumor cell lines.

Cells were exposed to various concentrations of selenite (Na_2SeO_3) for 24 and 48 hours and cell number (#), viability (trypan blue exclusion) and subsequent colony formation (CF) measured. In L1210 cells, doses of selenite between 5 and 20 µM had little effect on cell # or viability but significantly reduced CF. This effect was both time and dose dependent. Morphologically, cells treated with sub-toxic doses of selenite were shrunken in appearance with vacuolated cytoplasm and darkly stained, condensed chromatin. "Apoptotic bodies" defined as subcellular, membrane-bound fragments of condensed nuclear and cytoplasmic material were also observed.

We studied DNA damage induced by selenite using agarose gel electrophoresis and alkaline elution (AE). Cells treated with selenite showed non-random DNA cleavage. A banding pattern with regular size intervals of approximately 180 base pairs was observed on agarose gels. This observation is indicative of apoptosis and is considered due to the action of a specific Ca^{2+}-dependent endonuclease. AE profiles of DNA extracted from L1210 cells treated with selenite were distinctly different from control, X-ray damaged L1210 cells. AE profiles from X-ray damaged cells were linear, whereas selenite treated cells displayed multiphase profiles. These results further indicate that selenite induces non-random DNA cleavage and again, both the DNA laddering and AE profiles were dose dependent. We have extended these observations to the human breast tumor cell line, MCF7, and results indicate that selenite also induces apoptosis in this cell line.

Modulation of Carcinogen Metabolism by Diallyl Sulfide

C.S. Yang, J.H. Brady and J.-Y.Hong
Laboratory for Cancer Research, College of Pharmacy, Rutgers University, Piscataway, NJ 08855-0789

Diallyl sulfide (DAS), a component of garlic oil, has been shown to inhibit carcinogenesis by several chemicals. The present work suggests that inhibition of cytochrome P450-dependent carcinogen activation is a likely mechanism for this action. DAS, when given to rats orally, produced a time- and dose-dependent inactivation of hepatic cytochrome P450IIE1. Diallyl sulfoxide also produced similar effects and diallyl sulfone produced a more rapid response in the inactivation of P450IIE1. The inactivation appeared to be specific to P450IIE1. The same DAS treatment caused an induction of P450IIB1 and little charge on other P450 isozymes. When added to the incubation mixture, DAS also inhibited competitively the hepatic microsomal metabolism of N-nitrosodimethylamine (NDMA), an activity displayed by P450IIE1. Preincubation of diallyl sulfone with microsomes and NADPH caused a metabolism-dependent inactivation of P450IIE1 suggesting a possible mechanism of P450IIE1 inactivation *in vivo*. The inhibition and inactivation of P450IIE1 activity could explain the protective action of DAS against colon carcinogenesis induced by 1,2-dimethylhydrazine. Consistent with this concept is our observation that DAS pretreatment protected against hepatotoxicity induced by NDMA and CCl_4. Pretreatment of rats with DAS also inhibited the metabolism of NDMA and N-nitrosodiethylamine by kidney and nasal microsomes, and the metabolism of 4-(methylnitrosamino)-l-(3-pyridyl)-l-butanone (NNK) by lung and nasal microsomes. The metabolism of these carcinogens can also be inhibited by DAS added *in vitro*. The results suggest that DAS may inhibit carcinogenesis related to the aforementioned tissues and nitrosamines.

Supported by the American Institute for Cancer Research grant 88B18 and NIH grant CA 37037.

Effect of Dietary Arginine-Methionine Balance on Growth of Hepatoma

R.M. Millis and C.A. Diya
Department of Physiology and Biophysics, College of Medicine, and Department of Human Nutrition, School of Human Ecology, Howard University, Washington, DC 20059

Prior studies have shown that urinary polyamines may be indicative of tumorigenesis. Since arginine and methionine are precursors for polyamines, we hypothesized that alteration of dietary arginine and methionine may inhibit tumor growth and suggest nutritional strategies for cancer therapy. Groups of healthy adult male host ACI rats (n=8, 255-300g) were subjected to subcutaneous transplantation of viable Morris hepatoma inoculum from donor rats. Control groups were fed mixtures of amino acids in replacement of protein (22%), carbohydrate (61%) and fat (10%) with normal levels of minerals, fiber and vitamins. Choline was decreased (0.2%) to ensure that it would not be used as a supplementary vitamin for methylation in animals fed methionine-deficient diets. Compared to the control diet, experimental diets were made up of combinations of deficiencies in arginine (-65%) or methionine (-50%) and excesses of arginine (+20%) or methionine (+24%). Animals were fed the diets and water ad libitum. Daily food intake and body weight were measured for 28 days, after which tumors were excised, weighed and polyamines were measured. Statistical significance ($P<0.05$) of differences between controls and experimentals was analyzed using Duncan's multiple range test (SPSS). Results showed that (mean ± SEM) daily food intake (5.56 ± 0.95 to 7.66 ± 0.42g) was unaffected by the experimental diets. The control group gained body weight (26.39 ± 2.77 g). Small body weight decrements of experimental groups were detected (3.5 ± 0.9% to 4.8 ± 0.6%). Tumor weight of controls was found to be 8.49 ± 1.48% of body weight. The experimental diets which produced significant decrements in tumor weight were: (1) the arginine-methionine-deficient diet, (2) the arginine-excess/ methionine-deficient diet, and (3) the excess arginine diet. Decreased tumor growth was associated with nonspecific changes in tumor polyamines. Groups fed diets deficient in arginine had no significant changes in either body weight or tumor weight, but had significant decreases in tumor polyamines. The group fed the excess arginine diet had significant decreases in tumor weight, had no significant change in tumor putrescine, but had significant decreases in tumor spermine and spermidine levels. It is concluded that there is an association between inhibition of hepatoma growth and dietary deficiency of methionine in combination with either deficient or excess arginine, but changes in polyamines are not reliable markers for subcutaneous growth of transplanted Morris hepatoma in rats.

Prevention of Photocarcinogenesis and Immunosuppression by Vitamin E

H.L. Gensler
Department of Radiation Oncology and Cancer Center, University of Arizona, Tucson, AZ 85724

Ultraviolet irradiation of C3H/HeN mice induces skin cancer and an immunosuppression which prevents the host from rejecting antigenic UV-induced tumors. The capacity of topical vitamin E (dl-α-tocopherol) or dietary β-carotene to prevent photocarcinogenesis in haired mice was assessed. Skin cancer incidence in UV-irradiated mice was 81%, at 33 weeks after the first UV exposure; administration to mice of 25 mg dl-α-tocopherol thrice weekly, or 1% dietary β-carotene, for 3 weeks before UV irradiation, and throughout the experiment, reduced this incidence to 42% ($p=0.0065$, log rank test) and 67% ($p=0.05$), respectively. UV irradiated mice fed β-carotene underwent a 37% decline in plasma α-tocopherol levels and an 80% reduction in skin concentrations, suggesting that β-carotene may influence the actions of another lipid-soluble antioxidant. Immunoenhancement by vitamin E, was assessed by comparing levels of immunosuppression by splenocytes from normal or UV irradiated mice, with and without topical vitamin E treatment. Transfer of splenocytes from UV irradiated mice to naive mice prevented the recipients from rejecting a UV-induced tumor challenge, whereas splenocytes from UV irradiated mice treated with vitamin E did not prevent recipients from rejecting a similar tumor challenge. Phenotypic analysis of splenocytes used in the passive transfer assay, using a biotin-avidin-immunoperoxidase technique, revealed that α-tocopherol treatment of mice undergoing UV irradiation prevented the UV-induced down regulation of Ia expression in splenocytes, and increased the proportion of Lyt-2^+ and L3T4^+ splenocytes. Therefore, chronically applied vitamin E can effectively reduce cancer formation and immunosuppression induced by UV irradiation. Prevention of downregulation of Ia expression may have contributed to this immunomodulation. Dietary β-carotene was ineffective in preventing photocarcinogenesis in this haired mouse model, and led to a reduction of α-tocopherol in skin and plasma.

Effect of Refined Dietary Cellulose on Dimethylhydrazine Induced Colon Cancer in the Rat

M.H. Penner and J.-C. Hsu
Food Science and Technology, Oregon State University, Corvallis, OR 97331-6602

Results from studies analyzing the effect of refined cellulose on dimethylhydrazine induced colon carcinogenesis in the rat appear contradictory. Several studies have reported an apparent protection against colon carcinogenesis while others have found no effect. There are a number of factors which may influence the results of such studies: including the strain, sex and age of the rats, the time, dose and route of carcinogen administration, the non-cellulose composition of the basal diet, the amount of cellulose incorporated into the diet and the chemical and physical properties of the cellulose preparation utilized.

It is apparent from the discrepancy in published results that more information is needed regarding the factors that impart this variability. Studies attempting to provide this information must systematically modify specific experimental parameters using a "standard" experimental protocol. Our laboratory is currently involved in such a study which is designed to determine the importance of the structural properties of cellulose preparations used in experimental cancer studies. The experimental approach is to utilize cellulose preparations with significantly different physicochemical properties. The celluloses are characterized by physical and chemical methods to determine their degree of crystallinity, degree of polymerization, and non-cellulosic components. The degree of crystallinity, which reflects the relative amount of crystalline and amorphous character of a fiber, is potentially important in terms of influencing the fermentability and water holding capacity of the fiber. Non-cellulosic components of cellulose preparations are predominantly hemicelluloses and lignin. The extent of these contaminants is relevant due to the relative ease of fermentation of the hemicellulosic contaminants and the different physicochemical properties of lignin relative to cellulose. The ability to study the importance of cellulose structure relative to inhibition of colon carcinogenesis is dependent on the availability of structurally unique celluloses. In this regard, we have recently developed a method to prepare a unique hydrochloric acid-regenerated cellulose. This cellulose preparation, which maintains its linear beta-1,4-glucose structure, is structurally distinct from commercially available cellulose preparations and is more readily accessible to cellulolytic enzymes, factors which may affect cellulose fermentation and colonic pH.

Supported by the American Institute for Cancer Research grant 89A25.

Immunological and Nutritional Evaluation of Cancer Patients

R.W. Iafelice, W.L. Simonich, O.G. Rasmussen, R.G. Crispen, R.D. Levin and R.M. Williams
Departments of Nutrition and Immunology, Cancer Treatment Centers of America—American International Hospital (AIH), Zion, IL 60099

Serum zinc levels, T-cell subsets, and mitogen responsiveness were analyzed among cancer patients. We tested four hypotheses relating to zinc and immune function in cancer patients. These were that as serum zinc levels decrease, CD4, the CD4/CD8 ratio, Concanavalin A (Con A) -stimulated T-cell function, and phytohemagglutinin (PHA)-stimulated T-cell function each decrease. We retrospectively analyzed data on 119 patients. Data examined included plasma amino acids, vitamins, trace minerals, T- and B-cell number and function, and immunoproteins. Each hypothesis was tested using multiple regression with forward stepping. Nutrition/immune values, primary site, stage, age, and sex were each used as possible explanatory variables. We found that the helper cell levels of cancer patients covary directly with their serum zinc levels, other things being equal. For each one µg/ml decrease in the serum zinc level, the CD4 count drops by about 733 cells ($p<0.001$) and the CD4 percentage drops about 7.5 percent ($p=0.002$). However, serum zinc is not associated with CD4/CD8 ratio, Con A response, or PHA response.

Effects of Varying Ratios of Dietary n-3/n-6 Lipids on Growth and Metastasis of CT-26 in BALB/c Mice

F. Cannizzo, Jr. and S.A. Broitman
Departments of Microbiology and Pathology,
Boston University School of Medicine, Boston, MA 02118

This laboratory has demonstrated that increased levels of polyunsaturated fat in isocaloric diets cause increased growth rates in tumors implanted in the descending colon of mice. This study deals with the effect of dietary marine oil on growth and metastasis of bowel tumors. Male, weanling BALB/cByJ mice were fed one of five experimental diets containing various ratios of safflower oil (n-6 fat source) and marine oil (n-3 fat source) 30 days prior to the study commencement. Diets contained 24.5% fat w/w (46.9% kcals as fat), identical amounts of protein, carbohydrate, fibre, vitamins, minerals. Fat ratios: I - 100% marine oil, II - 93.0%, III - 69.75%, IV - 58.15%, and V - 0.0%. Mice were divided into three groups: bowel tumor, pulmonary colonization, and uninoculated weight gain controls. Bowel tumor assay: anesthetized animals were inoculated with 10^6 CT-26 cells (from tissue culture) in descending colon subserosally. Animals were sacrificed 21 days post-operative and tumors measured *in situ*. Tumor measurements: I - 40.85mm^3 ± 9.26mm^3 (diet – mean ± std. err.), II - 33.49 ± 7.53, III - 54.29 ± 12.24, IV 309.29 ± 58.05, V - 434.11 ± 77.16. By ANOVA: I, II, III differed from IV, V ($p<0.0001$). Pulmonary colonization assay: mice were injected with 10^5 CT-26 via tail vein and killed after 21 days. Lungs were insufflated with India ink and preserved in Fakete's to visualize tumor colonies. Colony Counts: I - 14.35 ± 3.9 (diet: mean colony number ± std. err.), II - 20.4 ± 6.1, III - 27.1 ± 6.9, IV - 23.8 ± 7.1, V - 41.8 ± 9.1. By ANOVA I, II differ from V ($p<0.05$). Repeat studies using identical diet formulations with fully hydrogenated coconut oil (saturated fat) showed no differences between diets in bowel tumor or pulmonary colonization assays. Mice and diet were weighed regularly; none of the diet groups weighed differently or consumed different amounts of diet/day before or after tumor inoculation compared to uninoculated controls. These findings demonstrate: 1. marine oils inhibit growth and metastasis of CT-26 tumors *in vivo*; 2. this inhibition results from more than simple displacement of dietary essential fatty acids. Marine oil may inhibit tumor growth by interfering with production of prostaglandins (growth and immune mediators) since n-3 fats inhibit cyclooxygenase or by interfering with transmembrane signaling systems which rely on membrane lipids for anchorage and bioactive metabolites (diacylglycerol). Both of these postulates are currently under study in our laboratory.

Radioprotection by Vitamin E: Injectable Vitamin E Administered Alone or in Combination with the Phosphorothioate WR-3689 Enhances Survival of Irradiated Mice

V. Srinivasan and J.F. Weiss
Radiation Biochemistry Dept., Armed Forces Radiobiology Research Institute, Bethesda, MD 20889-5145

The radioprotective effects of vitamin E may be related to its antioxidant properties and/or modulation of immune functions. In general, published data on radioprotection by vitamin E in rodents are inconsistent, probably due to differences in route of administration, chemical forms of the vitamin, basal diet composition, influence of nonaqueous vehicles, etc. In the current study, we determined the effectiveness of an injectable free form of vitamin E (α-tocopherol) in a vehicle containing solubilizer. Male CD2F1 mice were irradiated with ^{60}cobalt (theratron, unilateral exposure, 0.20 Gy/min). Increases in postirradiation 30-day survival were observed when vitamin E was administered SC at 50 and 100 IU/kg body weight either before or immediately after radiation exposure. After 9 Gy, 81% of the mice treated with vitamin E (100 IU/kg) survived, compared to 38% of controls (saline or vehicle). After 10 Gy, 47% of the vitamin-E-treated mice survived, whereas all irradiated controls died.

We further investigated whether vitamin E injected before or after radiation exposure could enhance the radioprotective effect of WR-3689, S-2-(3-methylaminopropylamino)ethylphosphorothioic acid. Phosphorothioate derivatives, such as WR-2721 and WR-3689, are among the best radioprotective and chemoprotective agents, but their use is limited by their toxicity. Improvement in protection was obtained when vitamin E (100 IU/kg) was injected SC 1 hr before irradiation, with WR-3689 (150 mg/kg) injected IP 30 min before irradiation. After 13 Gy, 81% of mice with the combined treatment survived, whereas there were no survivors after WR-3689 treatment alone. Effects of the vehicle were noted under certain experimental conditions. The data suggest that lower doses of phosphorothioates can be administered together with vitamin E to obtain the same effect as higher doses.

Will Nutrients that Prevent Neurogenic Intestinal Ischemia Decrease Colon Carcinogenesis?

E. Seifter, J. Mendecki, H. Dawson and J. Weinzweig
Department of Surgery, Albert Einstein College of Medicine, Bronx, NY 10461

Hypotheses regarding causation of colon cancers in humans emphasize the role of diet (lack of fiber, high fat content, presence of dietary carcinogens). Eating patterns and life style (mainly a lack of physical exercise resulting in increased digestion transit times) have also been implicated. Endogenous factors (bile sterols, proteolytic pancreatic enzymes) and the intestinal flora interact with compounds of dietary origin and their metabolites and produce digesta having high concentrations of both initiators and promoters that act locally for extended periods of time. Hypotheses advanced by workers in the behavioral fields deal with the effects of problems related to bowel habit development and predisposition to later intestinal diseases, including colon cancer.

Variants of this hypothesis attribute the predisposition to societal factors (acquisitiveness) that may be expressed by altered digestive functions.

We hypothesize that, in addition to diet and bowel habits, psychologic or neurologic factors influence colon carcinogenesis by affecting intestinal mucosal blood supply and by altering the activity of the bowel muscularis itself. These factors contribute to the development of a micro environment that favors carcinogenesis. Psychologic as well as other stressors cause vaso-constriction of submucosal vessels, producing ischemia of the mucosa and atony of the muscularis. Mucosal ischemia diminishes synthesis and secretion of mucus and weakens the barrier to bacteria and carcinogenic compounds. Repetitive stressful stimuli produce frequent incidents of mucosal sloughing followed by periods of reperfusion and oxidative injury. Atony of the muscularis tends to focus the site of exposure. We have found that supplemental β-carotene, Vitamin A and choline prevent mucosal ischemia and bowel atony. These nutrients that inhibit dedifferentiation and later stages of carcinogenesis are the very ones that block stress-induced actions that would otherwise produce an intestinal milieu favoring the accumulation of carcinogens and favoring their local action on mucosal cells. Beta-carotene plays a special role in preventing the reperfusion oxygen injury, thereby lessening promotion due to inflammation.

Biochemical and Morphological Effects of Dietary Carotenoids In Rats Fed a Choline-Deficient Diet

M.Y. Jenkins, N.M. Sheikh, G.V. Mitchell, E. Grundel, S.R. Blakely and C.J. Carter
Food and Drug Administration, Washington, DC 20204

Carotenoids have been shown to inhibit carcinogenesis in a number of experimental systems. The induction in rats of hepatocellular proliferative changes leading to neoplasia by a choline-deficient and low methionine diet affords a model system for evaluating effects of substances potentially modulating carcinogenesis. In this study, canthaxanthin (CA), β-apo-8′-carotenal (BA) or β-carotene (BC) in an extract of *Spirulina-Dunaliella* algae was fed at 0, 0.1 or 0.2% in a choline deficient (CD) diet. In each of 8 groups, 10 adult male Fischer 344 rats were fed diets with designated carotenoid source and level for 12 weeks. Carotenoids altered some of the changes induced by the CD diet. Increases in enlargement of fatty livers and low plasma cholesterol levels occurred with 0.2% BA feeding. Plasma retinol was further reduced 35% by BA or BC. BA and BC increased liver retinyl palmitate approx. 80 and 305%, respectively. Liver lipid peroxidation was enhanced and plasma α-tocopherol was reduced further by 0.2% BC. BC, BA and CA depressed liver α-tocopherol approx. 49, 67 and 78%, respectively. The decreased liver α-tocopherol was concurrent with an increase in carotenoid stores of CA> BA >BC. Hemoglobin levels were reduced in all rats fed carotenoids. Sections of liver tissue were examined histopathologically by light microscopy. All rats fed CD diets showed fatty and cirrhotic changes similar to those reported in the literature. Histochemical evaluation based on a semi-quantitative assay revealed a marked increase in peroxisome enzyme activity in the liver of all CD rats. None of the carotenoids appeared to affect the development of morphological changes in the liver of choline-deficient rats. Although carotenoids can function as antioxidants, they did not prevent changes observed in rats fed CD diets.

Comparison of Parenteral with Enteral Nutrition of Tumor-Bearing Rats

T. Foley-Nelson, W.T. Chance, F.-S. Zhang, A. Stallion and J.E. Fischer
Department of Surgery, University of Cincinnati and V.A. Medical Center, 231 Bethesda Avenue, Cincinnati, OH 45267-0558

Although the development of cachexia may complicate cancer therapy, controversy exists concerning its nutritional management. For example, utilization of total parenteral nutrition (TPN) may not be appropriate due to gut atrophy, possible stimulation of tumor growth, and lack of protein repletion. In the present experiment, host and tumor response were compared following identical parenteral or enteral (EN) nutritional supplementation. Eighteen days after sc. inoculation of adult male Fischer 344 rats (TB) with fresh methylcholanthrene-induced sarcoma, catheters were placed into either the external jugular vein or the stomach. Four days later, rats were begun on a 12-day course of either TPN or EN employing a Freamine III-based formula (amino acids = 6%, dextrose = 21.5%, lipid = 1.5%). At sacrifice, there was no difference in tumor weight between the various TB groups (Table 1). Although carcass weight was increased significantly in the TB-TPN group, there was no elevation in gastrocnemius protein content in either the TB-TPN or TB-EN groups as compared to the TB-chow group. Small intestine weight was preserved in the TB-EN group, but only to the level observed in the TB-chow rats. Total lipids in the liver were increased in both TB-TPN and TB-EN groups; however, the magnitude of the increase was less in the TB-EN rats.

Table 1

Group	N	Tumor Wt.(g)	Carcass Wt.(g)	Muscle Wt.(g)	Muscle Protein (mg)	Liver Wt.(g)	Liver Fat(mg/g)	Gut Wet Wt.(g)
Control-chow	12	--	283±9	0.39±0.01	330±5	3.25±0.1	65±2	7.3±0.2
TB-chow	10	80±4	212±9[a]	0.27±0.02[a]	214±13[a]	2.75±0.1[a]	70±3	5.4±0.4[a]
TB-TPN	12	72±4	246±4[a,b]	0.32±0.01[a,d]	236±8[a]	4.12±0.2[a]	101±10[a]	4.0±0.3[a,d]
TB-EN	5	63±6	243±0	0.31±0.01[a]	247±11[a]	3.93±0.3[b,c]	81±3[a]	5.4±0.3[a]

[a]$p<0.01$ vs control; [b]$p<0.05$ vs control; [c]$p<0.01$ vs TB-chow; [d]$p<0.05$ vs TB-chow

These results suggest that EN may be more beneficial than TPN in that gut mass is preserved and liver fat may be reduced. Neither of these treatments, however, resulted in significant protein repletion of tumor-bearing rats.

Supported by the American Institute for Cancer Research grant 90A44.

A High Potassium Diet Prevents Transepithelial Depolarization in Experimental Colon Cancer

S.M. Thompson and R.J. Davies
Department of Surgery, University of California, San Diego, CA 92103

Studies of cancer epidemiology have suggested that a diet in which the ratio of potassium (K) to sodium (Na) is elevated may be protective against development of cancer. Previous studies using a mouse model of experimental colo-rectal cancer have shown that transepithelial and cell membrane depolarization are associated with the initiated state following carcinogen administration. We have examined whether a diet high in K and low in Na might prevent the depolarization associated with the pre-malignant or malignant state and ultimately might affect the development of colon cancer.

Saline or dimethylhydrazine (DMH), a carcinogen known to cause colonic cancer in rodents, was administered to adult female CF_1 mice in a dose of 20 mg/Kg for 6 weeks by subcutaneous injection. One group of animals was maintained on a regular diet for which the ratio K:Na = 1.3 (molar ratio) whereas another group was maintained on a high K/low Na diet where K:Na = 4.9. Animals were sacrificed one week after their sixth injection and the distal colon was removed, opened and mounted in a modified Ussing chamber for measurements of I_{SC} (short-circuit current), V_T (transepithelial potential difference) and transepithelial ion fluxes.

In animals maintained on a regular diet, the V_T of DMH treated animals were depolarized relative to saline treated controls (-2.8 ± 0.4 mV, n = 23 compared to -3.7 ± 0.2 mV, n = 21 (mean ± SEM)). The V_T of DMH animals on the high K/low Na diet were also depolarized relative to their saline controls (-4.2 ± 0.5 mV, n = 41 versus -8.0 ± 1.0 mV, n = 39, respectively), but both were augmented compared to their counterparts on the normal diet and the V_T of the DMH animals was returned to near normal.

A high K/low Na diet results in relative transepithelial hyperpolarization despite DMH treatment when compared to animals fed a diet with a lower K:Na ratio. It remains to be determined whether this diet is protective in preventing colo-rectal cancer. The ionic and cellular mechanisms for this protective effect will be presented.

Supported by American Institute for Cancer Research grant 89A56.

The Effect of Glutathione Depletion on the Inhibition of Cell Colony Formation by Selenite

P.B. Caffrey and G.D. Frenkel
Department of Biological Sciences,
Rutgers University, Newark, NJ 07102

Selenium is an essential trace element which has been shown to have anticarcinogenic activity. One mechanism which has been proposed for this activity is a cytotoxic effect on tumor cells. As a means of assessing its cytotoxicity, we have examined the effect of selenite on the ability of tumor cells to form colonies. We have found that brief exposure of HeLa cells to micromolar concentrations of selenite resulted in significant inhibition of colony formation, indicating that this is a sensitive assay for selenite cytotoxicity. In order to investigate the influence of cellular sulfhydryl (SH) compounds on selenite cytotoxicity, we treated cells with buthionine sulfoximine (BSO) prior to selenite exposure. This treatment caused a five-fold reduction in the level of intracellular glutathione, the predominant cellular SH compound. This depletion of cellular glutathione resulted a significant decrease in the inhibitory effect of selenite on colony formation. A likely explanation for these results is that selenite must react with glutathione to form the selenodiglutathione derivative for it to exert its cytotoxic effect. This conclusion is supported by our finding that when cells were exposed to selenite which had previously been reacted with glutathione the BSO-induced decrease in cytotoxicity was eliminated. In contrast, prior reaction of selenite with other SH compounds such as cysteine and mercaptoethylamine did not restore cytotoxicity in BSO-treated cells.

Effect of Sodium Selenite on Initiation of Methylnitrosourea (MNU)-Induced Mammary Cancers

C.J. Grubbs, M.M. Juliana and L.M. Whitaker
University of Alabama at Birmingham, Birmingham, AL 35294

It is well established that selenium supplementation of the diet will inhibit the promotional stage of mammary carcinogenesis in rodents. Several experiments have also indicated that selenium supplementation for a short time (2-4 weeks) before and after carcinogen treatment will also inhibit mammary tumorigenesis. In this study, we evaluated the effect of feeding selenium for two months prior to the administration of MNU, a direct-acting carcinogen. Sodium selenite was incorporated into AIN-76A diet at dose levels of either 3.0 or 1.5 mg/kg of diet, and was fed to female Sprague-Dawley rats from 40 to 100 days of age. MNU (50 mg/kg BW) was administered by IV injection at 100 days of age. At termination of the study (six months after MNU), the incidence and av. no. of mammary cancers/rat were as follows: AIN-76A diet only, 40% (1.2); high dose sodium selenite, 63% (1.9); low dose sodium selenite, 63% (1.9). The effect of selenium on the promotional stage of MNU-induced mammary carcinogenesis was also determined to confirm previously reported data. MNU (40 mg/kg BW) was administered to female Sprague-Dawley rats at 50 days of age. Beginning at 52 days of age and continuing until the end of the study, diets were supplemented with either 3.0 or 1.5 mg sodium selenite/kg of diet. The study was terminated six months after MNU. The incidence and av. no. of mammary cancers/rat were as follows: AIN-76A diet only, 100% (7.1); high dose sodium selenite, 90% (4.4); low dose sodium selenite, 97% (5. 1). Under the conditions of these studies, sodium selenite caused an enhancement of mammary cancer initiation by MNU, but resulted in a suppression of mammary cancers when fed during the promotional phase. Additional studies are warranted to determine whether other inorganic and organic selenium compounds will also enhance cancer initiation when administered for a long time prior to carcinogen treatment.

Supported by National Cancer Institute grants CA44615 and CA28103.

Effects of Limonin and Nomilin on Glutathione S-Transferase Activity and Benzo(a)pyrene-Induced Neoplasia in the Lung and Forestomach of A/J MICE

L.K.T. Lam, B.L. Zheng and S. Hasegawa
Gray Freshwater Biological Institute,
University of Minnesota, Navarre, MN 55392 and
Fruit and Vegetable Chemistry Laboratory,
ARS, USDA, Pasadena, CA 91106

Limonin and nomilin are two of the bitter principles found in common edible citrus fruits such as lemon, lime, orange, and grapefruit. Both citrus limonoids have been found to induce increased glutathione S-transferase (GST) activity in laboratory animals. Many inducers of GST have been correlated with their ability to inhibit carcinogenesis. In this study the inhibition of chemically induced tumor formation in the lung and forestomach of A/J mice by dietary limonoids was investigated. Benzo(a)pyrene, an environmental carcinogen, was used as the tumor inducer. The results showed a reduction of tumor multiplicity in the forestomach by 40% (1.9 vs 3.2 tumors/tumor bearing mouse) with 0.27% dietary nomilin. Limonin at 0.5% did not significantly protect the animals. Both limonin and nomilin, when given in the diet, were able to reduce the number of lung tumors per animal in a dose dependent manner. The carcinogen control group had 11.9 tumors per animal with 100% tumor incidence. The limonin treated groups, with 0.5, 0.25 and 0.125% limonin, had 6.1, 8.1, and 10.8 tumors per animal, respectively. The nomilin treated groups, with 0.27, 0.135 and 0.068% nomilin, had 2.9, 5.7, and 14.9 tumors per animal, respectively. These results indicate that both limonoids tested can reduce lung tumor multiplicity in mice. Similar to the effects in the forestomach nomilin is a better inhibitor of lung tumor formation than limonin.

Supported by American Institute for Cancer Research grant 88A27.

Selenium and Immune Cell Function

L. Kiremidjian-Schumacher, M. Roy, H.I. Wishe, M.W. Cohen and G. Stotzky
New York University, College of Dentistry and Graduate School of Arts and Science, New York, NY 10010

This study examined the effects of dietary selenium (Se) modulation on the ability of a host to generate tumor-cytotoxic cells and to destroy tumor cells. Spleen or peritoneal exudate cells were removed from immunized (i.p. P815 cells) or non-immunized 14-week old, male C57Bl/6J mice maintained for 8 weeks on Se-deficient (0.02 ppm Se), normal (0.20 ppm Se), or Se-supplemented (2.0 ppm Se) *Torula* yeast diets. Se supplementation significantly increased spleen lymphocyte proliferation in response to stimulation with mitogen (PHA) or alloantigen (P815; mixed lymphocyte reaction), while Se-deficiency had the opposite effect. The production of Il-1 and Il-2 in control and experimental animals remained the same. Dietary and *in vitro* (5 x 10^{-8} M to 5 x 10^{-7} M) supplementation with Se resulted in the generation of higher numbers of cytotoxic lymphocytes (allogeneic stimulation), enhanced tumor cytotoxicity, and lymphotoxin production, whereas Se deficiency inhibited the responses. Similarly, dietary supplementation with Se enhanced tumor cytodestruction and tumor necrosis factor-α production by peritoneal macrophages elicited by allogeneic stimulation *in vivo*, while Se deficiency inhibited tumor cytodestruction. The augmentation of macrophage-mediated cytotoxicity appeared to be related to an increase in the number of cytotoxic cells and was not related to the ability of the cells to become activated, nor to changes in the endogenous levels of interferon-γ. ^{125}I-Il-2 binding studies showed that dietary or *in vitro* (1 x 10^{7} M) supplementation with Se resulted in enhanced expression of high affinity Il-2-receptors on activated lymphocytes, whereas Se deficiency inhibited the response. It appears that Se affects the development and magnitude of immune responses through modulation of the density of Il-2-receptors on the surface of responding cells.

Supported by American Institute for Cancer Research grant 86A08.

Vitamin A Inhibits Covalent Binding of Radiolabelled 3,4-Benzo(a)pyrene to DNA in Isolated Mouse Liver Nuclei

M.B. Baird, J.L. Hough, G.T. Sfeir and A.S. Guerra
Masonic Medical Research Laboratory, Utica, NY 13501

Vitamin A and related compounds, the retinoids, exert anti-tumor activity against a variety of cancers through inhibition of tumor growth. However, several previous studies have demonstrated and confirmed that retinoids inhibit both the mutagenicity of chemical carcinogens in bacterial/liver microsome assays, and also the *in vitro* microsomal activation of chemical carcinogens. Thus, retinoids may also inhibit tumorigenesis by depressing tumor initiation. Previous studies of chemical carcinogen activation have utilized microsomal membranes as the source for carcinogen activation. However, those membranes comprising the nuclear envelope may be of greater importance in generating carcinogens which bind to DNA. Therefore, the capacity of the nuclear envelope to activate 3,4-benzo(a)pyrene (BP) to forms capable of covalently binding to genomic DNA, as well as the capacity of all-*trans* retinol to modulate activation, was examined.

Liver nuclei were prepared from C57BL/6J male mice by sucrose gradient ultracentrifugation. Nuclei were preincubated aerobically for 15 minutes with retinol ranging in concentration from 0-400 µg. NADPH and ^{3}H-BP (53 µM) were added, and the incubations were continued for one hour. Nuclei were harvested, lysed, digested with RNAse followed by proteinase K, and the DNA collected by ion-exchange chromatography. DNA content and purity was estimated by UV spectrophotometry, and aliquots of the DNA samples were counted for radioactivity.

BP was readily metabolized by the nuclear envelope as evidenced by the incorporation of ^{3}H-BP into nuclear DNA. Increasing amounts of retinol in the incubation medium linearly decreased incorporation of ^{3}H-BP into DNA reaching maximal inhibition of 50% at 100 µg. These results confirm that the nuclear envelope readily generates short-lived, highly reactive metabolites of BP which covalentlv bind to nuclear DNA. Furthermore, 50% of the binding of metabolites of BP to DNA in isolated mouse liver nuclei can be inhibited by retinol, which suggests that the binding unaffected by retinol is mediated by a mechanism inaccessible to perturbation with retinol, or to yet an additional mechanism.

Diacylglycerol Accumulation During Choline Deficiency—Mechanism for Hepatic Carcinogenesis

S.H. Zeisel, J.K. Blusztajn,
E. Cochary and K. daCosta
Department of Nutrition, University of North Carolina at Chapel Hill, Chapel Hill, NC 27599-7400

Choline deficiency causes fatty liver and is associated with hepatocarcinogenesis. We have previously reported that 1,2-sn-diacylglycerol (1,2-DAG) concentrations within livers from choline deficient rats are markedly elevated (Febs Lett. 243:267-270, 1989) and have suggested that the carcinogenic effect of choline deficiency is mediated by 1,2-DAG activation of protein kinase C (PKC). In these experiments we report upon the subcellular localization of 1,2-DAG within choline deficient liver, and we present preliminary data on PKC activity in these fractions.

Rats were pair-fed for six weeks with control (0.2% choline), or choline deficient (0.002% choline) diets. Choline deficiency was verified by measuring hepatic choline and phosphocholine content. Hepatic DAG was determined by a radioenzymatic assay in which DAG was phosphorylated by a specific 1,2-sn-diacylglycerol kinase in the presence of [^{32}P-γ]ATP to [^{32}P]phosphatidic acid (PA). PA was purified and its radioactivity determined. Hepatic cytosolic and membrane-associated (plasma membrane, nuclear and endoplasmic reticular membranes) PKC activities were determined by a radioenzymatic assay in which the radioactivity transferred from [^{32}P-]ATP to histone in the absence of phosphatidylserine and 12-O-tetradecanoyl-phorbol 13-acetate was subtracted from that occurring in the presence of those activators.

1,2-DAG concentrations in livers from choline deficient rats were three-fold higher than in livers from controls. Most of this 1,2-DAG was localized in the lipid droplets that accumulate in the cytoplasm of hepatocytes. In deficient animals this fraction contained more than 700 nmol DAG/g liver, while in controls it contained 15 nmol DAG/g liver. Only plasma membrane was associated with significantly more 1,2-DAG in deficients than in controls (3-fold higher). Increased PKC activity was observed in several subcellular fractions prepared from choline deficient liver (plasma membrane & endoplasmic reticulum, endoplasmic reticulum, microsomes). Assays of PKC activity in plasma and nuclear membranes are pending.

Supported by American Institute for Cancer Research grant 89A14.

Prophylaxis by Butylated Hydroxytoluene (BHT) of Carcinogen-Induced Lung Tumors in Strain A/J Mice

A.M. Malkinson
Molecular Toxicology Program and Colorado Cancer Center, School of Pharmacy, University of Colorado, Boulder, CO 80309

BHT causes numerous deleterious effects to mouse lung by dietary, injection, and gavage routes of exposure. When administered by itself, BHT brings about a reversible toxicity in which Type I pneumocytes die and repair occurs by Type II cell compensatory hyperplasia. Chronic exposure to BHT following carcinogen treatment (tumor promotion protocol) increases the multiplicity of primary lung tumors in some strains. These tumors arise from Type II cells and bronchiolar Clara cells. In strain A/J mice, BHT administered a few hours prior to the carcinogen, urethane (tumor prophylaxis protocol), reduces tumor multiplicity. In other inbred strains tested, however, this same protocol either has no protective effect, is co-carcinogenic, or is lethal. We have studied genetic, metabolic, and biochemical aspects of this protection by BHT which appears uniquely to occur in A/J mice.

Genetic: In hybrid progeny produced following a cross of A/J with strains in which a BHT/urethane protocol is co-carcinogenic, the prophylactic effect of BHT was dominant in one case but BHT/urethane had no effect on tumor multiplicity compared to urethane alone in another hybrid. This suggests involvement of more than one gene in the tumor modulatory actions of BHT.

Metabolic: Old mice (>1 year old) are resistant to the pneumotoxicity of BHT but are sensitive to the prophylactic effect. Cedrene, a cytochrome P450 inducer, abolishes all pulmonary effects of BHT including prophylaxis in A/J mice. Piperonyl butoxide, a mixed function oxidase inhibitor, prevents toxicity, promotion, and prophylaxis, but not co-carcinogenesis. The BHT metabolites found after biotransformation of BHT in A/J mice do not differ from those produced in other mice. These results suggest that while the BHT metabolite responsible for prophylaxis may be different from that causing pneumotoxicity or co-carcinogenesis, it is not uniquely made in A/J mice.

Biochemical: Both the lungs and freshly isolated Clara cells of A/J mice have a lower protein kinase C (PKC) content than those of 14 other strains tested. This is important because BHT treatment of mice reduces pulmonary PKC activity.

Hypothesis: A metabolite of BHT lowers PKC activity in certain lung cell populations. Decreasing an already low PKC concentration in A/J mice protects against subsequent lung tumor development. One of the genes responsible for lung tumor prophylaxis in A/J mice regulates the cellular PKC concentration.

Supported by USPHS Grant CA33497 and American Institute for Cancer Research grant 86A80.

Glutathione Content in Food

D.P. Jones, E.W. Flagg, R.J. Coates and J.W. Eley
Dept. Biochem., Dept. Epidemiol. Biostat. and
Winship Cancer Center, Emory University,
Atlanta, GA 30322

The overall goal of measuring GSH in foods is to gain a better understanding of GSH as a potential nutrient in humans. GSH is one of the most important known anticarcinogens and antioxidants. GSH is absorbed intact in rat small intestine (T.M. Hagen and D.P. Jones, Am. J. Physiol. 252:G607-G613, 1987) and oral GSH increases plasma GSH concentration in humans. We are studying GSH contents in the normal human diet by measuring the GSH levels in foods listed in the National Cancer Institute's Health Habits and History Questionnaire. Foods were purchased locally and prepared as most commonly consumed in the U.S. GSH analyses were performed using an HPLC technique in which GSH was derivatized with iodoacetic acid and 1-fluoro-2,4-dinitrobenzene. A method of additions was used to correct for losses during sample preparation and a separate set of samples was run following treatment with dithiothreitol to measure total glutathione (reduced plus oxidized forms). Results showed that fresh fruits and vegetables have 50-150 mg GSH/kg wet weight. Cooking resulted in oxidation and formation of some products that were not recovered by treatment with dithiothreitol. Treatment of cooked meats and fish with dithiothreitol yielded values of total GSH in the range of 25-180 mg/kg. Commercially prepared foods, dairy products and most grain products were relatively low in GSH. Thus, GSH is likely to be bioavailable for humans and considerable variation is likely to occur in human ingestion of GSH. With the availability of this data base, it will be possible to begin to assess whether dietary GSH is an important determinant of the incidence of specific cancers.

Supported by American Institute for Cancer Research grant 87A53 and funds from the Department of Human Resources, State of Georgia.

The Effect of the Dietary Compound, Queuine on Some Enzymes Protective Against Oxidative Stress: Studies with Tissue Culture Cells and Germfree Mice

W.R. Farkas and L. Szabo
Program in Environmental Toxicology
University of Tennessee, College of Veterinary Medicine 37901-1071

Queuine is a 7-deazapurine that is found in the first position of the anticodons of some tRNA. It cannot be synthesized by eukaryotes. We depend on our diets or intestinal microflora for our queuine. The original transcripts of the tRNA genes contain guanine instead of queuine in their anticodons. This guanine is enzymatically excised and replaced by queuine. Unlike the other post-transcriptional modifications which occur in the nucleus, queuine insertion occurs in the cytoplasm. Queuine is not essential for life but there is evidence that it plays a beneficial role when organisms are stressed. We studied several enzymes involved in protection against oxidative stress and found that tissue culture cells growing in the absence of queuine have 50% less Mn-SOD than do cells growing in a medium that contained 1 µM queuine. We also studied the effect of queuine *in vivo*. We fed two groups of germfree mice either a queuine-deficient diet or an identical diet that contained queuine. Both liver and lung of queuine-supplemented (Q+) mice had higher superoxide dismutase than the (Q-) mice. There was no significant difference in the catalase in liver, kidney or lung between the two groups, but the levels of glutathione peroxidase was higher in liver and kidney from (Q+) mice. We found that the amount of malondialdehyde reactive material was significantly higher in (Q+) mice than (Q-) mice. The presence of dietary queuine had no effect on the levels of cytochrome P-450 and cytochrome b5. We also found that the enzyme is inhibited by bicarbonate. Preliminary evidence indicates that the inhibitor is actually the CO_2 that is in equilibrium with the bicarbonate. These observations may be the explanation for the low levels of queuine-containing tRNAs and Mn SOD found in tumor cells.

Supported by American Institute for Cancer Research grant 89A30.

Retinoic Acid and 1,25 (OH)2 Vitamin D3 Regulate the RB Tumor Suppressor Gene in Cell Differentiation: Role as a "Status Quo" Gene

A. Yen, S. Chandler and M.E. Forbes
Department of Pathology, Cornell University, Ithaca, NY 14853

In human promyelocytic leukemia cells induced to terminally differentiate, the relative cellular content of the Rb gene product varies with cell cycle phase and with progression toward the differentiated state. HL-60 cells were induced to undergo myeloid or monocytic differentiation due to retinoic acid or 1,25-dihydroxyvitamin D_3 respectively. The total amount of the Rb gene product per cell, including both unphosphorylated and phosphorylated forms, was correlated with cell cycle phase and progression of cell differentiation using multiparameter flow cytometry. The total amount of the Rb gene product progressively increased as cells advanced through the cell cycle. But the amount of Rb gene product relative to the total cell mass remained approximately constant, indicating that there was no apparent relative enrichment. When cells were induced to undergo either myeloid or monocytic terminal differentiation, an early progressive decrease in cellular content of the Rb gene product occurred well before any overt cell cycle modulation or phenotypic differentiation. The reduction in the amount of Rb gene product relative to the total cell mass was similar for cells in all cell cycle phases. The amount of cellular Rb gene product thus undergoes early down regulation during the processes of myeloid or monocytic terminal differentiation of these cells. In the instance of a variant HL-60 cell line which was defective in its capability to functionally differentiate in response to a specific inducer, the failure to differentiate was preceded by a failure to down-regulate cellular levels of the Rb gene product. When the same variant subline underwent myeloid or monocytic differentiation in response to other inducers, down regulation of the cellular Rb protein levels anteceded differentiation. The results suggest that the gene may have a function as a brake against cellular change, or as a "status quo" gene. As such its down regulation may be an essential component of early events leading to terminal cell differentiation, as well as neoplastic transformation.

Supported by American Institute for Cancer Research grant 87A59.

HPV16-Immortalized Human Keratinocytes Are More Sensitive than Normal Human Keratinocytes to Growth and Differentiation Control by Retinoids

L. Pirisi,[1] A. Batova,[2] J. Hodam,[2] E. Gandy[1] and K.E. Creek[2]
Department of Pathology, University of South Carolina School of Medicine,[1] and Department of Chemistry, University of South Carolina,[2] Columbia, SC 29208

Vitamin A deficiency is associated with an increased risk for cervical cancer and studies indicate that a diet rich in the precursor to vitamin A, β-carotene, reduces the risk of cervical cancer. Human papillomaviruses (HPV) are possible causative agents for cervical cancer. In particular, HPV16 is associated with most cervical malignancies and HPV16 DNA immortalizes human cervical cells and normal human foreskin keratinocytes (NHKc) *in vitro*. The transforming ability of the virus resides primarily in the open reading frames (ORF) E6 and E7. Retinoic acid (RA), the active metabolite of vitamin A, is a potent modulator of growth and differentiation of keratinocytes and has been shown to reverse lesions resulting from HPV infection. To investigate the role of RA in the control of HPV-induced lesions, we investigated the sensitivity to growth control by RA of five different keratinocyte lines (each derived from a single individual) immortalized by transfection with HPV16 DNA (HKc/HPV16). All the HKc/HPV16 lines were more sensitive than NHKc to growth inhibition by RA in both mass culture and clonal growth assays. In mass culture HKc/HPV16 exhibited about 45% growth inhibition at 10^{-7} M RA, which produced 8% growth inhibition of NHKc. β-Carotene (10^{-6} M) did not affect growth of either NHKc or HKc/HPV16. Retinol (10^{-6} M) inhibited growth of HKc/HPV16 but not NHKc. In clonal growth assays, a marked inhibition of HKc/HPV16 growth was evident at 10^{-8} M RA, while NHKc were inhibited only at 10^{-6} M RA. Clonal growth assays of HKc/HPV16 repeated at late passages (up to 160, approximately 670 population doublings) showed that the cells maintained RA sensitivity. In addition, HKc/HPV16 are more sensitive than NHKc to modulation of keratin expression by RA. No differences were observed in the rate of uptake or metabolism of RA or retinol between NHKc and the HKc/HPV16 lines. Dot blot and Northern blot analysis of mRNA extracted from two different HKc/HPV16 lines cultured in the absence or presence of 10^{-7} M RA showed that the expression of the HPV16 ORF E6 and E7 is 2 to 3-fold lower in the presence of RA. These results suggest that the increased sensitivity of the HKc/HPV16 lines to growth control by RA may be mediated by an inhibition of the expression of the HPV16 gene products required for the maintenance of continuous growth.

Supported by American Institute for Cancer Research grant 88A05.

The Role of Vitamin A and Analogues in Prevention of Radiation Toxicity During Radiotherapy of Cancer

E. Friedenthal, J. Mendecki, L. Davis and E. Seifter
Department of Surgery, Albert Einstein College of Medicine
Bronx, NY 10461

Damage to normal tissue and systemic toxicity are often the limiting factors in delivery of therapeutic doses of ionizing radiation. A possible protective effect of Vitamin A against radiation esophagitis and ileitis was tested in 2 groups of animals. One was fed laboratory chow with 3 x RDA of Vit A (control group) and the other was fed the same diet supplemented with 150,000 IU Vit A/Kg of food (Vit A group).

1. *Radiation Esophagitis.* 20 control and 20 Vit A fed rats were irradiated to the length of the esophagus with 2900 cGy delivered in one dose. During the first 2 weeks post-irradiation, control animals reduced their food intake by 65% and lost over 16% of their weight. The Vit A group showed only minor deviations. Histological sections of esophagus showed much less damage and more repair in the Vit A group.

2. *Radiation Ileitis.* a. Two groups of 20 C3HOu mice (control and Vit A) received whole body irradiation (WBI) of 1300 cGy 6 days after initiation of diet. Four days later the animals were sacrificed and microcolony survival assay was performed on cells of intestinal mucosa. b. A segment of jejunum isolated and attached to the abdominal wall was irradiated with 1300 cGy. Surviving jejunal crypts were counted. In both experiments the count of surviving crypts was about 60% higher in the Vit A group.

3. *WBI Depletion of Blood Elements.* 30 male C 57 BL/6 mice were placed on regular chow and 30 on diet supplemented with 90 mg β-carotene/kg. of chow. After 3 days and preliminary WBC and platelet counts the mice received 450 cGy WBI. Cell counts were made every 4 days for 25 days. About 30% higher WBC and platelet counts were seen in the supplemented group.

Our experiments suggest that Vitamin A and β-carotene have a significant potential for application in clinical radiation therapy as radioprotective agents.

Supported in part by American Institute for Cancer Research grant 84A08.

Dietary Sodium Deprivation Inhibits Cellular Proliferation: Evidence for Circulating Factor(s)

B.P. Fine, K.A. Hansen, T.R. Walters and T.N. Denny
Department of Pediatrics, UMDNJ-New Jersey Medical School, 185 South Orange Avenue, Newark, NJ 07103

Restriction of dietary sodium has long been known to inhibit normal tissue growth in animals. We have shown recently that restriction of dietary sodium intake also inhibits the cellular proliferation of solid tumors *in-vivo* (i.e., lymphoma and B16 melanoma [Cancer Res 48:3445-3448, 1988]). The present study is designed to detect the occurrence of circulating factors in the serum from salt-deprived C57BL/6 mice that influence mitogenesis in cultured B16 melanoma cells.

As a preliminary study we have examined the effects of serum from 5 week old male Sprague-Dawley rats, deprived of dietary sodium (SD), on proliferation of fibroblasts in culture. A control group (C) was fed the same low sodium food (<2 μg/g) ad-libitum and was offered 0.45% NaCl as drinking water. After three weeks on the specific diets the increase in body weight was C=96 g, SD=44 g. Blood was collected and a piece of skin was taken for culturing of fibroblasts. The serum from both groups was used to stimulate growth in quiescent rat skin fibroblasts from the C group. Using the fluorescent probes, BCECF and Fura-2, early membrane events that are coupled with cellular proliferation, such as cytoplasmic alkalinization and increased intracellular calcium, showed a greater response to serum from sodium-deprived animals. Cell cycle phases were determined by FACS apparatus and showed a slower rate of exit from G0/G1 and a slower rate of entry into S after the addition of serum from the SD group. The latter finding was confirmed by thymidine uptake (as compared to stimulation by fetal bovine serum: C=98%, and SD=69%).

These studies indicate that serum from sodium-deprived rats causes a dissociation between the early membrane events and the later nuclear phenomena.

Supported by American Institute for Cancer Research grant 89B19.

Chemoprevention of Cervix Cancer: Nutrient Intervention

S.L. Romney, P.R. Palan, J. Basu, A. Kadish, G. Goldberg and M. Mikhail
Departments of Obstetrics / Gynecology and Pathology, Albert Einstein College of Medicine, Bronx, NY 10461

Antioxidant vitamins have recently been postulated to have protective properties in active oxygen species-induced carcinogenesis. For more than a decade, we have been investigating whether essential micronutrients, particularly antioxidant vitamins A, E, C, and β-carotene are linked to the etiology and pathogenesis of cervix cancer. A double blinded placebo-controlled clinical trial of women diagnosed to have moderate uterine cervical dysplasia (CIN II) is being conducted. The protocol involves daily ingestion with informed consent of a nutrient formulation of β-carotene (18 mg), vitamin C (1.0 gm), and folic acid (800 μg) for a 6 month period. A total of 71 women have been enrolled (mean age 28.5 years). To date, there are no significant differences in age, race, educational background and smoking habit among the placebo versus the nutrient groups who are randomly assigned. Of 29 women who completed the therapeutic arm, an end point biopsy at 9 months was completed to determine whether regression occurred to mild dysplasia or normal cervical histology. The results suggest that 53% of the patients had no evidence of dysplasias; 21% were unchanged and described as moderate dysplasia; and one patient progressed to severe dysplasia and was treated. HPLC analyses at fixed intervals of coded samples for plasma retinol (ROH), β-carotene (BC), α-tocopherol (AT) and ascorbic acid (AA) were carried out. The data reveal significant increases in the plasma BC and AA levels which were 4 and 6 times higher in the treated group than placebo group at 1, 3, and 6 months after supplementation. These levels gradually declined to the base line values after the completion of the protocol. The plasma ROH and AT levels do not show any significant changes between the 2 groups during the study period. No clinical side effects were noticed among any participants. The compliance of the subjects and the safety of the protocol in monitoring a precancer lesion establish the feasibility for conducting a multi-institutional clinical trial.

Supported by American Institute for Cancer Research grant 87B62 and a Grant in Aid from Hoffmann LaRoche, Inc. Nutley, NJ.

Vitamin D_3 Binding by B700 Melanoma Antigen and Its Comparison to Other Albuminoid Molecules

D.M. Gersten, T.L. Walden, V.J. Hearing and N.K. Farzaneh
Department of Pathology, Georgetown University, Washington, DC 20007 and Laboratory of Cell Biology, National Cancer Institute, Bethesda, MD 20892

B700, a murine melanoma-specific antigen, is a member of the serum albumin protein family. Other members of this family include serum albumin, alpha fetoprotein, and vitamin D-binding protein. The complete primary structure and biochemical functions of B700, as well as its *in vivo* metabolic fate are largely unknown. We examined the functional characteristics of murine serum albumin, vitamin D-binding protein, and B700 for their ability to specifically bind [^{3}H]-1,25-dihydroxyvitamin D_3. Scatchard analysis revealed a single binding site for B700 with a Kd of 51,000M and a Bmax of 4.51 x 10^{-7}. There were no significant differences between the Kd and Bmax values among the albuminoid proteins under these experimental conditions. However, differences in the binding sites could be distinguished by competition of the 1,25-dihydroxyvitamin D_3 with other steroids. 2nM of vitamin D_3, vitamin D_2, or estrogen competed for the specific binding of 1, 25-dihydroxyvitamin D_3, by B700 but not by vitamin D-binding protein. The murine serum albumin binding site for 1,25-dihydroxy-vitamin D_3 more closely resembles vitamin D-binding protein than B700. These data indicate that the binding function of the albuminoid proteins is conserved in the B700 melanoma antigen, and suggest that vitamin D therapy for melanoma tumors might be antigen-mediated.

A Model System to Study Dietary Influences on Extension of a Murine Melanoma

J. Weinzweig, N. Weinzweig, H. Dawson, E. Friedenthal and E. Seifter
University of Chicago Medical Center, Department of Surgery; Wayne State University Medical Center, Department of Reconstructive Surgery; Albert Einstein College of Medicine, Department of Radiation Oncology and Department of Surgery

Studies with rodents demonstrated that supplements of vitamin A, β-carotene, arginine, ornithine and choline, cause increased collagen accumulation in dermal wounds, in subcutaneously implanted polyvinyl alcohol sponges, and in such implants containing C3HBA tumor cells. Moreover, these nutrients enhance subcutaneous collagen accumulation when accumulation is inhibited by stress, tumor, radiation, alkylating agents, anti-inflammatory steroids, or some states of dysnutrition. Because we likened the metabolic responses to tumors to those of injury (and thought of tumors as non-healing wounds), we studied the influence of dietary supplements on collagen accumulation in the capsule of C3HBA tumors following inoculation of female C3H mice with graded doses of tumor cells in the nipple line. An inoculum of 1×10^4 cells produced tumors in 50% of the mice with a latent period of 28 days. Groups of animals received chow diets supplemented with the following nutrients/kg: (a) retinyl palmitate, 150,000 IU; (b) β-carotene, 90 mg, choline chloride, 3 g; (c) arginine hydrochloride, 10 g; (d) ornithine dihydrochloride, 10 g. These treatments had the following effects: (1) the TD_{50} was increased from 1×10^4 to 5×10^4 and the latent period lengthened from 28 to 63 days; (2) the lifespan of tumor-bearing mice was increased from 52 to > 115 days; (3) at the time of death, untreated mice demonstrated tumors weighing 5-10 g and extensive metastases to the lungs and brain; treated animals did not demonstrate visibly evident tumors, but examination of the inoculation site revealed well encapsulated tumors weighing 0.1 g. The agents studied inhibit the growth of some tumors by influencing endocrine, exocrine, paracrine and autocrine function, thereby influencing systemic and cellular immunity. They also stimulate encapsulation which further inhibits tumor growth, invasion and metastasis. Thus, treatment alters tumor morphology and growth patterns; however, it does not affect the ability of the tumor cells to metastasize once they are removed from the collagenous capsule. We think that the anti-tumor properties of these nutrients are of general application and also may have special application to the control of melanoma growth, the staging of which is related not to lateral extension of tumor but to extension through the collagenous basement membrane and subsequent metastasis. In the model currently being studied [Cloudman S91 melanoma], mice are treated by one of several methods to create a blister or bleb at the dermal-epidermal junction. Melanoma cells are then injected into the raised blebs and the animals are subsequently evaluated, both histologically and by electron microscopy, for extension of the melanoma cells through the dermal basement membrane. Influences of the nutrients on basement membrane penetration by the melanoma cells are then studied.

The Effect of Vitamin A on Moderation of Oncogenesis and Tumor Growth

J. Mendecki, E. Friedenthal and E. Seifter
Albert Einstein College of Medicine, Bronx, NY 10461

Three types of experiments were conducted on 2 groups of animals. One group (control) was fed regular chow with 3 times RDA of Vitamin A (Vit A) and the other group (Vit A) was fed regular lab chow supplemented with 150,000 IU Vit A/Kg of food.

The objective was to determine the role of Vit A in inhibition of:

1. *Radiation Induced Oncogenesis*. Whole body irradiation (WBI) of C57BL mice causes lymphatic tumors associated with activation of a latent virus. Two groups of 60 female C57BL mice (control and Vit A) were subjected to 800 cGy WBI at 4 fractions of 200 cGy every 4 days. For radiation per se LD/30 was 0. Deaths from tumors began at about 3 months post-irradiation but proceeded twice as fast in controls.

2. *Oncogenesis of Spontaneous Tumors*. Two groups (control and Vit A) of fifty female C3H/HEJ (MTV+) 6 weeks old mice were established. In this strain 95% of the animals developed mammary tumors by 12 months of age. Mice began to develop mammary tumors at about 27 weeks and in the unsupplemented group 70% of mice exhibited tumors at 48 weeks of age, vs only 28% of mice in the experimental group.

3. *Growth of Metastases*. Two groups of 60 C57BL mice (control and Vit A) were inoculated with 10 cells of Lewis Lung Carcinoma (LLC) into a hind leg immediately above the ankle. When the tumor grew to 5 mm the leg was amputated at the hip. LLC deaths are usually due to lung metastases. At 30 days all surviving animals were sacrificed. During autopsies performed on animals dead from their tumors and on the sacrificed animals the lungs were inflated with a solution of India ink and metastases counted. Survival of animals fed Vit A at 30 days was 88% and the average number of lung metastases was 14 while in the control group only 58% of animals survived and an average of 31 metastatic nodules was found in the lungs.

The experiments suggest that Vit A may be of value in cancer prophylaxis.

Supported in part by American Institute for Cancer Research grant 84A08.

Plasma and Tissue Levels of the Antioxidants β-Carotene and Vitamin E in Women with Uterine Cervix Cancer

P.R. Palan, J. Basu, C. Runowicz, E. Bloch and S.L. Romney
Dept. of OB / GYN, Albert Einstein College of Medicine, Bronx, NY 10461

Highly active oxygen species are hypothesized to be involved in carcinogenesis. Two essential nutrients, β-carotene (BC) and α-tocopherol (AT), are major antioxidants potentially protecting cells from carcinogens. To investigate the association between the levels of vitamins and cervical neoplasia, we have assayed the BC and AT levels by HPLC in plasma and cervical cancerous and non cancerous tissues obtained from hysterectomized uteri from patients being treated for cervix cancer and benign uterine disease. Blood samples were also collected from normal women (free from any gynecologic diseases) and assayed for BC and AT levels. Plasma BC and AT levels were significantly reduced in the cancer patients. Cancer tissues had 1OX increased AT levels and significantly decreased BC levels. The data are;

Histology	(N)	Tissue BC	Tissue AT	(N)	Plasma BC	Plasma AT
		[Mean μg/g±SD]			[Mean μg/dl±SD]	
Normal	(10)	0.21±0.14	2.68±0.87.	(28)	31.1±9.6	649±275
Carcinoma	(10)	0.07±0.01	25.9±21.6.	(10)	11.1±7.2	358±111

t-test, $p < 0.01$ in all four comparisons.

The reduction of BC concentrations in plasma and tissue seen in this study confirms our previous observations (JNCI,1988; AJOG, Dec.1989). Increased AT levels in breast and liver cancer have been reported. This is the first study to report AT in human cervical tissue and its increase in cervix cancer. The findings suggest that the antioxidants BC and AT may have independent roles in the pathogenesis of cervix cancer.

Supported by American Institute for Cancer Research grant 87B62 and a Grant in Aid from Hoffmann-La Roche, Inc., Nutley, NJ.

Cross Sectional Study of Selenium Status in Patients Undergoing Colonoscopy

L.C. Clark, L.J. Hixson, N. Petel,
G.F. Combs, Jr. and R.E. Sampliner
Departments of FCM & Medicine, University of Arizona College of Medicine, & VAMC, Tucson, AZ 85716

This cross sectional study examined the micronutrient status of 100 patients (pts.) undergoing sequential outpatient colonoscopies at the Tucson VA Hospital. This is the first study, to our knowledge, that demonstrates a statistically significant association between plasma selenium (Se) status and the prevalence of neoplastic polyps of the colon. The primary hypothesis was that pts. with low Se status would have a higher prevalence of polyps than pts. with high Se status. In this review, 47 pts. did not report a prior history of cancer, neoplastic polyps, or prior colonoscopy. In these pts., a statistically significant association exists between plasma Se level and the risk of benign colonic neoplasms. The age adjusted odds ratio (OR) for neoplastic polyps is 3.6, 95% confidence intervals of 1.06, 12.5, for pts. with low versus high plasma Se. The strength of this association was stronger for pts. above 70 years of age (OR=5.4) versus those less than 70 (OR=2.3), suggesting a potential effect modification of this association by age. Pts. without polyps had an average Se level of 0.134 mcg/ml, while pts. with only diminutive polyps (<6mm) (n=13) had Se level of 0.127. Pts. with only large polyps (n=7) had a Se level of 0.125, while pts. with both (n=7) had a Se level of 0.121. Cigarette smokers were also found to have more neoplastic polyps <6 mm (74%) than non-smokers (30%) or ex-smokers (46%). Since this study was a feasibility trial, additional information on dietary factors was not collected, and, therefore, cannot be excluded as the underlying cause of this observed association (27 pts. with polyps, 20 without).

Supported in part by American Institute for Cancer Research grant 84B01.

N-Nitrosoproline Excretion in Volunteers Who Take Nitrate and Proline with a Standard Meal; or Who Live in Rural Nebraska, Drink High- or Low-Nitrate Water, and Eat Near-Normal Diets

S.S. Mirvish, A.C. Grandjean, S. Fike, T. Maynard, L. Jones, S. Rosinsky and G. Nie
Eppley Inst. Res. Cancer, University of Nebraska Med. Center, and Center Human Nutr., Omaha, NE 68105

The N-nitrosoproline (NPRO) test was applied in 2 related studies. The first was designed to examine conditions in the stomach that affect NPRO formation. The subjects followed a low NPRO diet for 5 days by avoiding nitrite-preserved meats and beer. On days 4 and 5, chewing gum and eating high-ascorbate foods were not allowed and a standard 650-calorie test lunch was eaten. L-Proline (500 mg) was given with the meal and sodium nitrate (400 mg nitrate) was given 5 min-2 h before the meal. Urines (24 h) and 5-ml saliva samples were collected. Urines were analyzed for NPRO (by GC-TEA after preparing methyl ester with BF3/methanol), nitrate (by nitrobenzene method), specific gravity and creatinine. Salivas were analyzed for nitrite and nitrate.

With nitrate given just before and proline with the meal, mean NPRO was 2.1 μg, significantly more than the 0.6 μg in controls receiving only the standard meal. Giving 1 g ascorbic acid with the proline and nitrate reduced NPRO to 1.2 μg. NPRO yield was 11.1 μg when nitrate and proline were taken while fasting, 5 x higher than when taken with a meal, demonstrating that food in the stomach inhibits nitrosation. Mean NPRO yield was 2.1, 4.9 and 2.3 μg when nitrate was taken 5 min, 1 h and 2 h before the meal, consistent with a model where NPRO is formed for 1 h after-taking proline.

In the second study, 44 rural Nebraska men with high- or low-nitrate drinking water from private wells underwent similar NPRO tests. The 5-day test included avoidance of high-NPRO foods and other practices as in the first study, urine collection on day 4 while following usual activities and near-normal diets, and urine collection on day 5 after an overnight fast, drinking 2 glasses of water, taking 500 mg proline and continuing the fast till 1 p.m. Basal NPRO for no nitrate in water was 1 μg/day. The 15 highest NPRO values were in the range 3-6 μg/day. The group with >18 ppm nitrate-N water showed significantly more NPRO than that with <18 ppm nitrate-N on day 4 but not on day 5. The high-nitrate group showed elevated urine nitrate on both days. Correlations between parameters for all results on each day revealed significant correlation for both urine NPRO and urine nitrate versus water nitrate on both days, for both saliva nitrite and saliva nitrate versus water nitrate on day 5, and for urine creatinine versus urine NPRO and urine nitrate on day 4. Hence increased water nitrate did indeed increase NPRO formation. Urine NPRO may have begun to increase above 30 ppm nitrate-N in the water, 3 times the EPA-recommended limit.

Supported in part by American Institute for Cancer Research grant 89B36.

Antimetastatic Effects of Tyrosine and Phenylalanine Restriction in Melanoma

C.A. Elstad, G. Raha and G.G. Meadows
College of Pharmacy and the Pharmacology/Toxicology Graduate Program, Washington State University, Pullman, WA 99164-6510

We have previously shown that dietary restriction of tyrosine (tyr) and phenylalanine (phe) inhibits growth of primary B16 melanoma, increases survival of tumor-bearing mice, and augments chemotherapy (Cancer Res. 42:3056, 1982; Cancer Res. 43:2047, 1983). Additionally, dietary restriction of these amino acids is effective in blocking spontaneous metastasis in rodents of not only melanoma but also L1210 leukemia (Nutr. Cancer 3:94,1981), Lewis Lung carcinoma, and RT74bs hepatocarcinoma (J. Natl. Cancer Inst. 78:759, 1987). We report here that exposure of B16-BL6 melanoma cells to low levels of tyr and phe both *in vivo* and *in vitro* suppresses the metastatic phenotype by directly affecting the tumor. This effect is specific for tyr and phe and the *in vivo* response is not related to decreases in food intake, body weight, or caloric intake. Cells modulated by the amino acid restriction are defective in their ability to colonize the lung after intravenous inoculation, and decreased colonization is associated with increased survival. The change in phenotype is immediate and is induced after one *in vivo* passage in mice fed the tyr- and phe-restricted diet and after one passage *in vitro* in culture medium reduced in these amino acids. Recent efforts to identify the mechanism(s) responsible for the altered phenotype indicate that tyr- and phe-modulated cells are less heterogeneous and are suppressed in their ability to establish metastatic tumor foci (Clin. Expl. Metastasis 8:393, 1990). One parameter associated with the phenotypic alteration is a reduced ability of the cells to degrade type I collagen. Preliminary studies indicate that this dietary approach is feasible in humans (Am. J. Clin. Nutr. 51:188, 1990).

Supported by American Institute for Cancer Research grant 85B79.

Modulation of Procarbazine-Induced Mammary Carcinogenesis in Female Rats by Dietary Lipotropes

R. Akhtar and A.E. Rogers
Mallory Institute of Pathology, Boston City Hospital and Boston University School of Medicine, Department of Pathology 02118-2394

Certain cancer chemotherapeutic agents, such as procarbazine (PCZ), are carcinogenic in laboratory animals. Susceptibility to them may be enhanced by nutritional deficiencies. Lipotrope deficiency increases mammary carcinogenesis by PCZ in male rats. The effects of moderate or borderline dietary lipotrope deficiency or of lipotrope hypersupplementation on mammary gland carcinogenesis by PCZ were studied in female, Sprague-Dawley rats. Rats were fed control (C, 0.045 mMols methyl per gram of diet), deficient (D, 0.026 mMols/g), borderline (B, 0.033 mMols/g) or hypersupplemented (H, 0.11 mMols/g) for 3 weeks from weaning and then given 20 doses of PCZ, 15 mg/kg each by i.p. injection. There were 32 rats per group. The cumulative probability of palpable mammary tumor development and final gross tumor incidence and number were inversely proportional to the dietary lipotrope content. The final tumor incidences were: H, 62%; C, 66%; B, 69%; and D, 78%. The average tumor numbers per tumor-bearing rat were: H, 2.5; C, 2.6; B, 3.5; and D, 4.0. In rats fed C, B and D diets, there was a significant ($P = 0.04$) inverse correlation between dietary methyl content and tumor number; individual group comparisons showed significant differences in tumor number between DPCZ and CPCZ ($p = 0.0008$). Hypersupplementation (Group H) did not influence tumorigenesis significantly. The results are consistent with earlier results in male rats and confirm the observation that lipotrope deficiency enhances PCZ-induced mammary carcinogenesis in rats.

Supported in part by American Institute for Cancer Research grant 87A65.

Lower Levels of Folates in Oral Mucosal Cells of Smokers Do Not Appear to Result from Differences in Dietary Folates

C.J. Piyathilake, R.J. Hine, E.W. Richards and C.L. Krumdieck
University of Alabama at Birmingham, and Baptist Medical Centers, Birmingham, AL

We recently reported lower levels of folates in oral mucosal cells (OMC) of cigarette smokers (S) than in non-smokers (NS). Those results support the hypothesis that exposure of cells of the respiratory tract to smoke creates a localized deficiency of folates which is likely to render these cells more vulnerable to neoplastic transformation by carcinogens in smoke. The present study was conducted to establish to what extent variations in dietary folate intake folic acid supplementation and alcohol use might account for differences in OHC folates. Blood and OMCs were collected from 15 S and 15 NS. The Health Habits and History Questionnaire (Block, Hartman and Dresser et al., 1986) was completed by each subject. A 96 well plate L. casei assay micro method was used to quantitate plasma and OHC folates. Cells were preincubated with folate-free pteroyl-gamma-glutamyl hydrolase. OMC folates are expressed as pg per mg wet weight of the pellet. The S group's mean OMC folate level (177 ± 55 pg/mg) was significantly lower than that of the NS (636 ± 117 pg/mg), $p < 0.003$. The S group's mean plasma folates (6.70 ± 1.33 ng/ml) was also significantly lower than that of the NS (12.87 ± 2.37 ng/ml). In contrast, there was no significant difference between the mean dietary folates for the two groups (291 vs 358 µg/day, S and NS respectively). Likewise, there were no differences in folate supplementation or alcohol consumption between the two groups. These findings suggest that the lower folates in OMC of smokers is related to exposure to cigarette smoke.

Supported in part by American Institute for Cancer Research grant 90SG12.

Effects of n6 and n3 Plasma Free Fatty Acids (FFA) on ^{3}H-Thymidine Incorporation (^{3}H-TI) in Hepatoma 7288CTC

L.A. Sauer and R.T. Dauchy
Bassett Research Institute, Cooperstown, NY 13326

Ingestion of dietary oils containing either n6 or n3 fatty acids increase or decrease, respectively, the growth rates of transplantable tumors. The mechanism for these effects is not yet known. In this study we examined the uptake of plasma FFA *in vivo* in tissue-isolated hepatoma 7288CTC growing in Buffalo rats fed either an essential fatty acid-deficient (EFAD) or -sufficient diet. Hepatoma 7288CTC removed FFA from the arterial blood in proportion to the rate of supply; about 40 to 60% of each FFA was utilized during one pass through the tumor. Uptakes were similar in tumors growing in rats fed the two diets. The effects of n6 and n3 FFA on the rate of tumor ^{3}H-TI were measured in hepatoma 7288CTC growing in EFAD rats. Tumors weighing about 5 g were perfused *in situ* for 2 hours with whole blood from donor EFAD rats that contained either no or added n6 and/or n3 FFA. ^{3}H-T (1 µC/g estimated tumor weight) was administered 20 min before the end of the perfusion. Baseline rates (no added n6 or n3 FFA) of ^{3}H-TI were 44±4 dpm/µg tumor DNA. Perfusion with blood containing 0.5mM linoleic [18:2n6], gamma-linolenic [18:3n6] or arachidonic [20:4n6] acids increased ^{3}H-TI to 475±15, 147±15 or 122±12 dpm/µg tumor DNA, respectively. The effects of the n6 FFA were additive. Sigmoid-shaped dose versus response curves were observed for linoleic and arachidonic acids indicating that the stimulative effects were saturable. The linoleic acid utilized was incorporated into tumor triglycerides and phospholipids. Alpha-linolenic [18:3n3] and eicosapentenoic [20:5n3] acids had no effect on the rate of tumor ^{3}H-TI when administered alone but inhibited the stimulative effect on linoleic acid by competitively inhibiting linoleate uptake. The data indicate that increased plasma free linoleic acid concentrations increased tumor uptake of linoleate and the rate of tumor DNA synthesis. Increased plasma n3 FFA concentrations, however, decreased tumor linoleic acid uptake, linoleate incorporation into tumor lipids and DNA synthesis.

Supported by National Cancer Institute grant CA27809-10 and American Institute for Cancer Research grant 90A42.

Effect of High and Low Fat Diets on Fecal Steroids and Mutagenic Activity in Colon Cancer-Prone Cotton-Top Tamarins (*Saguinus oedipus*)

L.M. Ausman, J.A. Johnson, C. Guidry, S. Shami and P.P. Nair

USDA-HNRCA, Tufts University, Boston, MA; School of Nutrition, Tufts University, Medford, MA; NERPRC, Harvard Medical School, Southborough, MA; Department of Biochemistry, Johns Hopkins University, School of Hygiene and Public Health, Baltimore, MD; and LNL-BHNRC ARS USDA, Beltsville, MD

Forty cotton-top tamarins (CTT), monkeys susceptible to spontaneous colitis and colon cancer in captivity, are being fed either a high-fat (40% kcal), low-fiber diet (HF), or a low-fat (20% kcal), high-fiber diet (LF). HF and LF diets contain equal amounts of saturated FA and cholesterol; however, HF contains 2-3 times more mono- and polyunsaturated FA and plant sterols than LF. LF contains 50% more dietary fiber (soluble and insoluble) than HF.

Fecal neutral sterols (FNS) and fecal bile acids (FBA) were measured every 4 months; also, feces were assayed for SOS inducing potency (SOSIP) by the SOS chromotest for genotoxicity. Concentrations of all FNS and conversion of cholesterol to secondary metabolites coprostanol and coprostanone were greater for HF. Fecal cholic, chenodeoxycholic, and lithocholic acid concentrations were similar for both diets; however, the fecal deoxycholic acid concentration was greater for HF and fecal ursodeoxycholic acid concentration was greater for LF. Conversion of FNS varied for both diets over time; conversion of FBA for both diets increased from 30 to 70% over the first year and then stabilized. There was no significant difference between diets for SOSIP; also, mutagenic activity showed no consistent pattern over time.

Dietary fat and fiber influence the concentration and conversion of FNS and FBA in CTT, and the extent of conversion varies widely among individual monkeys and over time. The concentration of fecal steroids and the production of secondary metabolites are thought to be markers of colon cancer risk in these animals.

Choline Deficient Enhancement of Aflatoxin B1 Adduct Formation in Rat Liver DNA

T.F. Schrager, P.M. Newberne, A.H. Pikul and J.D. Groopman
Mallory Institute of Pathology, Boston, MA 02118

A choline deficient methionine low (CMD) diet acts as a complete carcinogen when given chronically, and enhances the initiation and promotion of chemical carcinogenesis. Studies were conducted in this laboratory to identify an initiation effect of the CMD diet on aflatoxin B1 (AFB1) hepatocarcinogenesis in the F344 rat, and to identify a reliable molecular marker to investigate underlying mechanisms. Applying the CMD diet to a carcinogenic two week AFB1 dosing regimen (25 ug/rat/day, 5 days/week) significantly increased DNA adduct formation, a total of 41% over the two week dosing period. Covalent modification did not increase after a single dose, indicating the importance of using a chronic dosing model to observe an initiation effect. Because of the increased amount of dead and dying hepatocytes in CMD livers the 41% increase should be considered a minimal estimate of damage. Using liquid nitrogen to preserve livers caused a 10-12 fold loss of DNA in CMD livers, presumably due to greater fragility. Switching to ice to preserve livers greatly reduced DNA loss and adduct formation in the CMD livers was increased from the 41% level to 73%. All of these studies used a two hour time point after dosing to measure adduct levels since this is the time of maximal binding in control diet rats. Time course studies show that maximal binding is at one hour in hepatic DNA of CMD rats. Superimposing phenobarbital treatment on the CMD diet during AFB1 dosing prevents increased binding levels but does not reduce the levels further. Because PB protective effects are thought to be related to increases in detoxication enzymes, specifically glutathionine-S-transferase, PB may counteract a CMD inhibitory effect on GST, or protect against increased activation of AFB1. These possibilities are being investigated at this time.

Foodbase: International Food Consumption Database

J.S. Douglass, K.H. Fleming, S.K. Egan, B.J. Petersen and R.R. Butrum
Technical Assessment Systems, Inc.,
1000 Potomac Street, N.W., Washington, DC 20007

Technical Assessment Systems, Inc. (TAS) is working with the U.S. National Cancer Institute (NCI) on a three-year project to collect international food consumption survey data, and to enter the information into an IBM-PC compatible data management and analysis system. The database system, FOODBASE, is being created for NCI as a resource for investigating diet-disease relationships. The system will be equally useful for nutritionists, epidemiologists, and other health professionals to use in assessing the intake of foods and food constituents by populations throughout the world. FOODBASE will contain descriptive information about food consumption surveys conducted worldwide since 1940. The database will also contain summary data from many of these surveys. Food consumption and nutrient composition source data from three surveys (to be identified by NCI later in the project) will also be included in the system.

The system is designed for users with little or no computer experience, and will allow sorting and analysis of data to meet the needs of the user.

TAS is reviewing and coding information from survey documents collected thus far. We continue to collect survey data, and we welcome comments and recommendations from interested researchers. The system is expected to be completed in early 1992.

Effects of Alpha-Tocopherol and Beta-Carotene in EGF-Receptor Expression and Differential TNF-alpha Cytotoxicity Under AbLV Transformation

S. Mishra and H.P. Misra
Department of Biomedical Sciences, VMRCVM, Virginia Tech, Blacksburg, VA 24061

Activation of growth factor regulatory system may play a role in virally-induced malignant transformation of cells. The transformation induced with RNA tumor virus such as Abelson Leukemia Virus (AbLV) provides an excellent model in elucidating the molecular events involved in malignant transformation. The cytotoxicity of the tumor necrosis factor-alpha (TNF-alpha), a macrophage derived polypeptide hormone, on murine lung fibroblast cell line CL.7 and its two AbLV transformed daughter cell lines AbLV 3R.1 and AbLV 6R.1 were studied. The cytotoxicity was determined using 3 (4,5-dimethylthiazol-2-yl)-2,5-diphenyl-tetrazolium bromide (MTT) reduction assay. Compared to L929 fibrosarcoma calls the % cytotoxicity for the CL.7, 3R.1 and 6R.1 cell lines were found to be 36.4 ± 0.6, 18.6 ± 0.7, 53.4 ± 1.4 percent, respectively. The lipid soluble antioxidants such as alpha-tocopherol and β-carotene at 1 mM inhibited the TNF-alpha cytotoxicity by 50 and 30 percent, respectively. To determine whether TNF-alpha cytotoxicity can be correlated with a growth factor receptor expression, we determined epidermal growth factor-receptor (EGF-R) levels in these cell lines using ^{125}I-EGF(6×10^4 dpm/ng EGF) binding assay. The EGF-R levels were found to be positively correlated with TNF-alpha cytotoxicity ($r = 0.99$). Alpha-tocopherol both at 0.1 and 0.5 mM levels enhanced the TNF-alpha inducible EGF-R expression significantly in both the AbLV transformed cell lines, 3R.1 and 6R.1. However, the induction of the EGF-R by TNF-alpha in the normal cells (CL.7) was not affected by these levels of alpha-tocopherol. β-carotene, at concentrations of 0.1 and 0.5 mM, on the other hand was found to suppress EGF-R expression in both normal and transformed cell lines in presence and absence of TNF-alpha. The suppression of EGF-R expression by β-carotene and its enhancement by alpha-tocopherol suggests a broader role of these vitamins as growth factor regulators. The modulation of EGF-R (found at an enhanced level in certain cancers) by these vitamins suggests an attractive dietary regimen in prevention of these cancers.

Supported in part by American Institute for Cancer Research grant 84B03.

Index

Index entries in Posters are italicized.